PULMONARY EMERGENCIES

PULMONARY EMERGENCIES

Edited by

Steven A. Sahn, M.D.
Associate Professor of Medicine
Division of Pulmonary Sciences
University of Colorado Health Sciences Center
Attending Physician, Medical Intensive Care Unit
University Hospital
Director, Pleural Space Laboratory
Webb-Waring Lung Institute
Denver, Colorado

Churchill Livingstone
New York, Edinburgh, London, and Melbourne 1982

Distributed in the United Kingdom by Churchill Livingstone, Robert Stevenson House, 1-3 Baxter's Place, Leith Walk, Edinburgh EH1 3AF and by associated companies, branches and representatives throughout the world.

First published 1982
Printed in U.S.A.

ISBN 0-443-08169-7

7 6 5 4 3 2 1

Library of Congress Cataloging in Publication Data

Main entry under title:

Pulmonary emergencies.

Bibliography: p.
Includes index
1. Lungs—Diseases. 2. Medical emergencies. I. Sahn, Steven A. [DNLM: 1. Lung diseases. 2. Emergencies. WF 600 P9834303]
RC756.P827 1982 616.2'00425 82-12963
ISBN 0-443-08169-7

To my parents,
Mildred and Irwin,

my wife,
Eleanor,

and my children,
Karen, Stacey, Jimmy, Michael, and Rachel

Contributors

Richard K. Albert, M.D.
Associate Professor of Medicine, University of Washington School of Medicine; Assistant Chief, Pulmonary and Critical Care Medicine, Director, Medical Intensive Care Unit, Veterans Administration Medical Center, Seattle, Washington

Roger C. Bone, M.D.
Professor of Medicine, Chief, Pulmonary Disease, University of Arkansas for Medical Sciences, Little Rock, Arkansas

John G. Brooks, M.D.
Associate Professor of Pediatrics, Director, Pediatric Pulmonary Medicine, University of Rochester School of Medicine and Dentistry, Rochester, New York

James T. Good, Jr., M.D.
Assistant Professor of Medicine, Division of Pulmonary Sciences, University of Colorado Health Sciences Center; Attending Physician, Medical and Surgical Intensive Care Units, Associate Director of Respiratory Therapy, Denver General Hospital, Denver, Colorado

William H. Greene, M.D.
Associate Professor of Medicine, Infectious Disease Section, Department of Internal Medicine, Yale University School of Medicine, New Haven, Connecticut

Alan R. Hopeman, M.D.
Professor of Surgery, University of Colorado Health Sciences Center; Chief, Cardiac Surgery, Denver General Hospital, Denver, Colorado

Thomas M. Hyers, M.D.
Associate Professor of Medicine, Director, Pulmonary Division, St. Louis University Medical Center, St. Louis, Missouri

S. Lakshminarayan, M.D.
Associate Professor of Medicine, University of Washington School of Medicine; Chief, Pulmonary Section, Veterans Administration Hospital, Seattle, Washington

Richard A. Matthay, M.D.
Associate Professor of Medicine, Associate Director, Pulmonary Section, Department of Internal Medicine, Yale University School of Medicine, New Haven, Connecticut

Ernest D. Moritz, M.D.
Senior Investigator, Pulmonary Branch, National Heart, Lung and Blood Institute, Bethesda, Maryland

Thomas A. Neff, M.D.
Associate Professor of Medicine, Division of Pulmonary Sciences, University of Colorado Health Sciences Center; Chief, Pulmonary Division, Denver General Hospital, Denver, Colorado

David J. Pierson, M.D.
Associate Professor of Medicine, University of Washington School of Medicine; Director, Respiratory Therapy, Harborview Medical Center, Seattle, Washington

Eleanor E. Sahn, M.D.
Clinical Instructor in Medicine, University of Colorado Health Sciences Center; Instructor in Basic Cardiac Life Support, Denver, Colorado.

Steven A. Sahn, M.D.
Associate Professor of Medicine, Division of Pulmonary Sciences, University of Colorado Health Sciences Center; Attending Physician, Medical Intensive Care Unit, University Hospital; Director, Pleural Space Laboratory, Webb-Waring Lung Institute, Denver Colorado

Charles H. Scoggin, M.D.
Associate Professor of Medicine, Division of Pulmonary Sciences, University of Colorado Health Sciences Center; Institute Fellow, Eleanor Roosevelt Institute, Denver, Colorado

John L. Stauffer, M.D.
Assistant Clinical Professor of Medicine, University of California, San Francisco, School of Medicine, San Francisco, California; Chief, Pulmonary Disease Section, Veterans Administration Medical Center, Fresno, California

Foreword

It was a pleasant task to prepare this Foreword introducing a new book on pulmonary emergencies. The gratification came from two sources. When one considers the advances made in understanding and treating acute respiratory emergencies compared to where we were, say 10 or 15 years ago, it is clear that both science and its application, along with improved technology, represent real advances in our ability to meet and effectively manage sudden respiratory emergencies. An equal source of pleasure is that this book was organized and edited by a former fellow and current faculty member of the Division of Pulmonary Sciences and that most of the contributors were graduates of our training program and now contribute as faculty members of several institutions, including our own. These authors, along with other close friends and collaborators, have contributed succinct and authoritative chapters in areas of their special expertise, which gives this book the flavor of contemporary thought and practice. This, coupled with the fact that each contributor spends a substantial period of his academic life offering patient care services and teaching the art as well as studying and evaluating new methods of therapy, clearly makes this book dynamic and real.

Even though the practice of respiratory care is rapidly changing, Steven Sahn and his contributors have offered the very latest in technique and rationale for care of respiratory emergencies that can occur at any time and in any place—both in and out of hospitals.

Thomas L. Petty, M.D.

Preface

When the lungs or upper airway sustains severe injury, either through disease or trauma, the patient's life is in jeopardy. The physician responsible for the care of such a patient must act swiftly and correctly so that the patient has the greatest chance of survival. The purpose of *Pulmonary Emergencies* is to provide an update on the clinical presentation and pathophysiology of the most common pulmonary emergencies so that the clinician can institute the most rational treatment.

The first two chapters discuss the details of cardiopulmonary resuscitation and tracheal intubation, life-saving measures that become necessary in some pulmonary emergencies. The succeeding chapters, in general, provide the reader with the incidence, pathophysiology, clinical presentation, diagnosis, and management of these disorders of the lung. The mechanisms of disease leading to lung dysfunction are stressed, as the understanding of this provides a more scientific basis for therapy.

I am indebted to the contributing authors for their scholarly effort in bringing *Pulmonary Emergencies* to fruition. It is my hope that this volume will be of help to all of those who come in contact with pulmonary emergencies.

Steven A. Sahn, M.D.

Contents

1

Cardiopulmonary Resuscitation

James T. Good, Jr., M.D.
Eleanor E. Sahn, M.D.

INTRODUCTION

With impairment of normal cardiopulmonary function, oxygen delivery to the tissues is reduced, and if this process is not interrupted, cell death occurs. Maneuvers aimed at restoring both circulation and respiration so as to improve oxygen delivery are known as cardiopulmonary resuscitation (CPR).

While CPR is considered a relatively new practice, medical historians have discovered accounts of artificial respiration being performed in early biblical times.[1] Moreover, the techniques and styles of artificial respiration as it has been practiced varied greatly; by the early 1700s the standard approach to a comatose patient was to sling him over the back of a trotting horse in an effort to initiate spontaneous breathing. In 1904 the Schafer method of artificial respiration was introduced.[2] This prone-pressure method consisted of compressing the lower back, thus pushing the abdominal contents against the diaphragm and so forcing air from the lungs. While controversial, this method remained the "gold standard" of artificial respiration until 1946, when the technique of mouth-to-mouth resuscitation was reintroduced.[3] By 1948 a National Research conference on resuscitation formally recommended modification of the mouth-to-mouth method to replace the Schafer prone-pressure method. But while the mouth-to-mouth method appeared superior, many physicians remained reluctant to accept it. Undoubtedly, the concern of contracting infectious diseases, such as polio and tuberculosis, delayed the acceptance of the method. It was not until 1954, when an effective polio vaccine and specific antituberculous chemotherapy were available that this method of artificial respiration was accepted universally. Currently, mouth-to-mouth resuscitation combined with closed-chest cardiac compression comprise the two most important aspects of effective cardiopulmonary resuscitation.[4]

Table 1–1. Etiology of Cardiac Arrest

	No.	%
Primary heart disease	528	81.4
Cancer	26	4.0
Neurologic	18	2.8
Respiratory	17	2.6
Drowning	14	2.2
Sudden infant death syndrome	10	1.5
Alcoholism	10	1.5
Suicide	7	1.1
Accidental overdose	6	.9
Other (smoke inhalation, anaphylaxis, electrocution, etc.)	13	2.0
	649	

(From Eisenberg MS, Bergner L, Hallstrom A: Epidemiology of cardiac arrest and resuscitation in a suburban community. JACEP 8:2, 1979.)

INCIDENCE AND ETIOLOGY OF CARDIOPULMONARY ARREST

The incidence and etiology of cardiopulmonary arrest may vary, depending on the geographic area, but generally remains constant from series to series. In all reported studies, ischemic heart disease is the most common etiologic factor, and is responsible for approximately 80 percent of acute episodes of cardiopulmonary arrest.[5,6] A review of an 18-month experience in King County, Washington revealed that 649 acute cardiopulmonary arrests occurred, yielding an annual incidence of 7.2 per 10,000 people.[5] In this study group, only 5 percent of the population were over 65 years of age, and 98 percent of the population were middle socioeconomic-class Caucasians with an average age of 61 years. Men represented 72 percent of all patients and 74 percent of the patients with primary heart disease, which is a figure representative of most studies. Other etiologic factors are listed in Table 1–1. ECG rhythm strips documenting the cardiac rhythms were available from 244 patients. The most common rhythms associated with cardiac arrest included: (1) ventricular fibrillation (57 percent); (2) asystole (28 percent); (3) idioventricular rhythm (11 percent); and (4) ventricular tachycardia (4 percent) (see Table 1–2).

Because the time between the onset of circulatory arrest and the initiation of CPR is critical, several studies evaluating the efficacy of bystander-initiated cardiopulmonary resuscitation have been undertaken. In evaluating their community experience, Thompson et al.[7] reported the outcome of resuscitation attempts on 316 consecutive patients with out-of-hospital ventricular fibrillation. Thirty-seven percent of these patients died at the scene, while 34 percent died subsequently in a medical facility. The survival was significantly improved if bystanders had initiated cardiopulmonary resuscitation immediately. Of the 109 patients who

Table 1–2. ECG Rhythm Associated with Cardiac Arrest

	All Etiologies	Primary Heart Disease
	(n = 244)	(n = 200)
Ventricular fibrillation	57%	63%
Asystole	28%	23%
Idioventricular/nodal	11%	10%
Ventricular tachycardia	4%	4%

(From Eisenberg MS, Bergner L, Hallstrom A: Epidemiology of cardiac arrest and resuscitation in a suburban community. JACEP 8:2, 1979.)

received bystander CPR, 43 percent survived to be discharged to their homes. Of the 207 who did not receive such therapy, only 21 percent ultimately returned home.

In a series of 100 consecutive victims of cardiopulmonary arrest treated by paramedical teams, 24 patients were successfully resuscitated.[6] However, only 7 percent of these individuals left the hospital. The most important factor related to survival was the local treatment time, with the best chance for successful resuscitation and survival correlating with the shortest total time for an initial response to the call, treatment at the scene, and transportation to a medical facility.

Similarly, Eisenberg et al.[8] demonstrated that a short time interval from collapse to the initiation of CPR and to the delivery of definitive care was associated with increased survival in cases of cardiac arrest. Forty-three percent of their patients in whom CPR was initiated within 4 minutes and definitive care was provided within 8 minutes survived. If either of these times were exceeded, the chances of survival decreased dramatically.

PATHOPHYSIOLOGY

The immediate purpose of CPR is to quickly re-establish oxygen delivery to the cerebral cortex. After this is accomplished, cardiovascular stability and spontaneous respiration must be restored. In his original description of closed-chest cardiac massage, Kouwenhoven and associates[4] proposed that perfusion of body tissues occurred as a result of compression of the heart against the vertebral column, which forced blood into the systemic and pulmonary vasculature. Until recently, this concept was accepted widely; however, it seemed inconsistent with a number of clinical and experimental observations. Criley and colleagues[9] observed that by continuous coughing, a victim of cardiac arrest could maintain a conscious state. They hypothesized that an important component to the cough was the increase in intrathoracic pressure. Thus, it appeared that the increase in intrathoracic pressure, rather than direct compression of the heart, was the most important aspect of closed-chest massage in supporting systemic blood flow.

The observations of Weisfeldt and Chandra support this concept.[10] Figure 1–1 demonstrates that during chest compression, all pressures within the thorax are

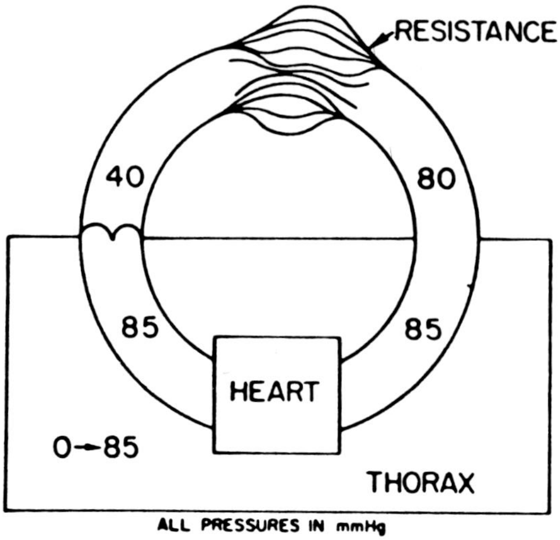

Figure 1–1. When conventional closed chest compression is applied during cardiopulmonary resuscitation, vascular pressures within the thorax approximate intrathoracic pressures. During compression there is no significant pressure gradient across the aortic valve and the extrathoracic aortic pressure is similar to intrathoracic aortic pressure. However, because of venous valve mechanisms, the extrathoracic venous pressure is markedly lower than simultaneous intrathoracic venous pressure. This extrathoracic arterial-venous pressure gradient results in "forward flow" and produces systemic arterial perfusion.

equal, and it is only the extrathoracic pressures that vary. The extrathoracic arterial pressure is similar to the intrathoracic aortic pressure; however, the extrathoracic venous pressure is markedly lower than the simultaneous intrathoracic venous pressure. At least three mechanisms are thought to be responsible for this generation of the extrathoracic arterial–venous pressure gradient. First, both intrathoracic and extrathoracic venous valve mechanisms are operating to prevent retrograde blood flow. Second, the venous capacitance of the peripheral circulation is greater than the arterial capacitance; thus, if equal amounts of blood were to simultaneously flow into both venous and arterial vessels, the arterial pressure would rise more than the venous pressure. Third, the arterial resistance to collapse is much greater than the venous resistance to collapse. Because of this, the veins would collapse readily at their point of entry into the thorax upon an increase in intrathoracic pressure, whereas the arterial vessels would not. Rudikoff et al.[11] have demonstrated in the dog model that increasing the intrathoracic pressure produces a differential in pressure between the arterial and venous sides, allowing for the extrathoracic arterial circulation to be perfused (forward flow).

Obviously, it is the cerebral circulation that is most important during the initial stages of CPR. Chandra et al.[12,13] have demonstrated that some measures which increase the intrathoracic pressure during CPR, such as abdominal binding and partial occlusion of the endotracheal tube, augment carotid blood flow. Abdominal binding improves carotid blood flow by two mechanisms: (1) increasing the effective circulatory blood volumes; and (2) directing blood flow away from intra-abdominal organs. The relatively new approach of augmenting carotid blood flow by high airway pressure ventilation combined with compression has been shown to improve not only hemodynamics but also survival in cases of cardiopulmonary arrest.[14] However, care must be taken to avoid continuous elevation of the intrathoracic pressure, for when this occurs, systemic blood flow will decrease because of: (1) impaired venous return; and (2) arterial vascular collapse. Thus, careful coordination of positive airway pressure methods with chest compression is imperative.

An additional problem with continuous positive airway pressure ventilation is elevation of the intracranial pressure.[15] Obviously, the combination of the elevated intracranial pressure with a lowered arterial pressure can result in a decrease in cerebral perfusion. Thus, the summation of many factors, including airway pressure, pleural pressure, intrathoracic pressure, and intracranial pressure must be considered when the ultimate driving force for producing cerebral blood flow is selected. Currently, it appears that positive-pressure ventilation combined with simultaneous closed-chest compression and abdominal binding yields the maximum carotid blood flow.

HYPOXIA AND BRAIN DAMAGE

As has been emphasized previously, because of the brain's extreme sensitivity to hypoxia, CPR must be initiated immediately to insure adequate cerebral perfusion. Normally, because of cerebral autoregulation, cerebral blood flow and oxygen delivery remain constant (50 to 60 ml/100 g of brain tissue per minute) until the mean arterial pressure (MAP) falls below 50 mmHg.[16] With cardiopulmonary arrest, the brain is deprived acutely of oxygen, and electroencephalographic changes have been noted to occur within 10 to 20 seconds. After exposure of the cerebral cortex to severe hypoxia for 3 to 5 minutes, extensive and irreversible neurologic damage occurs. Prolonged ischemia results in the softening of cortical tissues, with neurons becoming shrunken and necrotic.[16]

Earnest et al.[17] evaluated 38 survivors among 117 patients who were followed prospectively to discharge or death after admission following out-of-hospital cardiac arrest.[17] Three and a half years after the initial event, 20 of the 38 surviving patients were still living. Fifty-three percent of these 20 had resumed independent social activities, but only 32 percent of the 20 had returned to work. Eight of 14 patients tested were normal by limited neuropsychiatric testing. Earnest et al. found that a satisfactory long-term outcome was associated with patients being awake upon admission or awakening to follow commands within 48 hours of admission following acute cardiopulmonary arrest. None of the 9 patients with abnormal neurologic function at discharge subsequently resumed working or independent living.

Results similar to those of Earnest et al. were reported by Bates et al.[18] Of their 310 patients, 16 percent achieved an independent existence within a month after hospital discharge. Of those patients that remained comatose for at least 6 hours, 25 percent were severely disabled. Seventy-nine percent of the patients who were comatose after 1 week remained severely disabled. The chance of returning to an independent existence was greater in patients who by 24 hours after admission were capable of following commands and responding appropriately to verbal stimuli. The chance of regaining an independent existence was lower in individuals who had an extensor response of the limbs or who failed to move them in response to noxious stimuli. In general, the most important predictors of recovery following a cardiopulmonary arrest are: (1) duration of coma; (2) level of consciousness; (3) time elapsed prior to the initiation of CPR; and (4) level of consciousness at 24 hours.

TECHNIQUE OF CARDIOPULMONARY RESUSCITATION

The techniques of cardiopulmonary resuscitation[19] may be divided into basic life support and advanced cardiac life support. The basic life support techniques can be instituted immediately following an arrest by any trained person. The first steps are: (1) establishing the level of consciousness (shaking or shouting at the victim); (2) calling for assistance; and (3) positioning the victim correctly. The next steps include: (1) opening the airway, including relieving obstruction; (2) establishing breathing; and (3) establishing circulation.

Opening the Airway

The most important factor for successful resuscitation is establishing an open airway. While foreign material may cause airway obstruction, airway obstruction is most commonly caused by the tongue. In the unconscious victim, lack of muscle tone, combined with negative pressure created in the airway during efforts at inspiration, causes the tongue to fall back into the hypopharynx and obstruct the airway. Moving the mandible forward lifts the tongue away from the back of the throat and in many cases will open the airway. This is accomplished with either the head tilt–neck lift or head tilt–chin lift maneuver (see below). If these maneuvers do not open the airway, the head tilt combined with the jaw thrust may be used, since this provides greater forward displacement of the mandible and tongue.[20]

The head tilt–neck lift is accomplished, with the rescuer kneeling at the victim's side, by placing the hand nearest the victim's feet under the neck to lift and support it, and by placing the other hand on the forehead and applying back pressure with the palm. (Fig. 1–2A and B).

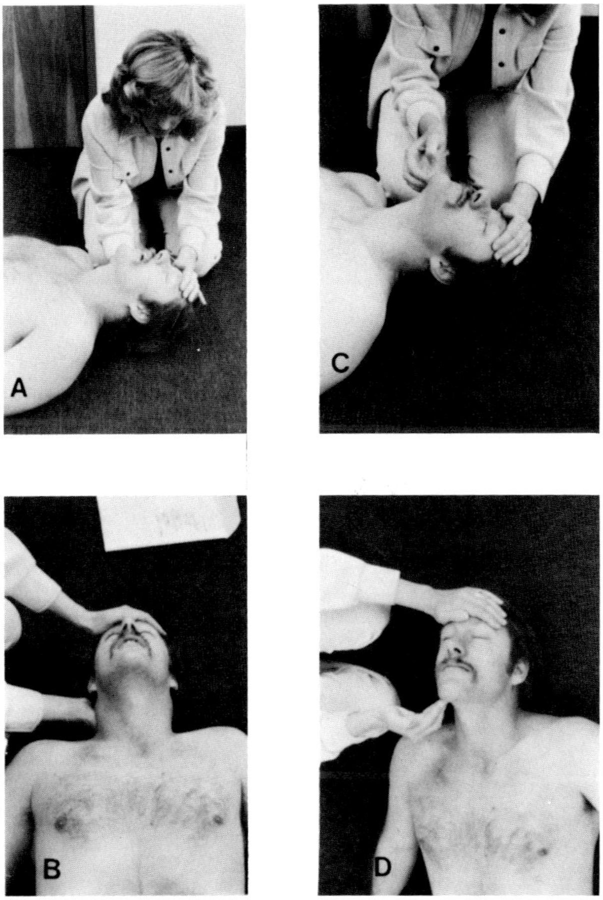

Figure 1–2. Opening the airway. (A) Head tilt–neck lift (side view). (B) Head tilt–neck lift (top view). (C) Head tilt–chin lift (side view). (D) Head tilt–chin lift (top view).

The head tilt–chin lift is accomplished by tilting the head back with one hand on the forehead while lifting and supporting the mandible with the fingertips of the other hand. (Fig. 1–2C and D). The chin is lifted so that the teeth are brought nearly together, but the mouth should not be closed completely. Care must be taken not to compress the soft tissues under the jaw, which might cause additional obstruction.

The head tilt–jaw thrust is initiated by placing the hands at the sides of the victim's head with elbows resting on the surface on which the victim is lying. (Fig. 1–3A and B). Grasping the angles of the mandibles, the rescuer lifts the jaw forward with both hands, at the same time tilting the head backwards. If the victim has a suspected neck injury, the jaw thrust is performed without any head

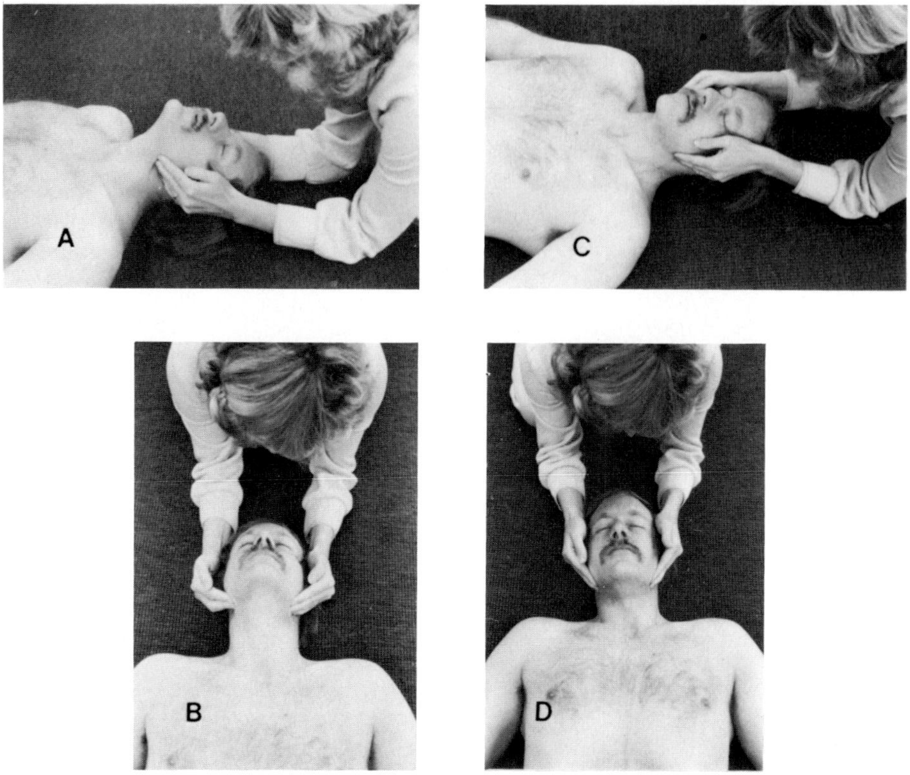

Figure 1–3. Opening the airway. (A) Head tilt–jaw thrust (side view). (B) Head tilt–jaw thrust (top view). (C) Jaw thrust without head tilt; (used with neck injury) (side view). (D) Jaw thrust without head tilt (top view).

tilt (Fig. 1–3C and D.) Any overzealous movement is avoided in opening the airway, in order to avoid inducing or worsening a cervical spine injury.

Once the airway is opened, the rescuer should determine if the patient has spontaneous respirations. In order to do this, the rescuer, with the victim's airway maintained in the open position, should listen and feel over the victim's mouth and nose while observing the victim's abdomen and thorax (Fig. 1–6B). If the chest rises and falls and air movement is noted, the rescuer should continue to maintain the patent airway. If respiratory efforts are initiated but no air movement is detected, then the airway may still be obstructed.

Foreign bodies, laryngospasm, and pharyngeal and tracheal tumors all may produce upper airway obstruction requiring acute management.

Management of the Obstructed Airway

The back blow, the manual thrust, and the finger sweep are the three basic maneuvers recommended for relieving foreign-body airway obstruction.[21] If the choking victim is conscious and adequate air exchange continues, he or she should

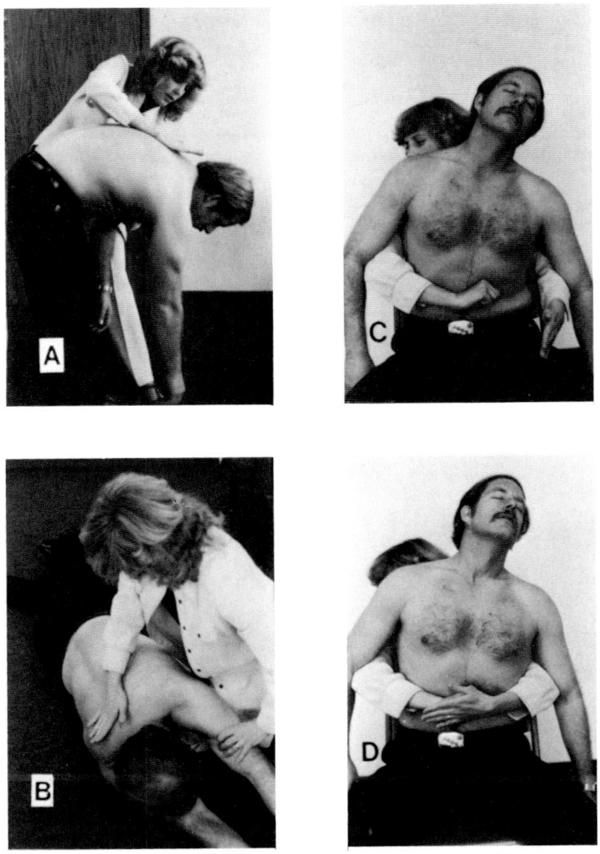

Figure 1–4. Managing the obstructed airway. (A) Back blow in conscious choking victim. (B) Back blow in unconscious choking victim. (C) Abdominal thrust (also known as Heimlich maneuver) in sitting choking victim (fist placement). (D) Abdominal thrust in sitting choking victim (placement of second hand over fist.)

be allowed and encouraged to persist with spontaneous coughing and breathing efforts. However, if the conscious victim cannot maintain air flow adequately and becomes cyanotic, the three manual maneuvers should be employed.

Back Blow

Back blows (Fig. 1–4A and B) may be applied with the victim in the standing, sitting, or supine position. If the victim is standing or is sitting and conscious, the rescuer should position himself at the side and slightly posterior to the victim. With the heel of the hand, the rescuer should deliver four sharp blows over the spine between the shoulder blades (Fig. 1–2). The other hand should be placed on the anterior thorax to support the victim. Each blow should be administered with

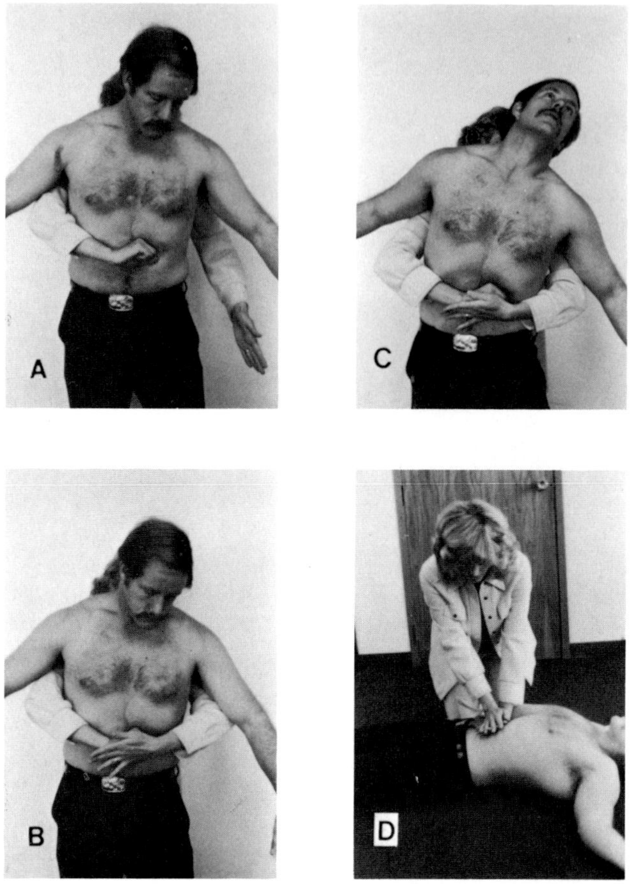

Figure 1–5. Managing the obstructed airway. (A) Abdominal thrust in standing choking victim (fist placement). (B) Abdominal thrust in standing choking victim (placement of second hand over fist). (C) Abdominal thrust in standing choking victim (inward and upward thrust). (D) Abdominal thrust in supine, unconscious choking victim.

full force. An unconscious victim should be rolled onto his or her side, facing the rescuer, with the victim's chest against the rescuer's thigh. The four back blows should be delivered as described above.

Manual Thrust

The manual thrust (Figs. 1–4C and D; and 1–5A through D) is a maneuver which creates an artificial cough and is intended to remove a foreign body from the upper airway. Manual thrusts should be applied either to the upper abdomen (abdominal thrust) or to the lower chest (chest thrust). To minimize the chance of rupture or laceration of abdominal or thoracic viscera, the rescuer should take care not to

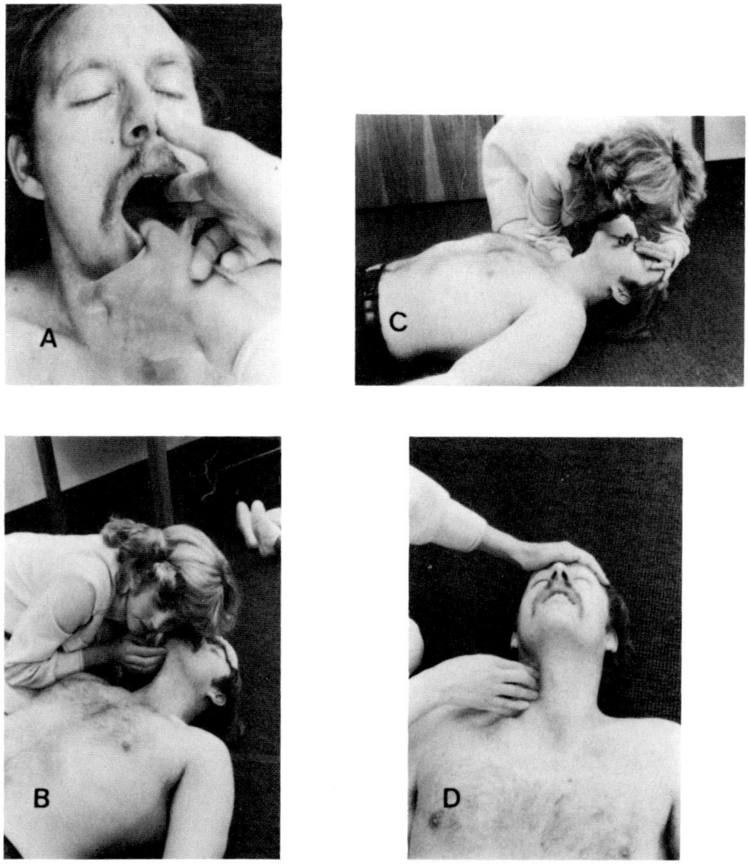

Figure 1–6. Managing the obstructed airway and initiation of artificial respiration. (A) Tongue-jaw lift with finger sweep in unconscious choking victim. (B) Observing, listening, and feeling for spontaneous breathing. (C) Administering mouth-to-mouth respiration (note that head tilt–neck lift is maintained while nostrils are pinched shut). (D) Maintaining open airway with head tilt while palpating carotid artery.

place his hand on the xiphoid process; instead, the hand should be placed either below the rib cage (abdominal thrust) or above this area (chest thrust).[22] As with the back blows, four manual thrusts should be delivered in succession, each one intended to relieve the obstruction. All four thrusts are delivered only if the obstruction is not relieved.

With an unconscious victim, the rescuer should place one hand against the victim's abdomen well below the xiphoid process (between the rib cage and the umbilicus), with the second hand resting on top of the first. With the shoulders directly over the victim's abdomen, an upward-inward thrust is applied with the rescuer's hands.

These manual thrusts can also be applied to the chest, using the same guidelines given for the abdominal thrust. Hand position is the same as for closed-chest cardiac massage (see below). The question of whether the manual thrust (Heimlich maneuver) or the back blow is superior in relieving upper airway obstruction remains controversial. It is generally accepted that the combination of the two is superior to either method alone.

Finger Sweep

If both the back blow and the Heimlich maneuver are unsuccessful in relieving upper airway obstruction and the victim becomes unconscious, the victim's mouth should be opened by grasping the tongue and lower jaw and lifting (tongue–jaw lift) (Fig. 1–6A). Not only does this action draw the tongue away from the back of the throat, but it allows the rescuer to examine the upper airway. The index finger should be inserted along the cheek, deeply into the posterior pharynx. If a foreign body is encountered, it should be dislodged and removed, being careful not to force the object deeper into the airway.

If four back blows, four manual thrusts, and the finger sweep do not relieve an upper airway obstruction, these three maneuvers should be repeated in sequence until the obstruction is relieved or more advanced medical help becomes available.

Breathing

If, once the victim's airway is patent, breathing does not resume, the rescuer should initiate respiration. Using the index finger and the thumb of the hand that is on the victim's forehead, the rescuer should close the nostrils by pinching them (Fig. 1–6C). After taking a deep breath, the rescuer should then open his mouth widely, cover the victim's mouth with his own mouth, and blow air into the victim's mouth while simultaneously watching to see if the victim's chest is rising. Mouth-to-nose ventilation may be more effective than mouth-to-mouth ventilation. Small children need to have both their nose and mouth covered by the rescuer's mouth. If the victim has had a laryngectomy, mouth-to-stoma artificial ventilation is required. In single-rescuer CPR, two full breaths without allowing full exhalation after the first breath are given after each cycle of fifteen chest compressions. With two-rescuer CPR, one breath every five seconds is given.[23] This should be given during the upstroke of the fifth chest compression.

Artificial Circulation

After establishing the airway and initiating respiration, the rescuer must determine if a pulse is present by palpating the carotid artery (Fig. 1–6D). If there is no pulse, external cardiac compression must be initiated. This technique consists of

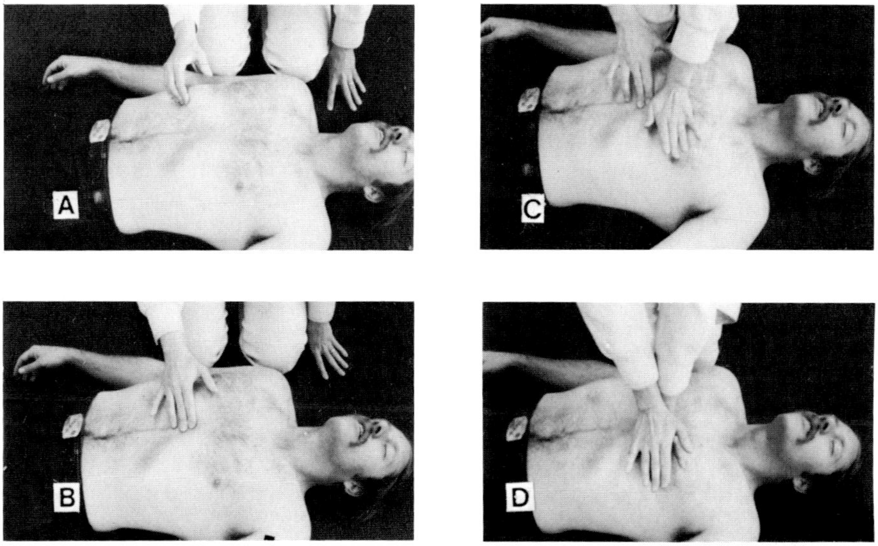

Figure 1–7. Initiation of closed-chest massage: landmarks and hand placement. (A) Run fingers along lower rib margin using hand closest to victim's feet. (B) Place middle finger in notch where lower ribs meet sternum. (C) Place heel of hand nearest the victim's head adjacent to index finger on sternum. (D) Place first hand (hand closest to victim's feet) atop second hand.

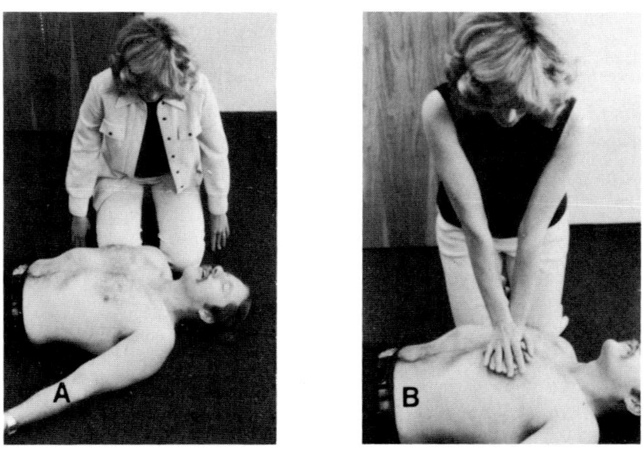

Figure 1–8. Performing closed-chest massage. (A) Rescuer kneeling close to victim's side. (B) Performing closed-chest massage (note position of fingers off chest wall and locked elbows).

rhythmically applying pressure over the lower half of the sternum. The cardiac arrest victim should be placed in a horizontal position, taking care to make sure that the head is not above the level of the heart. Effective external cardiac compression requires a 4- to 5-cm depression of the sternum of an adult. This commonly generates a pressure of between 80 and 90 mmHg.[24] Successful compression also requires that the victim be on a firm surface, such as the ground. A board may have to be placed under a victim who is lying on a soft surface, such as a bed.

TECHNIQUE OF EXTERNAL CARDIAC COMPRESSION

External cardiac compression[19] involves the following steps:

1. The rescuer should take a position close to the patient's chest, and should kneel over the victim (Fig. 1–8A).
2. Using the hand closest to the victim's feet, the rescuer locates the notch where the lower rib margins meet the sternum and places the middle finger on this notch, with the index finger on the sternum just next to the middle finger (Fig. 1–7A and B).
3. The heel of the hand closest to the victim's head is then placed on the sternum, just next to the index finger of the first hand. (The location of the xiphoid process is irrelevant) (Fig. 1–7C).
4. The first hand is removed from the notch and placed on top of the hand on the sternum (Fig. 1–7D).
5. The rescuer's fingers must be kept off the chest wall; they may either be extended or interlaced.
6. The rescuer then straightens his arms with the elbows in a locked position. Next, the rescuer positions his shoulders directly over his hands so that the thrust for external chest compression is straight down (Fig. 1–8B).
7. The rescuer must depress the sternum approximately 4 to 5 cm, and then release the pressure completely to allow for diastolic filling.
8. With two-man CPR, a compression rate of 60 per minute should be sustained, with each compression lasting 0.5 to 0.6 seconds. The compression cycle should be uninterrupted, regular, and smooth.
9. The rescuer's hands should not be lifted off the chest wall, nor should their position be changed during CPR.

In the case of single-rescuer CPR, artificial ventilation and artificial circulation must be performed—as specified earlier—using a ratio of 15 chest compressions to 2 respirations. Once CPR is initiated, it should not be interrupted for more than 5 seconds, except for tracheal intubation or transportation. Under *no* circumstances should CPR be interrupted for more than 30 seconds for either transportation or intubation.

SPECIAL RESCUE SITUATIONS

Electric Shock

Of paramount importance is that the rescuer be certain that resuscitation efforts will not put him in danger of electric shock. Specific problems that one may expect to encounter in an electric-shock victim include: (1) tetany of the respiratory muscles, which usually is limited to the duration of the electric exposure; (2) prolonged paralysis of the respiratory muscles, which can last for minutes after an electric shock has terminated; and (3) cardiac arrest secondary to ventricular fibrillation. Because of the frequency of ventricular arrhythmias in cases of electric shock, some sources advocate the immediate use of a chest thump prior to the CPR procedures previously outlined.

Drowning

In general, when a rescuer is attempting to save a drowning victim, mouth-to-mouth resuscitation, as well as external chest compression, should not be attempted in the water. These steps may be initiated if the rescuer has some flotation device. Recent reports using a modified scuba lung capable of delivering high flow rates (780 L/min) to a drowning victim appear encouraging.[25] With this high-flow regulator, occlusion of the victim's nose is not necessary, and simultaneous external chest compression can be performed. In the future, the modified scuba lung may prove to be an important means of in-the-water cardiopulmonary support for drowning victims.

Accident Cases

Accident victims, especially those in motor vehicle accidents, frequently sustain neck injuries. It is imperative that the rescuer produce no additional injury. If neck injury is suspected, the rescuer should use the jaw thrust without tilting or turning the victim's head to open the airway.

Without question, bystander-initiated basic CPR greatly improves survival in cases of cardiopulmonary arrest. The techniques of CPR are most effective when started immediately after such an arrest. While basic cardiac life support may sustain life temporarily, the special equipment available in ambulances and emergency rooms can improve survival by offering victims advanced cardiac life support. However, only well-trained personnel should attempt to use such support equipment, since its improper use can further jeopardize the victim's life.

THE USE OF DRUG THERAPY AND DEFIBRILLATION IN ADVANCED LIFE SUPPORT

Once artificial breathing and closed-chest cardiac compression have been initiated, an intravenous line must be established. It is recommended that a central line be placed, since in cases of circulatory collapse it is frequently impossible to establish peripheral venous lines. Either an internal jugular or a subclavian approach may be used. Because sterile technique is not observed during the emergent placement of a central line, it should be removed following resuscitation of the victim, and replaced by lines inserted with a sterile approach.

With the hypovolemic patient, the administration of intravenous fluids is critical. Those fluids which result in the greatest intravascular volume expansion are the crystalloid solutions, such as 0.9 percent saline or lactated ringer's solution. In addition, colloid solutions, such as the commercial albumin (Plasmanate or 5 percent albumin) can be used. Care must be taken if acute myocardial infarction is suspected, because volume expansion in this situation has been shown to potentiate cardiogenic shock.[26]

MEDICATIONS USED DURING CARDIOPULMONARY RESUSCITATION

Sodium Bicarbonate

With combined respiratory and circulatory collapse, anaerobic metabolism ensues rapidly and severe systemic acidosis occurs. Because the acidosis is of a combined metabolic and respiratory nature, the administration of sodium bicarbonate, as well as providing adequate alveolar ventilation, is essential in restoring a normal acid–base balance.[27] In general, the administration of 1 ampule of sodium bicarbonate (45 mEq) is reserved for arterial pH values of less than 7.25 with a normal or low PCO_2 ($PCO_2 \leq 40$). The potential hazards of excess bicarbonate administration include severe metabolic alkalosis, with impairment of oxygen release from hemoglobin because of a left shift of the oxygen-hemoglobin dissociation curve, and sodium and water overload resulting in both hypernatremia and hyperosmolality.[28]

In general, if normal cardiac rhythm can be restored rapidly, the patient is being ventilated adequately, and tissue perfusion appears good, sodium bicarbonate should not be given until the first arterial blood gas with pH measurement has returned from the laboratory. In situations in which the patient is acidemic, remains unstable, and has an irregular cardiac rhythm, 2 ampules of sodium bicarbonate may be given intravenously, each ampule being given over a 1½- to 2-minute period. Prior to giving additional bicarbonate, however, the arterial pH should be checked.

Drugs Used for Control of the Heart Rhythm and Rate

Lidocaine Hydrochloride

For patients suffering from ventricular ectopy, intravenous lidocaine hydrochloride and procainamide hydrochloride remain two of the most useful drugs. Ectopy associated with acute myocardial infarction should always be treated. The drug of choice in the initial treatment of such cases remains lidocaine. This should be injected immediately, using an initial bolus of 1 mg/kg body weight, followed by a continuous intravenous infusion of between 1 and 4 mg per minute via an infusion pump.[29] The administration of prophylactic lidocaine may reduce the incidence of ventricular ectopy associated with myocardial infarction. This is probably not necessary when a patient is being monitored in a coronary care unit. In the field, however, such administration appears reasonable. The toxic effects of lidocaine include seizures, altered states of consciousness, muscular twitching, and slurred speech.

Procainamide Hydrochloride

Procainamide is an effective drug, not only for use in suppressing ventricular ectopy, but also for recurrent ventricular fibrillation resistant to defibrillation. The usual dose of procainamide is 100 mg, given intravenously over a 5-minute period (20 mg/min) until the arrhythmia is abolished or hypotension ensues. Additionally, one should observe the QRS complex, and if the initial dose of procainamide widens it by more than 50 percent of its original width, no additional drug should be given. As with lidocaine, the procainamide maintenance dosage is between 1 and 4 mg/min.[30] Complications of procainamide administration include hypotension and prolongation of the QRS complex. If renal failure is present, the dosage of the drug should be reduced. The lupus syndrome associated with procainamide use has not been observed with acute administration of the drug.

Propranolol

Propranolol is a beta-adrenergic blocking agent. It acts by competing for the beta receptor sites with beta-adrenergic stimulators such as norepinephrine. Propranolol is most effective in the treatment of resistant ventricular tachycardia and in the treatment of supraventricular tachycardias. Its intravenous use must be done with care because of the potential for producing complete heart block and asystole. The usual dose is 1 mg given slowly for 5 minutes, with a total dose not exceeding 5 mg. Complications of propranolol administration include severe cardiac depression, and bronchospasm in those patients with asthma and chronic obstructive airways disease.

Bretylium Tosylate

The use of bretylium has been reserved for treating ventricular fibrillation and ventricular tachycardia unresponsive to other forms of therapy, including lidocaine, procainamide, electric shock, and propranolol. In situations in which a refractory ventricular fibrillation exists, 5 mg/kg of bretylium is given in a bolus, followed by electrical defibrillation. This may be repeated and increased to 10 mg/kg at 15- to 30-minute intervals if ventricular fibrillation persists.[31] Once a loading dose has been administered, the drug can be used by continuous infusion at a rate of 1 to 2 mg/min.

Atropine Sulfate

Atropine is a parasympatholytic drug that reduces vagal tone. It is most useful in the treatment of sinus bradycardia accompanied by marked hypotension. Atropine can be useful if a high-degree AV block is present at the nodal level, resulting in the ventricular asystoles.[32] If the patient has recovered and is not hypotensive or symptomatic from the bradycardia, atropine is generally not used. If it is to be used, the total dose should not exceed 2 mg.

Isoproterenol

Isoproterenol is a beta-adrenergic stimulator. It has both inotropic and chronotropic effects and its primary use is for the treatment of bradycardia resulting from heart block. However, isoproterenol may produce ventricular dysrhythmias, and the physician must be aware that this drug increases myocardial oxygen requirements, thus making its use in myocardial infarction limited. The recommended infusion rate is between 2 and 20 μg/min.

Drugs Used to Augment Cardiac Output and Maintain Blood Pressure

This group of drugs acts specifically on both alpha and beta receptors. In general, when peripheral vascular tone is decreased, alpha stimulation is required to increase the peripheral vascular resistance. In addition, if beta stimulation of the heart is depressed or reduced, a specific beta agonist may be necessary. It is important to realize that alpha and beta agonists have both peripheral and central (myocardial) effects, and that it is the summation of these effects that produces the end result.

Epinephrine

When asystole occurs and cardiac rhythm cannot be restored, epinephrine hydrochloride remains the drug of choice. This drug can elevate the perfusion pressure during chest compression, has both inotropic and chronotropic effects, and may make the myocardium more receptive to electrical defibrillation. In addition to direct myocardial stimulation, epinephrine produces an alpha effect systemically and can increase the blood pressure. In situations in which an intravenous line has not been established, the intracardiac injection of epinephrine may be used. While cardiac taponade and hemothorax are potential complications, the intracardiac injection of epinephrine has been found to be a relatively low-risk and lifesaving procedure.[33]

Norepinephrine

Norepinephrine is a more potent vasoconstrictor than epinephrine, as well as a powerful inotropic agent. Generally, norepinephrine also produces a more rapid blood-pressure response than other catecholamines. This drug must be given by continuous intravenous infusion. Because of the extreme potency of norepinephrine and the difficulties in using standard blood-pressure measurements to monitor patients, it is recommended that an arterial line be placed prior to its use. As with isoproterenol, myocardial oxygen consumption is increased with norepinephrine administration, and this can be deleterious in the case of an acute myocardial infarction. In general, this is a drug which is used only temporarily or in a "last ditch" situation.

Dopamine Hydrochloride

Dopamine is a natural precursor of norepinephrine, and depending upon its dose has dopaminergic, beta adrenergic, and alpha adrenergic effects. The infusion of dopamine is titrated according to the blood pressure, urine output, and CNS response. Generally, one starts with a dose of 5 to 20 μg/kg/min. In doses above 20 μg/kg/min, the pharmacologic effect of dopamine is almost purely alpha adrenergic.[34] Because of the multiple potential effects of dopamine, it is frequently necessary to monitor the left ventricular filling pressure (pulmonary capillary wedge pressure) to optimize dosage. Care must be taken not to administer an alkaline solution simultaneously with dopamine, since the drug is inactivated in this setting.

Dobutamine Hydrochloride

In contrast to dopamine, dobutamine is a direct beta adrenergic receptor stimulator which has little systemic arterial effect at usual doses (2.5 to 10 μg/kg/min). Because of this inotropic effect without an effect of increasing the peripheral vascular resistance, dobutamine is frequently helpful in augmenting cardiac output.[35]

Calcium Ion

Because calcium is an essential cation in muscular contraction, as well as in maintaining ventricular automaticity, it has been utilized in ventricular standstill. The drug is available in both the calcium gluconate and calcium chloride forms. In general, the calcium chloride form is preferred, although because of its extreme sclerosing nature, it can be given only through a central line. The usual dose is 5 to 10 ml of a 10 percent solution, which can be repeated at 10-minute intervals.

Sodium Nitroprusside

Nitroprusside is a rapidly acting peripheral vasodilator which produces immediate hypotension. Its use may be helpful in situations in which there is an extremely high peripheral vascular resistance and depression of cardiac output. It is mandatory that hemodynamic monitoring be done on patients who receive sodium nitroprusside. The usual dosage is less than 10 μg/kg/min and depends on the peripheral vascular response.

Diuretics

Diuretics should be given to patients with fluid overload and left ventricular failure. Furosemide should be given in a 40 mg intravenous bolus, and the dose should be doubled until a therapeutic response is observed. It has been noted that the administration of furosemide can lead to immediate improvement of acute pulmonary edema prior to the onset of diuresis. While the mechanisms for this is not well understood, it is probably related to changes in the pulmonary circulation. In general, furosemide should not be used during acute cardiac resuscitation, but only after the patient has been "stabilized."

COMPLICATIONS OF CARDIOPULMONARY RESUSCITATION

The potential complications of CPR are many and relate to: (1) overzealous closed-chest compression; (2) inadequate intubation, (3) intracardiac and subclavian punctures; and (4) excessive fluid administration. Specific complications include: (1) Intubation of the esophagus and right main-stem bronchus; (2) tracheal occlusion by an esophageal obturator airway (EOA); (3) fractured ribs; (4) pneumothorax and pneumomediastinum; (5) hemothorax; (6) costochondral separation; (7) flail chest; (8) hemopericardium; (9) pulmonary edema; (10) aspiration pneumonia; and (11) infection (sepsis) from contaminated intravenous lines.

Intubation of the esophagus, tracheal placement of an esophageal obturator, and prolonged intubation of the right main-stem bronchus all may result in inadequate ventilation and oxygenation. Of immediate concern is esophageal intubation with an endotracheal tube. Because auscultation of the chest and abdomen during assisted ventilation does not always delineate proper placement of the endotracheal tube, the tube position should be re-checked with a laryngoscope if there is any doubt about its location. The esophageal obturator airway (EOA) is a long, cuffed endotracheal tube with an occluded distal end (see Chapter 2). If this is put into the trachea rather than the esophagus, adequate assisted ventilation cannot be given. Theoretically, if the EOA tube were placed in the trachea, breath sounds would not be heard, and the tube would have to be removed and repositioned immediately.[35] However, this is not always the case, and tracheal obstruction is a potential hazard with this device.

Overzealous closed chest compression can produce rib fractures and can result in pneumothorax, pneumomediastinum, hemothorax, and in some cases a flail chest. With closed chest compression to the proper depth (4 to 5 cm), these complications should be minimal.

Immediate complications, which can result either directly or indirectly from the placement of venous lines or intracardiac punctures in CPR, include hemopericardium, pneumothorax, and hemothorax; a more remote complication is infection from the site of a catheter insertion.[32] A tension pneumothorax should be suspected when breath sounds suddenly disappear in association with bradycardia and hypotension. With excessive fluid administration, patients can quickly develop pulmonary edema. If fluid overload is of concern, a Swan-Ganz catheter should be placed to monitor fluid management.

An additional complication of CPR is aspiration pneumonia with subsequent respiratory failure. To prevent this, care must be taken to protect the patient's airway, and the cuff of the endotracheal tube should be inflated to prevent the aspiration of gastric and oral contents.

While the complications associated with CPR are many and severe, they should in no way prevent the aggressive implementation of advanced CPR by qualified individuals. When complications are recognized early, and there is appropriate therapeutic intervention, it is rare that they adversely effect the outcome.

References

1. The Holy Bible, Authorized (King James) Version, 2 Kings 4:32.
2. Schafer EA: Description of a simple and efficient method of performing artificial respiration. Med-Chir Trans R Med Chir Soc 87:609, 1904.
3. Comroe JH Jr, Dripps RD: Artificial respiration. JAMA 130:381, 1946.
4. Kouwenhoven WB, June JR, Knickerbocker GG: Closed-chest cardiac massage. JAMA 173:1064, 1960.
5. Eisenberg MS, Bergner L, Hallstrom A: Epidemiology of cardiac arrest and resuscitation in a suburban community. JACEP 8:2, 1979.
6. McSwain GR, Garrison WB, Artz CP: Evaluation of resuscitation from cardiopulmonary arrest by paramedics. Ann Emerg Med 9:341, 1980.
7. Thompson RG, Hallstrom AP, Cobb LA: Bystander-initiated cardiopulmonary resuscitation in the management of ventricular fibrillation. Ann Intern Med 90:737, 1979.
8. Eisenberg MS, Bergner L, Hallstrom A: Cardiac Resuscitation in the community. JAMA 241:1905, 1979.
9. Criley JM, Blaufuss AN, Kissell GL: Cough induced cardiac compression. JAMA 236:1246, 1976.
10. Weisfeldt ML, Chandra N: Physiology of cardiopulmonary resuscitation. Ann Rev Med 32:435, 1981.
11. Rudikoff MT, Marghan WL, Effron M, et al.: Mechanisms of blood flow during cardiopulmonary resuscitation. Circulation 61:345, 1980.
12. Chandra N, Snyder L, Weisfeldt ML: Abdominal binding during CPR in man. Circulation 60:11, 1979.
13. Chandra N, Rudikoff M, Tsitlik J, et al.: Augmentation of carotid flow during CPR in the dog by simultaneous compression and ventilation with high airway pressure. Am J Cardiol 43:422, 1979.
14. Wilder RJ, Weir D, Ruch BF, et al: Method of coordinating ventilation and closed-chest cardiac massage in the dog. Surgery 53:186, 1963.
15. Rogers MC, Nugent SK, Stidham GL: Effects of closed-chest cardiac massage on intracranial pressure. Crit Care Med 7:454, 1979.
16. Beeson PB, McDermott W: Textbook of Medicine, 14th ed, Philadelphia, WB Saunders, pp 647, 1975.
17. Earnest MP, Yarnell PR, Merrill SL, et al.: Long-term survival and neurologic states after resuscitation from out-of-hospital cardiac arrest. Neurology 30:1298, 1980.

18. Bates D, Caronna JJ, Cartlidge NEF, et al.: A prospective study of nontraumatic coma: methods and results in 310 patients. Ann Neurol 2:210, 1977.
19. National Conference on Cardiopulmonary Resuscitation: Standards and guidelines for cardiopulmonary resuscitation and emergency cardiac care (ECC). JAMA 244:453, 1980.
20. Guildner CW: Resuscitation—Opening the airway: A comparative study of techniques for opening an airway obstructed by the tongue. JACEP 5:588, 1976.
21. Committee on Emergency Medical Services, Assembly of Life Sciences, National Research Council, National Academy of Sciences: Report on Emergency Airway Management, 1976.
22. Visintine RE, Baick CH: Ruptured stomach after Heimlich maneuver. JAMA 234:415, 1975.
23. Cardiopulmonary Resuscitation: Conference Proceedings, May 23, 1966, Washington, DC, National Academy of Sciences, National Research Council, 1967.
24. March NF, Matthews RC: New techniques of external cardiac compressions; acquatic cardiopulmonary resuscitation. JAMA 244:1229, 1980.
25. DaLuz PL, Weil MH, Liu VY, et al.: Plasma volume prior to and following volume loading during shock complicating acute myocardial infarction. Circulation 44:98, 1974.
26. Bishop RL, Weisfeldt ML: Sodium bicarbonate administration during cardiac arrest. JAMA 235:506, 1976.
27. Mattar JA, Weil MH, Shubin H, et al.: Cardiac arrest in the critically ill: II hyperosmolal states following cardiac arrests. Am J Med 56:162, 1974.
28. Wyman MG, Lalka D, Hammersmith L, et al.: Multiple bolus technique for lidocaine administration during the first hours of acute myocardial infarction. Am J Cardiol 41:313, 1978.
29. Grengiardien E-GV, Heissenbuttel RH, Bigger JT: Intermittent intravenous procainamide to treat ventricular arrhythmias. Ann Intern Med 78:183, 1973.
30. Koch-Weser J: Drug therapy: Bretylium. N Eng J Med 300:473, 1979.
31. Brown BC, Lewis AG, Criley JM: Asystole and its treatment, the possible role of parasympathetic nervous system in cardiac arrest. JACEP 8:448, 1979.
32. Davidson R, Barresi V, Parker M: Intracardiac injections during cardiopulmonary resuscitation. JAMA 1110, 1980.
33. Goldberg LI: Dopamine—Clinical uses of an endogenous catacolamine. N Engl J Med 291:707, 1974.
34. Tuttle RR, Mills J: Dobutamine—development of a new catacolamine to selectively increase cardiac contractility. Circ Res 36:185, 1975.
35. Meislin HW. The Esophageal Obturator Airway. A Study of Respiratory Effectiveness. Ann Emerg Med 9:54, 1980.

2

Tracheal Intubation

John L. Stauffer, M.D.

INTRODUCTION

The establishment of a patent airway is the most vital aspect of life support and critical patient care. Basic life support begins with control of the airway by proper positioning of the head and neck. Intubation of the trachea with a cuffed tube, the definitive step in control of the patient's airway, is a fundamental aspect of advanced life support. Successful intubation of the trachea effectively isolates the airway, maintains its patency, and provides a route for oxygenation, ventilation, and the evacuation of tracheobronchial secretions and foreign material. Once the trachea is intubated, attention may be focused on correcting physiologic disturbances and treating underlying disease processes. In this chapter, intubation of the trachea and other life-saving methods of emergency airway care will be reviewed.

Definitions

Tracheal intubation is the insertion of a hollow tube into the trachea by one of several routes. The term "endotracheal intubation" is usually used to refer to translaryngeal insertion of a tube into the trachea by either the oral ("orotracheal") or nasal ("nasotracheal") route. The trachea also may be intubated through an incision into the larynx (laryngotomy) or into the trachea (tracheotomy). The opening (stoma) created by the tracheotomy is the tracheostomy. Laryngotomy is performed through the cricothyroid membrane and therefore is called cricothyroidotomy or cricothyrotomy. A "definitive airway" is a cuffed endotracheal or tracheostomy tube which isolates and protects the airway and provides a route for oxygenation, ventilation, and the removal of secretions. Other uncuffed artificial airways, such as tracheostomy cannulae and laryngectomy tubes, may be placed into the trachea but are not definitive airways.

Who Should Intubate?

No reliable data are available to indicate the frequency of endotracheal intubation and who performs it. Whenever tracheal intubation is necessary, it should be done by the most skilled and experienced person available. Usually, but not always, this is the physician. Ideally, an anesthesiologist or nurse anesthetist should perform every emergency endotracheal intubation, but this ideal cannot be achieved, since many emergencies occur in settings in which anesthesia personnel are not immediately available. Not all physicians are adept at intubation, but all critical-care physicians should be skilled in establishing a patent airway and intubating the trachea. Endotracheal intubation skills are learned first on manikins and later in the operating room with guidance by anesthesiologists and nurse anesthetists. Recent data suggest that respiratory therapists with proper training and experience can perform endotracheal intubation as well as or better than physicians.[1,2] Clearly, trained paramedical personnel can perform endotracheal intubation successfully, and this skill may save many lives.[3,4] In the hospital emergency room and intensive care unit, intubation of the trachea may be done by qualified physicians, nurses, nurse anesthetists, and other specially trained personnel. The important thing is not who does it but that it be done well. All critical-care and emergency departments should have provisions for training and retraining in endotracheal intubation.

Indications for Tracheal Intubation

Tracheal intubation may be classified as emergency, urgent, or elective. Elective intubation is done for the administration of general anesthesia. The general indications for emergency and urgent intubation of the trachea are: (1) relief of upper airway obstruction; (2) isolation and protection of the airway; (3) facilitation of suctioning the tracheobronchial tree; and (4) facilitation of assisted ventilation. In the emergency setting, tracheal intubation is attempted when prolonged ventilation is needed or when simpler methods of ventilation and oxygenation are not successful or feasible. Common medical conditions requiring emergency or urgent tracheal intubation include cardiopulmonary resuscitation, coma with an unstable airway, acute respiratory failure from a variety of causes, inhalation injury to the airway, risk of pulmonary aspiration, and the need for tracheobronchial suctioning. The victim of cardiac arrest and the patient with acute respiratory failure usually have several or all of the general indications for tracheal intubation. Common surgical conditions requiring tracheal intubation are shock, respiratory failure, and trauma to the mouth, head, neck, larynx, or trachea.

EQUIPMENT FOR TRACHEAL INTUBATION

All of the equipment necessary for tracheal intubation should be arranged conveniently in a single portable tray or basket which is readily available in the emergency area. The minimum essential equipment is listed in Table 2-1. A wide

Table 2–1. Equipment for Emergency Oral or Nasal Endotracheal Intubation

Nasal/oral endotracheal tubes (sizes 7, 8, and 9) with attached 15-mm male adaptors
Stylet for oral endotracheal tube
20 ml plastic syringe for cuff inflation
Four-way stopcock for cuff inflation
Two-way swivel adaptor
Water-soluble lubricant
Topical anesthetic spray with applicator
Topical vasoconstrictor (cocaine [10%] or phenylephrine [1%]) with applicator
Laryngoscope with curved (two sizes) and straight (two sizes) blades
Magill forceps
Adhesive tape or tracheostomy tape
Tincture of benzoin
4 × 4-inch gauze
Scissors
Oral pharyngeal airways (several sizes)
Endotracheal tube suction kit
Sterile gloves
Yankauer pharyngeal suction tube
Portable or wall suction apparatus
Self-inflating resuscitation bag with mask
High-flow oxygen source

variety of sizes of cuffed, disposable endotracheal tubes and laryngoscope blades should be included. Commercial kits containing the necessary equipment for intubation are available, but a tray or basket assembled to meet individual requirements is preferable. Periodic inspection of the intubation-equipment set with an affixed list of contents is necessary to ascertain that all equipment is present and functioning properly.

Endotracheal Tubes

The reusable, hard red rubber endotracheal tubes of the 1950s and 1960s have been replaced by cuffed, disposable endotracheal tubes made of synthetic materials. Reusable endotracheal tubes have no advantage and may be toxic if they are sterilized by ethylene oxide or gamma radiation. Modern endotracheal tubes incorporate standard features (Fig. 2-1) proposed by the Z-79 Committee of the American National Standards Institute.[5] Although a wide variety of tubes is available, only those approved by this organization and labelled "Z-79" should be used. A polyvinyl chloride or silicone rubber (silastic) composition allows the tubes to become more compliant at body temperature, adapting to the airway without kinking. Additionally, the tubes and their cuffs are made of nontoxic materials, proven to be safe by implantation testing in animals. The standard radius of curvature of both oral and nasal endotracheal tubes is 14 ± 2 cm. The bevel on the patient (distal) end of the endotracheal tube is angled at 30 degrees for nasal tubes and 45 degrees for oral tubes, and faces to the left when the tube is viewed from the concave aspect. The distal end of the endotracheal tube is rounded and smooth to avoid mucosal injury and has a radiographic marker for easy identification on the chest radiograph. The Murphy eye is a side-hole at the

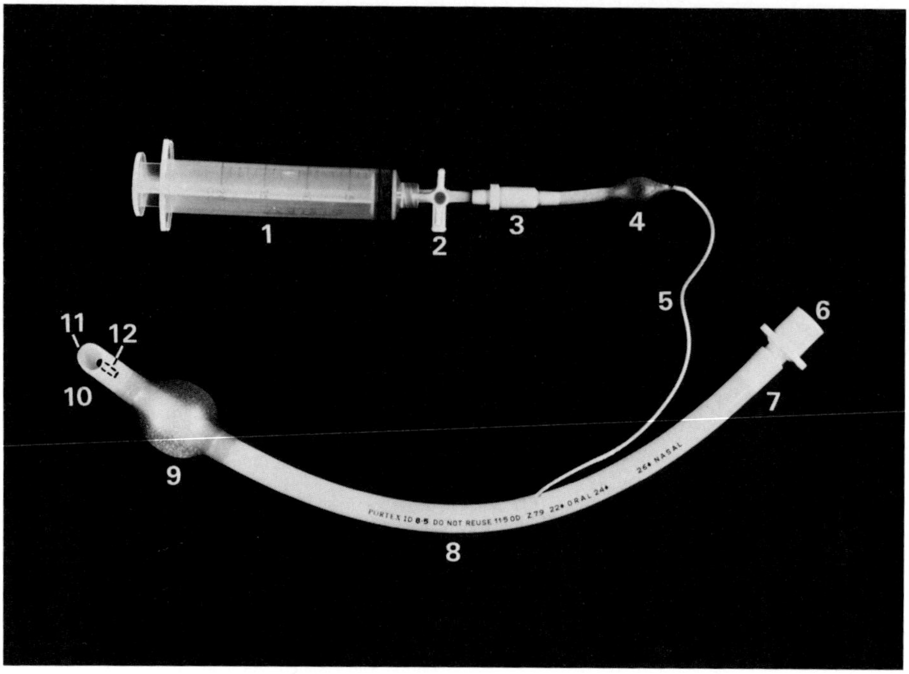

Figure 2–1. The Portex Blue Line disposable oral-nasal endotracheal tube (Portex, Inc., Wilmington, MA) is one example of a modern endotracheal tube. Features include: (1) inflating 20 ml syringe, (2) four-way stopcock, (3) inflating valve, (4) pilot balloon, (5) inflating tube, (6) 15-mm male adaptor, (7) proximal end, (8) label region, (9) soft cuff, (10) distal end, (11) bevel, and (12) Murphy eye.

patient end of the tube, opposite the bevel. The Magill endotracheal tube lacks the Murphy eye. An air-inflatable cuff is bonded tightly to the distal end of the tube just above the Murphy eye. The pilot balloon is an optional but highly desirable endotracheal tube feature that provides a rough estimate of cuff pressure. An inflating tube, recessed into the side wall of the endotracheal tube, connects the cuff to the pilot balloon and one-way inflating valve. A removable, 15-mm male adaptor is inserted into the machine (proximal) end of the tube.

Endotracheal tubes are either clear or opaque, depending upon their composition. Clear tubes permit the visualization of secretions and condensed water vapor and inspection of the tracheal mucosa with a fiberoptic bronchoscope. Markings on the shaft of the endotracheal tube in a label region indicate the size and type of the tube, nontoxicity by the letters "IT" (implant testing), and depth of insertion by centimeter markings. The tube lumen is perfectly circular, so as to avoid kinking and to maximize the cross-sectional area of the tube, and the tube wall is thin enough to maximize the internal diameter. The tubes should be packaged individually in see-through plastic packages that maintain the required curvature and indicate the size and type of the tube in large letters on the right hand corner. A peel-away backing is ideal for ease of opening the package. Most tubes are supplied in sterile packages. If the package is not sterile, the package information should state suitable methods of sterilization.

Selecting the proper size of endotracheal tube is very important. A tube that is too large increases the risk of laryngeal injury,[6] while one that is too small makes suctioning more difficult and increases airway resistance. The internal diameter (ID) of the tube in millimeters is the preferred way to refer to tube size. French size designations are confusing and vary from one manufacturer to the next. The outer diameter of an endotracheal tube is usually 2 to 4 mm greater than the internal diameter depending on the wall thickness. Most endotracheal tubes have walls about 1.5 mm thick. Adult males can be intubated orally with size 8.0 to 9.0 (millimeters of ID) tubes, whereas adult females usually tolerate size 7.0 to 8.5 (millimeter ID) oral tubes. A size smaller or larger may be needed, depending upon tracheal variation in the individual being intubated. Nasal intubation is usually done with tubes 1 mm smaller than are used for oral intubation. Elderly men with patulous tracheas may require a size 10 oral tube. The length of the endotracheal tube depends upon ID size and whether or not the tube is pre-cut. A size 7 endotracheal tube has a minimum tube length of 300 mm, with the minimum tube length increasing by 10 mm for each 0.5 mm increase in ID.

Although oral and nasal endotracheal tubes are fundamentally similar, there are a few minor differences. Nasal endotracheal tubes are longer and have a 30 degree bevel angle. Many tubes now are marketed for either transoral or transnasal insertion, but the intubator should select the tube that is manufactured for a specific route of insertion whenever possible.

An inflatable cuff makes the endotracheal tube a definitive airway. Uncuffed tubes have no advantage except for a slightly greater ease of insertion and for use in pediatric patients, in whom the glottis is small. Uncuffed tubes should not be used for emergency tracheal intubation of adults, since the cuff is necessary to seal the airway, to guard against aspiration, and to provide a closed system for assisted ventilation. Tubes with detachable cuffs are dangerous and should never be used. Hard cuffs (high pressure, low volume, low profile) have less bulk, may be easier to pass through a tight glottis, and are less likely to be lacerated by teeth and intubation equipment, but should be avoided because of the risk of serious tracheal injury. Soft cuffs (high volume, low pressure) minimize tracheal injury because lateral pressure on the tracheal mucosa, usually under 25 mm Hg, is below capillary perfusion pressure. Because the in vitro diameter of the fully inflated soft cuff greatly exceeds the diameter of the tracheal lumen, which ranges from 13 to 23 mm in adults,[7] some wrinkling of bulky soft cuffs occurs after insertion. The cuff contact area on the tracheal mucosa depends on the amount of cuff fabric and the pressure-volume relationship (compliance) of the cuff. Cuffs that are too bulky allow an up-and-down "pistoning" motion in the tracheal lumen, do not anchor the tube in the center of the lumen, and cause mucosal grooves at points where the cuff fabric wrinkles.[8] The Portex "Profile" cuff (Portex, Inc., Wilmington, MA) has been designed to avoid these problems. The cuff should be highly compliant to adapt to the shape of the patient's trachea. Because of considerable variation in the compliance of available cuffs,[9] careful examination of the inflated cuff before insertion is important. A cuff that is very firm and has a low profile after inflation probably is not compliant.

There is probably no "safe" cuff pressure, since any pressure on the delicate, ciliated epithelium of the trachea will cause some injury. Automatic cuff pressure control devices are available to limit the internal pressure in the cuff to a safe level, including the regulating valve and control balloon of the Lanz tube (Extracorporeal Medical Specialties, Inc., King of Prussia, PA) and the detachable pressure-relief adaptor (Shiley, Inc., Irvine, CA). However, automatic cuff pressure control devices are expensive and may preclude maintaining an increased cuff pressure for long periods if this becomes necessary, as in the patient on a mechanical ventilator with high airway pressures.

Several variations on the standard endotracheal tube are available, but none are advantageous for emergency endotracheal intubation. Uncuffed Cole tubes, Ring tubes, and Jackson-Reese endotracheal tubes are desirable for pediatric endotracheal intubation.[10] "Armored" endotracheal tubes with wire reinforcement of the shaft to prevent kinking are available but have no value in most emergency intubations. The foam cuff Kamen-Wilkinson tube limits lateral tracheal wall pressure to 15 mmHg, decreasing the risk of serious tracheal injury,[11] but the greater bulk of the foam cuff makes intubation potentially more difficult.

Accessory Equipment for Endotracheal Intubation

Several items from the intubation tray or basket merit attention; these are shown in Figure 2-2, and are as follows:

1. Laryngoscope. The laryngoscope is a lighted instrument with a handle and detachable blades which permits visualization of the larynx during either oral or guided nasal endotracheal intubation. The handles come in several sizes and contain one or two batteries. Both straight and curved (MacIntosh) blades are available, the latter being more popular. Several sizes of each type of blade should be available on the emergency intubation cart. Disposable plastic laryngoscopes are available in commercial intubation kits, but most emergency physicians prefer reusable laryngoscopes.
2. Oral pharyngeal airways. Oral pharyngeal airways may facilitate post-intubation care and protection of the airway. They may be placed in the mouth after oral or nasal endotracheal intubation to prevent biting and tube obstruction, to provide a route for suctioning secretions, and to buttress the oral endotracheal tube. When properly positioned, the oral pharyngeal airway displaces the base of the tongue from the posterior wall of the pharynx and ensures patency of the airway. Desirable features in such an airway include a nontoxic composition, a suitable curvature and length, smooth surfaces, labeled flanges, and enough rigidity to displace the tongue.[5] A bite block at the proximal end of the airway should be rigid enough to prevent obstruction by biting. The Guedel type of airway is made of polyvinyl chloride or rubber and has a central channel for suctioning. The

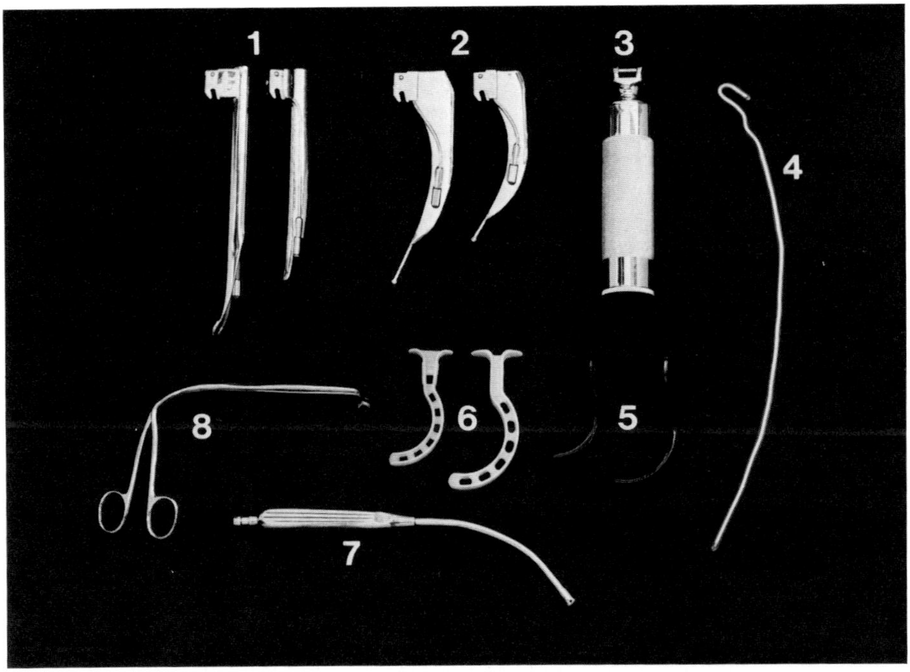

Figure 2–2. The intubation tray or basket includes: (1) two straight laryngoscope blades, (2) two curved (MacIntosh) blades, (3) laryngoscope handle, (4) wire guide, (5) two Guedel oral pharyngeal airways, (6) two Berman oral pharyngeal airways, (7) a Yankauer suction tip, and (8) a Magill angled forceps.

Berman type is a more rigid polyvinyl chloride strut, shaped like an I-beam on cross section, and with two side channels.

3. Other accessory items for endotracheal intubation. The Magill angled forceps is a useful device for guiding the tip of a nasal endotracheal tube into the glottis. Malleable wire guides or introducers are available to stiffen oral endotracheal tubes for insertion into the glottis. Suctioning equipment should be readily available. The Yankauer suction tip is a rigid, wide-bore, curved suction device that is particularly useful for clearning vomitus or thick secretions from the mouth and pharynx. A flexible suction catheter is used to clear the endotracheal tube after intubation. Catheters with multiple eyes at the tip are safer than those with only one eye.[12,13] Plastic two-way swivels attach to the 15-mm male adaptor of the endotracheal tube and decrease the transmission of mechanical forces to the tube. Endotracheal tube holders for both oral and nasal tubes are available to anchor the tube in proper position. If used, they should be soft and compliant and not exert undue pressure on the skin, mucous membranes, or teeth. Tube holders particularly are useful for anchoring oral tubes in edentulous patients, and for preventing "pistoning" motion of the tube.

Tracheostomy Tubes

Critical-care personnel should be familiar with the uses and limitations of tracheostomy tubes in the emergency setting. A tracheostomy tube may be inserted through a patent cricothyroid or tracheal stoma for emergency control of the airway. Only those tracheostomy tubes that meet the Z-79 Committee standards should be used. Soft-cuffed, disposable tubes of polyvinyl chloride or silicone rubber composition are the accepted standards in critical care; metal Jackson tubes and uncuffed tubes should be used in emergencies only if nothing else is available. A neck-plate or flange helps buttress the machine end of the tube and has two holes for securing by tape. The angle of the flange to the center shaft of the tracheostomy tube varies from 65 to 90 degrees, and the physician can select one of these angles on the basis of preference and anatomic considerations. Tracheostomy tubes are not beveled, but their features are otherwise similar to those of endotracheal tubes. Accessory tracheostomy equipment includes a plastic obturator to ease insertion of the tube, gauze tape to hold the neck-plate or flange in place, and a two-way swivel adaptor. A plastic wedge is useful for prying connecting tubing off the 15-mm male adaptor in order to minimize transmission of rotational forces directly to the trachea.

A removable inner cannula is an option that permits easy cleaning of a tracheostmy tube. Fenestrated tubes with or without inner cannulae allow the patient to talk and may facilitate weaning. Double-cuffed tracheostomy tubes and tubes with swivel neck-plates or flanges are available, but their value has not been established. Flexible, uncuffed silastic tracheostomy tubes are sometimes used for permanent tracheostomies, but are not advised for emergency use. Metal Jackson tracheostomy tubes have no application to emergency airway care. Special-purpose tracheostomy cannulae, including the Kistner tracheostomy tube[14] (G. P. Pilling & Son Co., Philadelphia, PA) and the Olympic tracheostomy button (Olympic Medical Corp., Seattle, WA), are sometimes useful for long-term care of the patient in whom access to the trachea is needed, but have no role in emergency tracheal intubation.

METHODS OF EMERGENCY OXYGENATION AND VENTILATION

Several methods can be used to oxygenate and ventilate the patient in a cardiac or pulmonary emergency. Tracheal intubation is one such method but is neither the first nor the most important in emergency establishment of an airway. To establish an emergency airway, the general sequence outlined in Table 2-2 is recommended.[15,16] Obstruction of the upper airway, usually caused by flaccidity of the muscles of the tongue and hypopharynx in the unconscious patient, can be relieved in about 70 percent of cases simply by extending the head (head tilt maneuver.)[15] This step may be facilitated by either the neck lift or chin lift maneuvers. The jaw thrust–head tilt maneuver may accomplish additional forward displacement of the jaw if the head tilt–neck lift or head tilt–chin lift maneuvers are unsuccessful (see

Table 2–2. Steps to Follow in Emergency Establishment of an Airway

1. Head tilt maneuver, along with chin lift, neck lift, or jaw thrust
2. Positive pressure ventilation (mouth-to-mouth or bag-and-mask)
3. Removal of any obstructing foreign material
4. Insertion of nasal or oral pharyngeal airway if necessary to maintain patency of the airway
5. Endotracheal intubation Alternative: Use of esophageal obturator airway
6. Cricothyroidotomy Alternative: Percutaneous translaryngeal or transtracheal catheter jet ventilation

Chapter 1). Positive pressure ventilation is then performed by the mouth-to-mouth technique or with a self-inflating resuscitation bag connected to an oxygen source. If effective ventilation is not possible, obstructing material is sought and removed. An oral or nasal-pharyngeal airway may then be inserted, if necessary, to facilitate ventilation and the evacuation of secretions, but the routine use of such an airway is not advised, since these devices may cause gagging, vomiting, and soft-tissue trauma. If a definitive airway is needed, oral or nasal endotracheal intubation is done. If endotracheal intubation is not possible or is unsuccessful, and if the victim is an unconscious, apneic adult with no airway reflexes, the esophageal obturator airway may be used. If none of the above methods is successful and if asphyxiation appears inevitable without intervention, an emergency cricothyroidotomy should be done. As a "last ditch" method, the cricothyroid membrane may be punctured or incised, or the trachea may be punctured with a large-gauge needle for jet ventilation with oxygen. Emergency tracheotomy is reserved only for rare situations in which cricothyroidotomy is not feasible.

Patients in respiratory failure may be oxygenated and ventilated successfully for extended periods without tracheal intubation through the use of a tight-fitting face mask and resuscitation bag,[17] as shown in Figure 2-3. "Bag-and-mask" ventilation is particularly suitable for patients who are awake, breathing spontaneously, and retaining CO_2. This life-saving technique can be used in the field by paramedical personnel not skilled in endotracheal intubation. Bag-and-mask ventilation is always performed before attemps are made to intubate the patient with an endotracheal tube. Endotracheal intubation is less hazardous if the patient is adequately oxygenated and ventilated beforehand. Occasionally, however, bag-and-mask ventilation is all that is necessary to resuscitate a patient. For example, a patient in light coma of short duration and with intact airway reflexes may be managed without intubation. Whenever bag-and-mask ventilation is performed, attention must be given to the adequacy of ventilation as determined by symmetrical expansion of the chest, relief of hypercapnia and hypoxemia, and the avoidance of complications such as gastric distention caused by the insufflation of air into the esophagus. Pulmonary aspiration is a constant risk, particuarly if protective airway reflexes are blunted.

Endotracheal intubation is considered after upper airway obstruction has been relieved and bag-and-mask ventilation has been initiated. Many factors must be considered in the decision to intubate, including the stability of the airway, the presence or absence of foreign material, the need for suctioning of tracheobron-

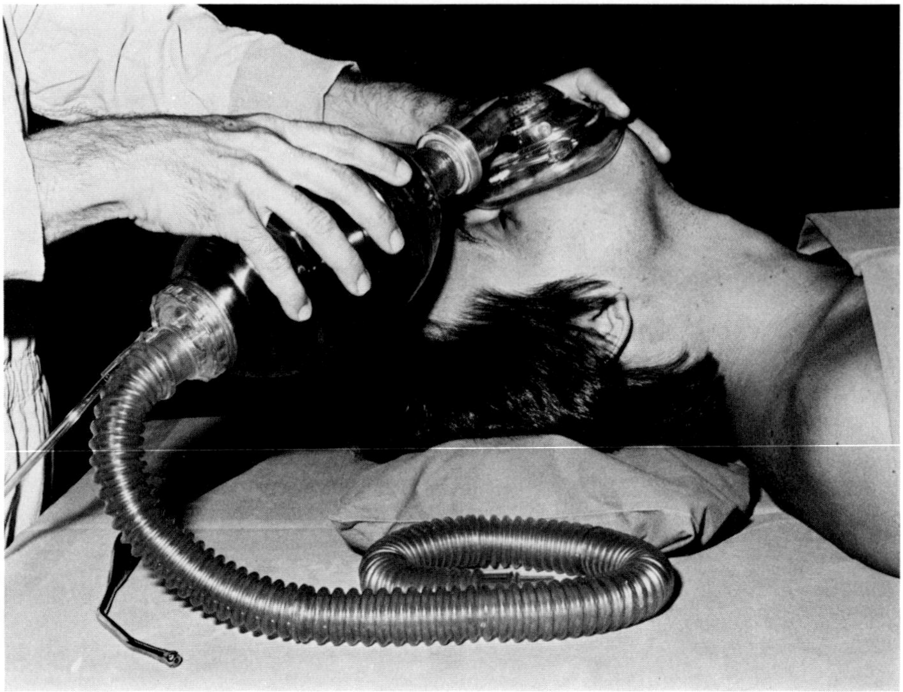

Figure 2–3. Bag-and-mask ventilation with the Laerdal self-inflating resuscitation bag (Laerdal Medical Corp., Armonk, NY) connected to an oxygen source. Note the flexion of the neck and extension of the head to maintain patency of the upper airway.

chial secretions, the risk of aspiration, the availability of skilled respiratory care, the need for mechanical ventilation and oxygenation, the nature of the underlying disease process, and the anticipated duration of the need for an airway. Like all procedures, tracheal intubation is a matter of clinical judgment and should never be performed as an automatic or "rote" procedure. However, unnecessary delay in intubation should be avoided, and the old adage, "When in doubt, intubate," probably is valid.

ENDOTRACHEAL INTUBATION

Endotracheal intubation for one or more of the indications previously discussed is usually necessary for patients requiring bag-and-mask ventilation. The urgency of endotracheal intubation depends upon the patency of the airway, the need to remove tracheobronchial secretions, the urgency to oxygenate and ventilate the patient in respiratory failure, and the need to protect the airway from aspiration. The obstetric patient with a full stomach who needs general anesthesia, the patient who has lost protective airway reflexes, and the comatose patient with an unstable airway should be intubated quickly. Endotracheal intubation with a cuffed tube should be performed before a nasal or oral gastric tube is inserted in the comatose patient, since these tubes impair function of the upper and lower esophageal sphincters and increase the risk of pulmonary aspiration.

Endotracheal intubation may be performed whether the patient is conscious or unconscious. In the conscious patient, it may be used in emergencies and elective situations[18]; it is often indicated when there is danger of upper airway obstruction or aspiration, such as in obstetric anesthesia. The patient with a full stomach should be intubated while awake if possible. Intubation of the conscious patient demands considerable skill, judgment, and effective topical anesthesia. It may be done either nasally or orally, but the nasal route is preferred because there is less stimulation of gagging and vomiting reflexes. In contrast, the unconscious patient is usually much easier to intubate. Here the oral route is preferred, especially if the muscles of the neck and jaw are relaxed. Greater difficulty is anticipated if the patient is apneic, if anatomic or mechanical problems prevent visualization of the glottis, or if vomiting occurs. If trismus prevents opening the mouth, as in the patient with status epilepticus, nasal intubation will probably be necessary.

Endotracheal Intubation versus Tracheotomy

With the increasing acceptance of prolonged endotracheal intubation for periods of as long as 2 to 3 weeks, endotracheal intubation now may be used initially in place of routine early tracheotomy in the management of patients with selected types of acute respiratory failure; among these are patients with flail chest and those with Guillain-Barré syndrome.[19] Additionally, many authorities now prefer endotracheal intubation to tracheotomy for managing patients with extensive third degree burns of the head and neck, even when laryngeal edema is present.[20]

Endotracheal intubation is the preferred method for establishing a definitive airway in most emergencies. In elective situations, early tracheotomy is sometimes considered if the prolonged need for an artificial airway is anticipated. Awareness of the advantages and disadvantages of endotracheal intubation versus tracheotomy may help the clinician select the most appropriate type of definitive airway. The main advantages of endotracheal intubation are ease and speed of placement of the tube, and the requirement for less experience and skill than is needed for tracheotomy. Endotracheal intubation also avoids the many complications of tracheotomy, is less expensive, and causes less morbidity and mortality. Comparative disadvantages of endotracheal intubation include its many complications, greater patient discomfort in long-term airway management, difficulty with feeding, possibly greater difficulty in suctioning the trachea, the potential for laryngeal injury, and the aesthetically displeasing aspects of prolonged oral or nasal intubation.

Tracheotomy avoids laryngeal and other airway complications of endotracheal intubation, causes less discomfort in long-term use, and permits easy suctioning of tracheobronchial secretions. It also allows mouth care, feeding, communication, and control of oral secretions. The disadvantages of tracheotomy versus intubation include numerous potential complications, a 3 percent mortality rate, the permanent scar which results, greater expense, and a high incidence of tracheal stenosis.[21]

Oral versus Nasal Endotracheal Intubation

Either the nasal or the oral route is acceptable for emergency intubation. The skilled intubator selects the best route for each particular patient rather than performing one method routinely. Rigid, "cookbook" guidelines for endotracheal intubation should be condemned. During cardiopulmonary resuscitation, oral intubation is preferred because it is faster and easier than nasal intubation. In patients with acute respiratory failure, the oral route is recommended if the patient is expected to be intubated for less than 5 days. The nasal route is selected if prolonged intubation is anticipated. Additional indications for the nasal route are trismus from a variety of causes (tetanus, seizures, and spasm of the masseter muscles), oral trauma, fracture of the mandible or other serious maxillofacial injuries, decerebrate rigidity, suspected fracture of the neck, obstructing lesions of the mouth and oropharynx (edema, carcinoma, paritonsillar abscess, macroglossia, and Ludwig's angina), ankylosis of the cervical spine, temporomandibular joint disease, and the need for oral surgery. As previously indicated, the obstetric patient, the patient with a stomach full of food or blood, and the patient with an upper intestinal obstruction may be intubated with less risk of vomiting and aspiration when the nasal route is selected. The patient with a short "bull" neck, the patient who gags excessively, and the uncooperative, struggling patient are all candidates for nasal intubation. The nasal route is avoided in the presence of nasal fracture or severe trauma, nasal obstruction, and paranasal disease such as sinusitis or otitis media.

Oral endotracheal intubation is easier, faster, less traumatic, and less painful than nasal intubation. Epistaxis and other nasal and paranasal complications are avoided. Additionally, a larger tube is tolerated through the mouth, facilitating suctioning and decreasing airflow resistance, and an oral tube is less likely to kink than a nasal tube. In contrast, nasal intubation causes less gagging. After a nasal tube is secured in place, it is more comfortable, better anchored, and less likely to be dislodged than an oral tube. The patient can swallow secretions and communicate with his or her lips. Mouth care can be performed, the complications of oral intubation are avoided, and the tube cannot be obstructed by biting. Another benefit of nasal intubation is that it also causes less laryngeal ulceration than oral intubation.[22]

The success rate of emergency nasal intubation varies from 80 to 95 percent.[23] Emergency nasal intubation can be done by the guided technique with the aid of a laryngoscope, or it may be done blindly. Blind nasal intubation, introduced by Magill in 1930,[24] has many merits as a means of establishing an emergency airway, particulary if the patient is conscious.[23,25,26] Blind nasotracheal intubation of the conscious patient is desirable because upper airway protective reflexes are maintained, and there is no need to use a laryngoscope, decreasing the risk of laryngospasm and cough. The only requirement is that the patient be breathing spontaneously. In a recent study of 300 patients on whom blind nasotracheal intubation was done by emergency department physicians, the success rate was 92 percent and the complication rate only 3 percent.[23]

Anesthesia for Endotracheal Intubation

Anesthesia of the airway is an important requirement for successful endotracheal intubation of the conscious or semiconscious patient. Unfortunately, emergency intubation is often done in such urgency that anesthesia is overlooked. However, anesthesia makes intubation more comfortable for the patient and may facilitate mechanical ventilation by preventing "bucking" and protracted coughing. The mucosa of the nose, pharynx, and hypopharynx can be anesthetized adequately with an atomizer containing 3 to 4 ml of lidocaine (1 percent or 4 percent) or cocaine (10 percent). An atomizer with a movable tip helps direct the anesthetic to the hypopharynx. A malleable laryngeal applicator or cotton swab on the end of a curved forceps can be used to apply anesthetic to the pyriform sinuses and glottis. If the patient is unconscious, topical anesthesia usually is not required but may help to block pharngeal reflexes.

Anesthesia of the larynx and trachea can be achieved by injecting anesthetic solutions through the cricothyroid membrane.[27] This technique, "translaryngeal anesthesia," is a useful adjunct to conventional oral or nasal anesthesia. Properly performed, it greatly facilitates intubation by "desensitizing" the larynx and trachea, preventing laryngospasm and cough. It is indicated only in selected urgent or elective intubations and should not be done if immediate intubation is needed. Translaryngeal anesthesia is particularly useful for blind nasotracheal intubation of the conscious patient, and some anesthesiologists prefer it for routine orotracheal intubation as well.[27]

Translaryngeal anesthesia is performed by identifying the cricothyroid space and puncturing the cricothyroid membrane with a 22 gauge, 1-inch needle.[23] A needle in the cricothyroid space lies about 1.3 cm below the true vocal cords,[27] and there is little risk of vocal cord injury. Two to 5 ml of lidocaine (4 percent) are injected rapidly into the subglottic space at end-expiration. The patient is instructed to cough to help distribute the anesthetic over the mucosa of the trachea and the inferior surface of the vocal cords.[28] Pressing firmly over the injection site decreases the risk of subcutaneous emphysema and hematoma. Complications are rare when the technique is done properly,[27] but it should be done only by someone with expertise. The procedure is contraindicated if the necessary anatomic landmarks are obscured by obesity, tumor, a large thyroid gland, or other factors, and if the patient has a bleeding tendency.

Several other methods of anesthesia for intubation are worthy of mention. Superior laryngeal nerve blockade is an effective way of blocking the sensory innervation of the larynx[28] but is usually unnecessary if successful topical anesthesia is obtained. Neuromuscular blocking agents and paralyzing drugs such as succinylcholine and pancuronium rarely are necessary in emergency endotracheal intubation. They should be used only by a skilled anesthesiologist with full support facilities available.[29] General anesthesia, also rarely needed to assist emergency endotracheal intubation, should obviously be done only by a trained anesthesiologist or nurse anesthetist. Oversedation and general anesthesia are in fact dangerous, because they depress protective glottic reflexes.[7]

Technique of Oral Endotracheal Intubation

The skilled practitioner approaches intubation with a calm demeanor and an attitude that is reassuring to the patient and to others. A controlled, orderly approach by the physician helps allay the anxiety which often surrounds the patient needing emergency tracheal intubation. Intubation attempts by inexperienced and anxious personnel often add more chaos to the emergency.

Careful preparation for endotracheal intubation increases the chance of successful tube placement. Ideally, two assistants should be in attendance. All necessary equipment should be assembled beforehand and checked for proper function while any upper airway obstruction is being relieved and bag-and-mask ventilation is being performed. If assisted ventilation is necessary, a mechanical respirator is prepared for use. Informed written consent is desirable but cannot be obtained unless the intubation is elective.

The length of oral tube needed is estimated based on the size of the patient. The distance from the lips to the carina is estimated by judging the distance from the incisor teeth to the angle of Louis, which is at the level of the carina. This distance is about 28 to 32 cm in adults.[7] Since the tip of the endotracheal tube should be approximately 4 cm above the carina, the oral tube is usually inserted about 24 to 28 cm beyond the teeth, markings on the tube indicating the depth of insertion. If the nasal route is selected, 2 to 3 cm are added to this estimate. Pre-cut tubes may be used after proper estimation of the needed length, but it is preferable to use uncut tubes 32 to 36 cm in length in adults and to trim them to the proper length after insertion. The 15-mm male adaptor is affixed to the endotracheal tube before insertion so that ventilation can proceed immediately following intubation.

The patient is examined with careful attention to the mouth, nose, neck, muscle relaxation, and mobility of the cervical spine and temporomandibular joint. Foreign bodies in the mouth and dental appliances are removed and secretions are suctioned from the mouth and pharynx. A variety of sizes of endotracheal tubes marked for oral (or nasal) insertion are made available, and several sizes of both curved and straight laryngoscope blades are assembled. The headboard of the bed is removed and the bed is raised to a high level. If the patient is unconscious, the head of the bed is elevated to reduce the risk of aspiration.

After topical anesthesia is obtained, a short-acting intravenous sedative drug (such as diazepam, 5 to 10 mg) is administered just prior to intubation only if needed to calm the patient and only if ventilatory support is immediately available. The patient is placed in the supine position with the neck flexed on the chest and the head extended at the atlanto-occipital joint. The upper incisor teeth are protected by a gauze pad or shield. The lips and teeth are opened with the left hand, using a crossed-finger technique to protect the lips during insertion of the laryngoscope blade. Care is taken to avoid pressure and leverage on the teeth and gums. The straight or curved (MacIntosh) laryngoscope blade is selected and lubricated with water. With the laryngoscope in the left hand, the blade is inserted along the right side of the mouth and down the right side of the tongue, displacing the tongue upward and to the left. If the straight blade is used, it is passed just beyond the tip of the epiglottis and the laryngoscope is lifted up and forward at a 45 degree angle.[7] The straight laryngoscope blade offers a better view of the larynx, since the epiglottis is moved out of the line of sight. Pressure on the thyroid cartilage of the larynx may expose the vocal cords. The vocal cords are visualized directly and continually. The endotracheal tube, lubricated with water-soluble plain or anesthetic jelly, is then grasped with the right hand and passed slowly and gently along the right side of the laryngoscope blade into the glottis and 5 to 6 cm beyond the vocal cords. If too much resistance is met at the glottis, a smaller tube is used. The tube is rotated in any direction necessary to enter the glottis. The concave portion is then brought forward after the trachea is entered. The endotracheal tube is *not* passed along the groove of the laryngoscope blade, an error frequently made by beginners.

The intubator should also be able to use the curved laryngoscope blade. The curved blade produces less laryngospasm and cough because it does not contact the laryngeal side of the epiglottis, which is innervated by the superior laryngeal branch of the vagus nerve.[30] The curved blade also may be easier to use in the patient who cannot fully open his or her mouth. The blunted tip of the curved blade is passed into the vallecula—the space between the base of the tongue and the epiglottis (Figs. 2-4(A) and (B)). The laryngoscope is then lifted forward and upward without leverage, stretching the hyoepiglottic ligament and exposing the glottis. If only the arytenoid cartilages are exposed and the vocal cords cannot be seen, the tip of the endotracheal tube may be directed blindly just anterior to the arytenoids. Gentle, steady pressure directs the tip of the tube into the glottis and past the vocal cords. Blind jamming of the endotracheal tube against firm resistance should be avoided because of the risk of hypopharyngeal perforation.

After oral intubation, the patient is oxygenated and ventilated with a resuscitation bag. The cuff pressure is then adjusted to the appropriate level, using the minimal-occluding-pressure or the minimal-leak technique. Tracheobronchial secretions are suctioned through the tube. The chest is auscultated and observed for symmetry of expansion to ascertain that the tube has not inadvertently entered a mainstem bronchus. Right mainstem bronchus intubation usually can be detected from the absence of breath sounds on the left or failure of the left chest to expand. However, auscultation of the chest is not a foolproof way to determine proper placement of the tube in the trachea, particularly in patients with emphysema who have diminished breath sounds. Right mainstem bronchus intubation may produce no clinical manifestations at all, and inappropriate hypoxemia may be the only clue. Esophageal intubation may be detected by the absence of chest expansion, the absence of breath sounds in the peripheral lung fields, and a loud bubbling noise on auscultation over the stomach. Excessive coughing or "bucking" after intubation may indicate that the tip of the tube is touching the carina, in which case the tube should be pulled back. After intubation, a chest radiograph is obtained to confirm proper tube placement. When the head and neck are in a neutral position, the tip of the tube should be at the level of the third or fourth vertebral body.[31] Flexion of the neck moves the tip about 2 cm toward the carina, while extension moves it about 2 cm away from the carina.[32]

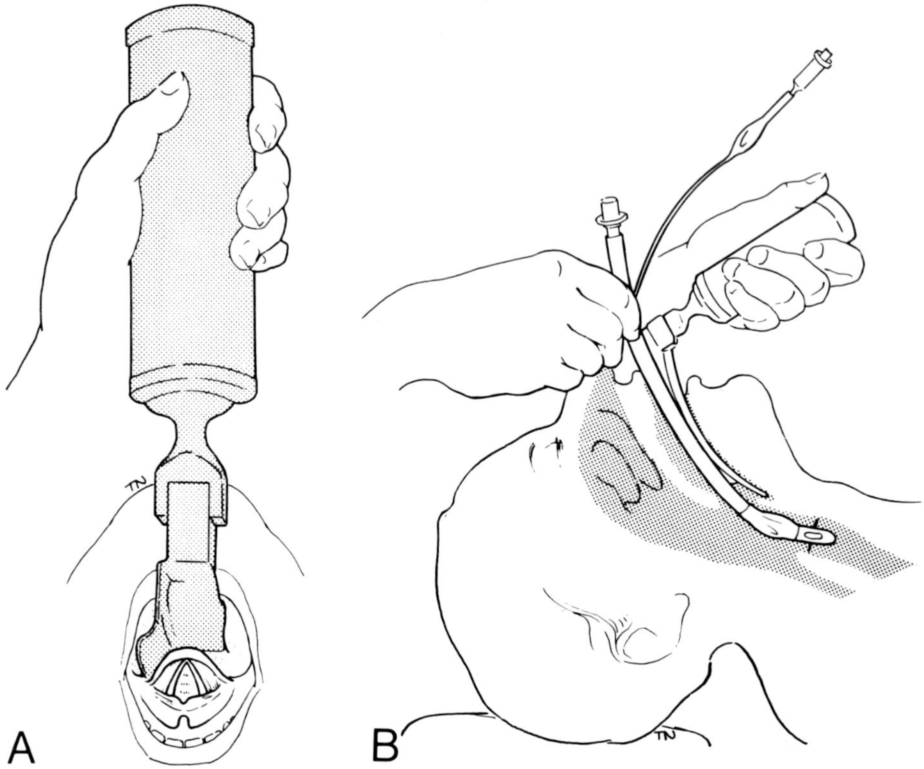

Figure 2–4. (A) Exposure of the vocal cords by proper use of the laryngoscope with a curved blade is illustrated. Note the tip of the blade in the vallecula, exposing the epiglottis. (B) Oral endotracheal intubation with a curved blade. The endotracheal tube is passed along the right side of the mouth and blade, past the exposed epiglottis, through the glottis, and into the trachea.

Following its insertion, the endotracheal tube is secured in the mouth with gauze tape, adhesive tape fixed to the skin with benzoin, or an endotracheal-tube holder. An oral pharyngeal airway is inserted only if necessary for reasons previously discussed. A nasogastric tube is usually passed to decompress the stomach or to provide nourishment. When the chest radiograph shows the endotracheal tube to be in proper position, excess tubing is trimmed at the mouth so that the 15-mm adaptor is just at the edge of the lip. A protruding endotracheal tube invites kinking, displacement into the right mainstem bronchus, and self-extubation. The trimmed tube allows a reference point to assure proper tube placement on a daily basis. Persistent coughing or "bucking" may be controlled by effective suctioning or, if necessary, by instilling 5 ml of lidocaine (1 percent) into the endotracheal tube. Finally, arm restraints are applied if necessary to protect the tube from spontaneous dislocation.

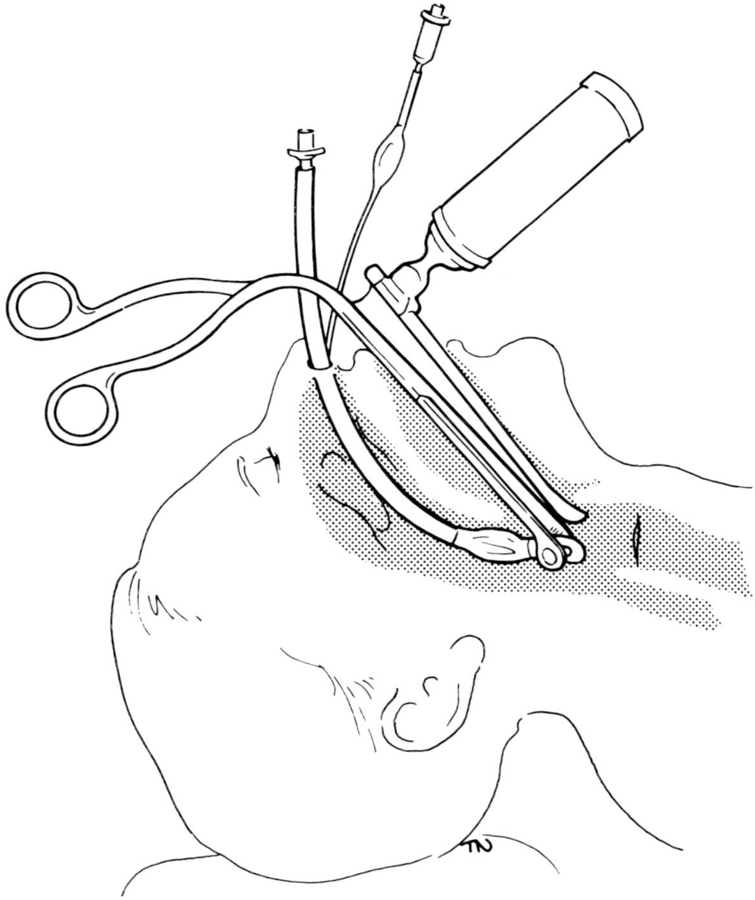

Figure 2–5. Guided nasal endotracheal intubation with the Magill forceps. The distal tip of the nasal tube is guided into the glottis with the Magill forceps. Note that the straight laryngoscope blade passes the epiglottis.

Technique of Guided Nasal Endotracheal Intubation

The patient is prepared for nasal intubation in much the same way as for oral intubation. The pharynx, hypopharynx, and laryngopharynx are fully anesthetized, with care taken to assure complete anesthesia of the pyriform sinuses and glottis. Topical anesthesia of the nasal mucosa is obtained with cocaine or lidocaine. Cocaine acts both as a vasoconstrictor and as an anesthetic, while lidocaine acts only as an anesthetic. Phenylephrine (1 percent) can be used in conjunction with lidocaine to shrink the nasal mucosa, producing a larger channel through which to pass the tube. Both sides of the nose are anesthetized in case attempted passage through one side fails; the nose is examined carefully and the more patent side is selected. The proper-sized nasal endotracheal tube is lubricated with plain or anesthetic water-soluble jelly, more lubricant being necessary than for oral intubation. The patient's chin is brought forward and the neck is flexed. The tube is then passed slowly and gently, with the curve directed anteriorly at first through the anterior nares and along the inferior meatus of the nasal cavity, rotation being used as much as necessary. If firm resistance is encountered, the tube is not jammed forward because of the risk of bleeding and turbinate bone injury. Once the tip of the tube reaches the oropharynx, less resistance is felt. The tube then is advanced slowly into the hypopharynx. Next, with the laryngoscope in the left hand, the intubator advances the tip of the tube under direct vision into the glottis with the right hand. The Magill forceps may be used to pick up the tip of the tube and pass it through the vocal cords, care being taken not to lacerate the cuff. (Fig. 2-5). External pressure on the thyroid cartilage of the larynx by an assistant may bring the glottis into view. After the glottis is entered, the procedure is identical to that in orotracheal intubation. The nasal tube is secured at the nose with tape, and protruding tube material is trimmed.

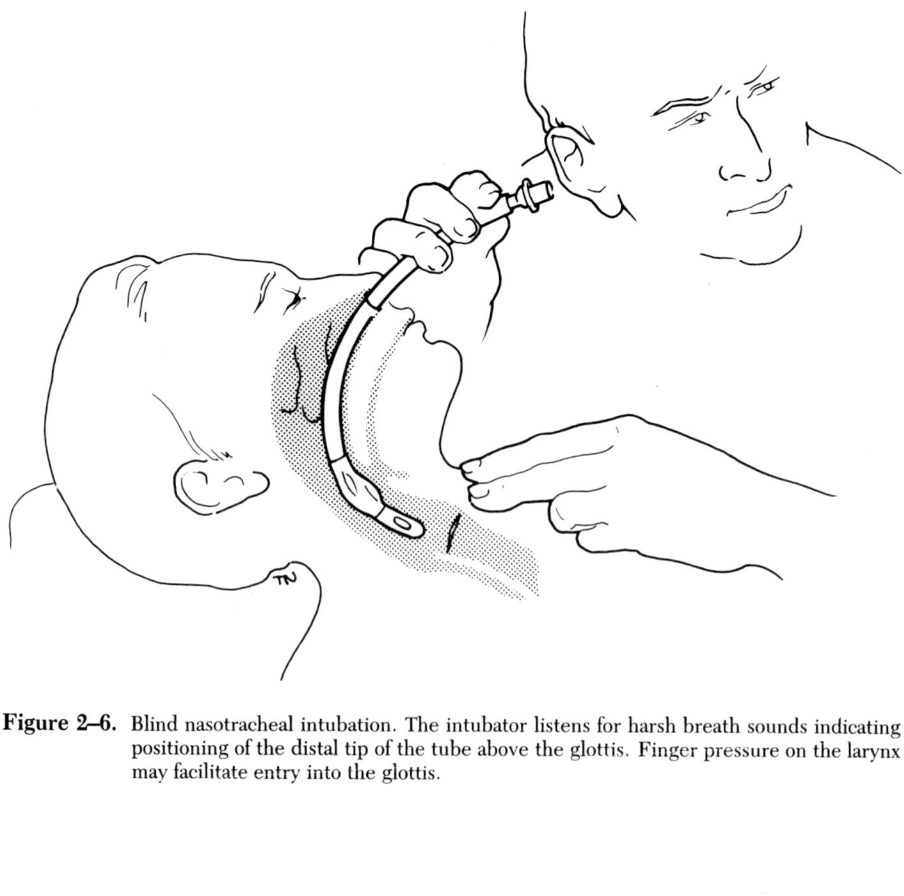

Figure 2–6. Blind nasotracheal intubation. The intubator listens for harsh breath sounds indicating positioning of the distal tip of the tube above the glottis. Finger pressure on the larynx may facilitate entry into the glottis.

Table 2–3. Common Errors in Endotracheal Intubation

1. Inadequate training, experience, and judgment
2. Failure to assemble needed equipment before starting intubation
3. Failure to pre-oxygenate and pre-ventilate the patient
4. Inadequate topical anesthesia, sedation, or muscle relaxation
5. Selection of improper route of intubation
6. Improper positioning and alignment of head and neck
7. Improper use of the laryngoscope
8. Jamming the tube forward against resistance
9. Prolonged or repeated intubation attempts
10. Endobronchial or deep tracheal insertion of the tube
11. Equipment malfunction

Technique of Blind Nasotracheal Intubation

Blind nasal endotracheal intubation is like guided nasal intubation with a few exceptions. Preoxygenation, ventilation, and topical anesthesia are done as described previously. If time permits, atropine (0.01 mg/kg i.m.) and a sedating agent such as diazepam (5 to 10 mg i.v.) are given. Oversedation is avoided. Paralysis with succinylcholine is recommended by some authorities.[15] Blind nasal intubation is performed in Fowler's position, with the head of the bed at 45 degrees, if the patient has a full stomach. The head is slightly extended in the "sniffing" position. If a nasogastric tube is in place, it should be removed since it may divert the nasotracheal tube.[25] A Magill forceps and a laryngoscope should be available and ready to use in case blind intubation fails. The nasal tube is passed as far as the epiglottis. Then, as the tube reaches the hypopharynx, the intubator's ear is placed at the proximal end of the tube (Fig. 2-6). When breath sounds indicate that the tube is above the glottis, it is advanced quickly, during deep inspiration, when the vocal cords are maximally abducted. Passage into the glottis is identified by the sudden appearance of harsh, raspy breath sounds, coughing, inability of the patient to phonate, and bulging of the larynx. Proper tube placement is confirmed by the methods discussed above.

Pitfalls in Endotracheal Intubation

The commonest pitfall in endotracheal intubation is inexperience (Table 2-3). Failure to assemble all of the necessary equipment prior to starting intubation is a mistake often made by the student. Oxygenation and ventilation before starting intubation often are overlooked. The conscious patient may not be adequately anesthetized, sedated, or premedicated. Muscle relaxation may be poor. Airway reflexes may be hyperactive and incompletely blocked by topical anesthetics. Failure to position the head and neck to maximize exposure of the glottis is a common error. The laryngoscope blade may be inserted too deeply or used as a lever rather than as an elevator of the tongue and neck. Most of these pitfalls in technique can be avoided through proper training, practice, and experience.

ALTERNATIVE METHODS OF ESTABLISHING AN EMERGENCY AIRWAY

The Esophageal Obturator Airway

Placement of an esophageal obturator airway (EOA) is an acceptable alternative to endotracheal intubation in selected circumstances, particularly cardiopulmonary resuscitation of the unconscious, apneic patient.[33–37] Introduced by Don Michael and associates in 1968 as a "mouth-to-lung airway,"[38] and modified by Gordon and Don Michael in 1973,[34] the EOA has become popular for the initiation of assisted ventilation by paramedical personnel in the field when tracheal intubation is not authorized or is unavailable.[38] It has been approved for use as an adjunct to artificial ventilation by the National Conference on Cardiopulmonary Resuscitation and Emergency Cardiac Care.[39] Adequate ventilation of the lungs may be achieved,[36, 40–42] and oxygenation may be as good as that obtained with endotracheal intubation.[35] The EOA is indicated for use only in unconscious, apneic, areflexic patients who have suffered cardiac or respiratory arrest. However, there is considerable controversy about the role of the EOA in cardiopulmonary resuscitation.[37] Some advocate its use in most cardiopulmonary resuscitation attempts in the field and even in the hospital,[42] but most experts would restrict its use to situations in which endotracheal intubation is not available for cardiopulmonary resuscitation.[43,44] Perhaps the EOA is used most appropriately when the patient does not need to be moved and ventilatory assistance is needed only for short periods.[44] It is contraindicated in children under the age of 16 because of uncertain depth of insertion, in patients with esophageal disease or damage, including trauma and ingestion of corrosive agents, and in patients who are conscious or semiconscious.

There are many advantages of the EOA, particularly its ease and speed of insertion by paramedical personnel; it may be inserted in less than 5 seconds[37] and without extension of the head, an advantage in patients with suspected fracture or immobility of the cervical spine. A laryngoscope is not needed. The esophageal balloon reduces the risk of pulmonary aspiration. Furthermore, the EOA may be inserted blindly with the patient in almost any position, and the glottis need not be visualized. The only additional equipment needed is a 35-cc syringe to inflate the esophageal balloon. External heart massage need not be interrupted during resuscitation attempts.[33] Finally, the technique is simple to teach and easy to learn.

However, there are many drawbacks to use of the EOA. Gastric and foreign-body aspiration can occur because the airway is not protected. For example, the EOA is undesirable in patients with oral or facial trauma, in which blood, teeth, and foreign material can be aspirated into the airway.[45] Tracheobronchial suctioning is precluded when the EOA is used. Additionally, at least two persons are needed to use the EOA: one to seal the mask tightly with both hands and the other to ventilate the patient, thus leaving no one to move the patient if only two paramedics are on the scene.[44] Other disadvantages of the EOA include the inability to provide an airtight seal around the mouth and nose, the inability to intubate the esophagus, and numerous reported complications which are re-

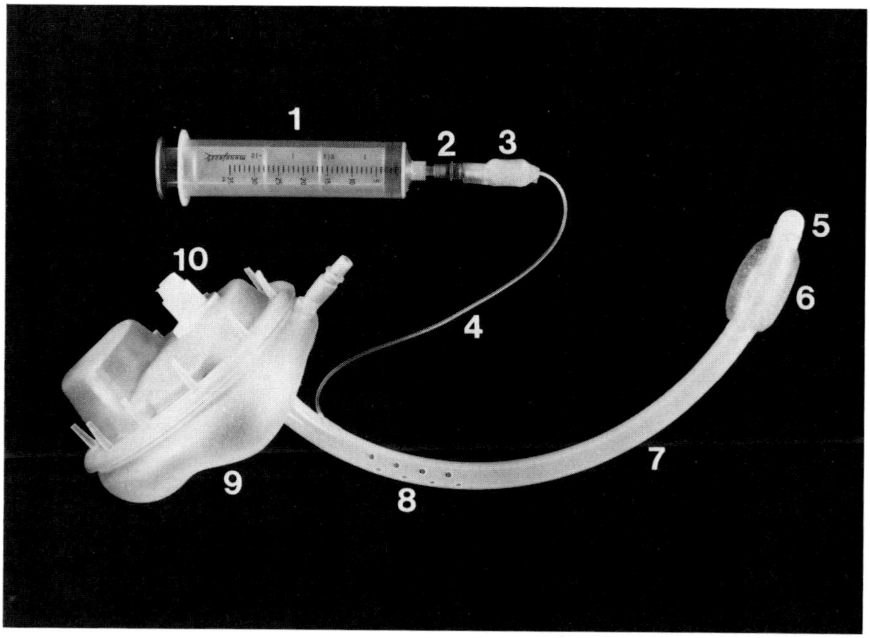

Figure 2–7. Features of the Gordon-Don Michael esophageal obturator airway (Brunswick Manufacturing Co., Inc., North Quincy, MA) include (1) 35 ml air syringe; (2) inflation valve; (3) pilot balloon; (4) inflating tube; (5) blunt distal tip; (6) inflatable esophageal obturator cuff; (7) esophageal tube; (8) air holes; (9) adjustable pre-inflated face mask; and (10) snap-lock connector with 15-mm male adaptor.

viewed below. Several variations of the original EOA have been designed to overcome some of these limitations, including the esophageal gastric-tube airway (Brunswick Manufacturing Company, Inc., North Quincy, MA), the Pilcher or "Vermont" adaptation,[46] and the tracheal-esophageal airway.[47]

There are no published standards for EOAs.[5] The device resembles an endotracheal tube, but its distal end is occluded by a blunt, pliable rubber obturator. Sixteen 3-mm openings are located along the shaft of the tube in the region which will lie in the hypopharynx. A clear plastic face mask with an airtight inflatable seal anchors the proximal end of the tube at the mouth. Features of the EOA include a 33 cm length, 9 mm internal diameter, smooth round edges to avoid mucosal injury, reusability, polyvinyl chloride composition, 16 cm radius of curvature, 35 ml cuff, and an inflating tube system which is similar to that of an endotracheal tube (Fig. 2-7).

Insertion of the EOA is very simple. The practitioner's left thumb and index finger lift the tongue and jaw forward while the head remains in a neutral position. The EOA is lubricated and passed blindly through the mouth and into the esophagus so that the cuff is just below the carina. Excessive force is avoided because of the risk of esophageal laceration. The mask is then seated tightly on the face with two hands, and the seal is inflated to make an airtight fit. The cuff is inflated with 25 to 35 ml of air. Overinflation of the cuff may rupture the esophagus. Positive pressure ventilation is performed with the mouth, a resuscitation bag, or an Elder valve, and proper function of the system is ascertained by confirming symmetrical chest expansion and auscultation. If the EOA has inadvertently been inserted into the trachea, no breath sounds will be heard, and the tube should be removed immediately. If endotracheal intubation is performed after insertion of the EOA, it should be done while the EOA is still in place to prevent vomiting and aspiration. After the endotracheal tube is placed successfully, the esophageal balloon may be deflated and the EOA removed. During this procedure, the head should be placed downward and turned to the side in case vomiting occurs. The reader is referred to the literature for descriptions of the use of newer modifications of the EOA.[40,46]

Cricothyroidotomy

Cricothyroidotomy is the preferred method of emergency surgical access to the trachea when bag-and-mask ventilation, endotracheal intubation, or use of the EOA are unsuccessful.[20,39,48,49] In an emergency, the cricothyroid membrane may be incised with a scalpel or other sharp instrument to open the airway. Alternatively, the membrane may be punctured with a cannula or catheter to relieve upper airway obstruction when the equipment and facilities for surgical cricothyroidotomy are unavailable. Cricothyroidotomy or cricothyroid membrane puncture are indicated in the event of impending asphyxia from partial or complete obstruction of the upper airway at or above the glottis when simpler methods of establishing an airway have failed. Examples of such an emergency include severe laryngospasm, laryngeal edema, laryngotracheal trauma, and foreign body obstruction that cannot be relieved by the Heimlich maneuver or back blows.[50] In situations in which blood, foreign matter, secretions, or edema prevent visualization of the larynx, or in which blind nasal endotracheal intubation has failed, cricothyroidotomy may be life-saving. Neither cricothyroidotomy nor cricothyroid membrane puncture is suitable for infants and small children.[49] Severe laryngeal trauma or acute laryngeal disease may also contraindicate the use of these techniques.[51]

As an elective procedure, cricothyroidotomy remains controversial; as an emergency procedure, however, it has considerable merit,[48,49] being faster, easier, and safer than emergency tracheotomy.[49,51,52] It avoids the thyroid gland and the vessels lower in the neck. The cricothyroid membrane is close to the skin, easily palpated, large (mean dimensions 0.9 × 3.0 cm),[27,49,53] buttressed by cartilage on two sides, and less vascular than the trachea. However, as an elective procedure for long-term airway maintenance, cricothyroidotomy has not replaced tracheotomy, because of limited experience and data comparing it with conventional tracheotomy.

A variety of tubes, catheters, and makeshift devices can be passed percutaneously through the cricothyroid membrane to provide emergency oxygenation and ventilation. The ideal tube for this purpose, of course, is a standard tracheostomy tube; but less sophisticated devices can be used. Indeed, any sharp or pointed object can be forced through the cricothyroid membrane to open the airway after a

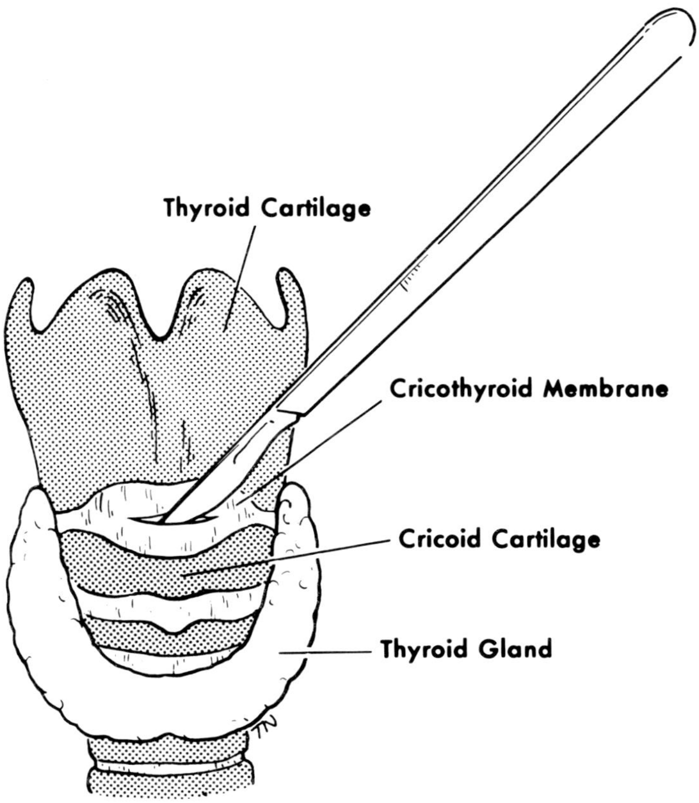

Figure 2–8. Cricothyroidotomy. The cricothyroid membrane is incised horizontally to permit passage of a tracheostomy tube or other makeshift device to open the airway.

small transverse incision is made in the skin.[48] The barrel of a ball point pen, a plastic connector from the male end of an intravenous line,[54] a piece of stethoscope tubing, two keys held apart, or other devices may be used.[48] To permit spontaneous ventilation, a tube with a minimum internal diameter of 4 to 5 mm is necessary.[15] A 14-, 16-, or 18-gauge plastic needle can be used if a high-pressure source of oxygen is available for jet ventilation, as discussed later in this chapter.[39,55–60]

Emergency cricothyroidotomy should be done by a qualified surgeon if possible. The head and neck are hyperextended and the skin is cleansed with antiseptic solution. The skin over the cricothyroid membrane is infiltrated with lidocaine (1 percent). The thyroid cartilage of the larynx is held firmly with the thumb and middle finger of the left hand, and the skin over the cricothyroid membrane is stabilized with the index finger. A transverse skin incision approximately 1.5 cm in length is then made over the membrane. A hemostat is used to dissect subcutaneous tissue. The cricothyroid membrane is exposed and incised horizontally (Fig. 2–8). Because the cricoid cartilage is circumferential, posterior perforation is unlikely. The incision can be enlarged with a Trousseau dilator. A size 7 to 8 (millimeter ID) tracheostomy tube is inserted. Elective conversion of a cricothyroidotomy to a tracheotomy for long-term airway management is controversial.[49,52]

Emergency Tracheotomy

Emergency tracheotomy is mentioned only to be condemned. Since the nineteenth century, when it became a popular procedure for the emergency relief of upper airway obstruction from diphtheria, croup, and foreign bodies, tracheotomy has carried a stigma as a life-saving emergency procedure. Now, however, tracheotomy should be regarded as an elective procedure and not as an emergency one. Indeed, emergency tracheotomy in an uncontrolled setting is rarely ever indicated. It may have a role in a few rare situations such as severe laryngeal trauma or severe acute laryngeal disease when emergency cricothyroidotomy is not feasible. Emergency tracheotomy may also be done in the operating room in a rare emergency in which there is life-threatening obstruction in the laryngeal or supralaryngeal airway. Tracheotomy should be attempted only by a trained surgeon and should never be done if the lighting, equipment, and support facilities are not optimal.

Translaryngeal and Transtracheal Jet Ventilation

Either the cricothyroid membrane or trachea may be punctured to oxygenate and ventilate a patient in acute respiratory distress or during cardiopulmonary resuscitation when simpler measures for establishing an airway are either not feasible or not successful. In the hands of experts, translaryngeal and transtracheal jet ventilation ("transtracheal ventilation" or "percutaneous ventilation") have the useful life-support role of buying time until intubation can be accomplished. The use of 14 gauge or smaller catheters necessitates the use of "jet" ventilation with high pressure oxygen or air.[61] Spontaneous breathing is possible only if a large enough catheter (10 gauge) is inserted into the trachea by use of a tracheotome.[62]

A report in 1956 by Jacoby[55] on the effectiveness of transtracheal ventilation demonstrated that an 18-gauge catheter and a high-pressure source of oxygen ("jet" ventilation) could provide adequate oxygenation for up to 30 minutes in patients with upper airway obstruction. Many subsequent studies have demonstrated that oxygenation and ventilation can be accomplished for short periods of time with transtracheal catheters of 14- to 18-gauge size connected to a high-pressure source of air or oxygen.[56,57,60,63–66] Transtracheal jet ventilation at high frequency (100 or 200 breaths per minute) has been described recently, and is an exciting area for further investigation.[58,67]

Transtracheal jet ventilation is rarely indicated in an emergency. It is a "last ditch" maneuver when simpler and safer means of oxygenation and ventilation are either unavailable or unsuccessful and the patient is likely to die of asphyxiation unless an airway is established immediately. It may, however, be useful in the patient with partial upper airway obstruction, such as by an aspirated foreign body.[68] It may also expel mucus and foreign material lodged in the upper airway, thereby clearing the airway before endotracheal intubation is done.[57,59] Transtracheal jet ventilation reduces the risk of gastric distention which sometimes occurs with bag-and-mask ventilation, and avoids the hazards of traumatic intubation.[57] In cardiopulmonary resuscitation, it eliminates the apneic period between the cessation of bag-and-mask ventilation and tracheal intubation.[57] Transtracheal jet ventilation is contraindicated in the uncommon event of complete upper airway obstruction,[57] in infants and small children,[49] and if identifying anatomic landmarks are obscure.

A transtracheal catheter can be inserted in 10 seconds.[57] The preparation for this is the same as that for cricothyroidotomy. A 14- or 16-gauge plastic intravenous catheter with an inside needle ("extracath") attached to a 5 or 10 ml aspirating syringe is passed, with the syringe bevel upward, through the cricothyroid membrane or through the trachea one or two rings below the cricoid cartilage. The tip of the needle is directed at a 45-degree angle caudally into the trachea.[55] Entry into the trachea is noted by a "pop" and the return of air into the syringe. The inner metal needle is then withdrawn and the plastic catheter is advanced into the trachea to the hub, and is tied into place. It is very important to aspirate air repeatedly in order to ascertain proper placement of the tip of the plastic catheter in the lumen of the trachea.[57,65] The plastic catheter is connected by extension tubing having a stopcock or simple hand valve to a high-pressure source of oxygen (50 psi), the hospital oxygen supply, an oxygen tank, a pressure-driven mechanical ventilator,[63] or a self-inflating resuscitation bag via an adaptor.[68] Insufflation of oxygen into the trachea inflates the lung and entrains air through the glottis, while expiration occurs passively by elastic recoil of the lung.[65]

There are obviously many limitations to transtracheal jet ventilation. Jet ventilation by a transtracheal catheter is impossible if there is complete expiratory airflow obstruction, unless a second catheter is passed for the escape of expiratory gas.[69] Hypercapnia may develop, particularly if the procedure is prolonged. Blood and mucus may obstruct the catheter and impair ventilation, making constant care of the catheter necessary to assure its patency.[61] There is little experience with transtracheal jet ventilation in the emergency setting, and most successful studies have been done on anesthetized and paralyzed patients. Nor are there any data comparing transtracheal jet ventilation with simpler measures such as bag-and-mask ventilation. Further studies and experience are needed before this technique becomes an accepted part of emergency airway care.

DIFFICULT ENDOTRACHEAL INTUBATION

Occasionally, endotracheal intubation may be extremely difficult.[20,69,70] In a recent prospective study of endotracheal intubation in critically ill adults, 20 percent of all intubations required four or more attempts for satisfactory placement of the tube in the trachea, and 31 percent required more than 2 minutes.[21] The difficulty of intubation, as perceived by the intubator, depends upon many factors, includ-

Table 2–4. Causes of Difficult Endotracheal Intubation

General
Airway occlusion by secretions, blood, foreign material
Patient not anesthetized, sedated, restrained
Motion of the patient
Gagging, biting, or "bucking"
Trauma to supralaryngeal airway
Oral-mandibular
Trismus
Ankylosis of temporomandibular joint
Fractured jaw
"Buck" teeth
Micrognathia
Nasal
Nasal obstruction
Nasal septal defect
Pharyngeal
Foreign-body obstruction
Epiglottitis
Croup
Large tonsils
Patulous epiglottis
Laryngeal
Laryngospasm
Foreign-body obstruction
Laryngeal edema
Carcinoma of larynx
Cervical spine
Ankylosing spondylitis
Rheumatoid arthritis
Fracture
Scar contracture of the neck

ing expertise, the setting and urgency of the intubation, various antomic and mechanical considerations, the state of relaxation of the patient, and the availability of the necessary intubation equipment. A difficult intubation may be relatively easy for the experienced anesthesiologist, while the easy intubation may be difficult and taxing for the novice emergency or critical-care physician. The trained, experienced intubator with a thorough knowledge of the anatomy of the upper airway encounters a "difficult" intubation infrequently. Examples of difficult intubation include intubation performed outside the hospital under suboptimal conditions, intubation during cardiopulmonary resuscitation, and intubation of the patient with hemoptysis, hematemesis, vomiting, or upper airway obstruction. Some of the anatomic and mechanical causes of difficult intubation are summarized in Table 2-4.

A difficult endotracheal intubation may often be prevented if the common pitfalls of intubation (Table 2-3) are avoided. Simple maneuvers, such as proper positioning of the head and neck and proper alignment of midline anatomic structures, should not be overlooked. If the problem is that the patient cannot open his or her mouth, nasal intubation may be successful. Intubation of the conscious patient should be tried if the patient is at risk for aspiration.[71] The patient who is moving excessively or resisting intubation may be cautiously sedated with diazepam (10 mg i.v.). The anesthesiologist may easily intubate the patient with trismus after administering an intravenous anesthetic agent followed by a short-acting muscle relaxant. A small (7 mm ID) endotracheal tube can be used if laryngospasm, laryngeal edema, or a tight glottis prevent insertion of a larger tube. Coughing and "bucking" during intubation can often be managed by improving topical anesthesia. The patient with a strong gag reflex should be intubated by the nasal rather than the oral route. Patients with anatomic deformities of the supralaryngeal airway may be managed temporarily on an emergency basis with a ventilating rigid bronchoscope before intubation. If the oral endotracheal tube becomes molded or bent during insertion, a malleable wire guide or stylet may solve the problem. Care must be taken to prevent the tip from protruding beyond the distal end of the tube. The intubator who is unable to visualize the vocal cords should check the positioning of the patient's head and neck, be certain that the laryngoscope is being used properly, and have an assistant apply external pressure on the larynx. Blind passage of the tube anterior to the visualized arytenoid cartilages sometimes works, or a flexible Salem plastic introducer may be used to guide the tube into the glottis.[70] The patient can attempt voluntary hyperpnea to produce optimal abduction of the vocal cords. The changing of an endotracheal tube that is already in place may be facilitated by the use of an intratracheal suction catheter as a guide.[69,72]

The flexible fiberoptic bronchoscope has become a valuable solution to the problem of difficult intubation.[69,70,73–75] This instrument is placed into the lumen of a size 8.0 or larger endotracheal tube after passage of the tube through the nose or mouth to the level of the hypopharynx. The bronchoscope is then passed directly through the glottis into the trachea, and the endotracheal tube is slid over the guiding bronchoscope into the trachea. Battery-powered, flexible fiberoptic laryngoscopes have also been developed for this purpose,[76] but have a number of limitations. A lighted flexible stylet for guided oral intubation in adults,[77] a special hook introducer for nasotracheal intubation,[78] and a retrograde transcricothyroid catheter technique[20,69,79,80] have been described as solutions to difficult intubation, but none have been popular since flexible fiberoptic instruments have become available.

Prolonged intubation attempts can lead to profound hypoxemia and should be avoided.[39] Because the anxious intubator is often unaware of the elapsed time during intubation attempts, he or she should be interrupted if more than 30 seconds elapse, and bag-and-mask oxygenation and ventilation should be resumed.[39] If none of the above solutions to difficult intubation are successful, the anesthesiologist should be called to assist. The anesthesiologist may anesthetize the patient, administer a short-acting muscle relaxant, and intubate the patient.[69]

COMPLICATIONS OF ARTIFICIAL AIRWAYS

Complications of Endotracheal Intubation

The establishment of an emergency airway may result in serious complications, and several studies suggest that complications are more likely in the emergency setting.[81,82] Clearly, "crash" endotracheal intubation invites serious complications.

In contrast, major complications of elective endotracheal intubation done by an anesthesiologist in the controlled setting of the operating room are rare.[83] Awareness of the complications of endotracheal intubation should reduce their occurrence and allow for their earlier recognition and successful management.

Complications of endotracheal intubation may occur during insertion of the tube, while the tube is in place, during extubation, or after extubation.[82,84] Table 2-5 summarizes a number of selected complications. Intubation trauma usually results from improper technique, poor preparation of the patient, and other variables, some of which may not be controllable. After the endotracheal tube is in place, many factors may contribute to complications, including the duration of intubation, the pressure of the tube on the mucosa, the size of the tube relative to the larynx and trachea, motion between the tube and the patient, compliance of the tube, chemical irritants, infection, hypotension, the use of corticosteroids, and the respiratory care provided for the patient. At the cuff site, additional possible determinants of complications include the pressure exerted laterally against the tracheal mucosa, the duration of cuff inflation, the size of the sealing area, and the conformity of the cuff to the trachea. With the exception of cuff pressure, the role of each of these variables in the pathogenesis of tracheal injury is poorly understood.

There are few prospective studies of the complications of endotracheal intu-

Table 2–5. Complications of Endotracheal Intubation

General Complications	Orotracheal Complications	Nasotracheal Complications
During Tube Insertion		
Pain	Dental trauma	Epistaxis
Trauma to eyes, face, neck	Oral soft-tissue trauma	Turbinate bone trauma
Vomiting and aspiration		Thrombotic occlusion of tube
Retropharyngeal perforation		Avulsion of adenoid tissue
Hypopharyngeal perforation		Bacteremia
Vocal cord hematoma or avulsion		
Laryngospasm		
Tracheal laceration		
Bronchial intubation		
Bronchospasm		
Subcutaneous emphysema		
Mediastinal emphysema, mediastinitis		
Pneumothorax		
Esophageal intubation		
Gastric dilatation		
Excessive coughing or "bucking"		
Accidental dislodgement of tube		
Malfunction of tube or cuff		
Overinflation of cuff		
Hypoxemia		
Hypotension or hypertension		
Cardiac arrhythmia		
Cardiac or respiratory arrest		

Table 2–5 (continued). Complications of Endotracheal Intubation

General Complications	Orotracheal Complications	Nasotracheal Complications
While Tube is in Place		
Discomfort	Obstruction of tube by biting	Obstruction of tube by kinking
Self-extubation	Dental trauma	Nasal septal necrosis
Malfunction of tube or cuff	Trauma to lips, tongue, oral soft tissues	Nasal alar necrosis
Dislodgement		Mucosal ulceration
Inadequate nutrition	Stomatitis	Rhinitis
Difficulty suctioning secretions		Sinusitis
Obstruction of tube by secretions		Otitus
Ineffective cough		
Aerophagia, gastric dilatation		
Increased work of breathing		
Laryngeal inflammation, ulceration, granuloma formation, synechiae		
Subglottic edema		
Tracheal inflammation, ulcerations, granuloma formation		
Tracheomalacia		
Tracheal dilatation		
Carina irritation		
Aspiration		
Pneumonia		
Atelectasis		
Impairment of mucociliary transport		
Squamous metaplasia of respiratory epithelium		
During Extubation		
Discomfort		
Stridor (laryngospasm, laryngeal edema)		
Bronchospasm		
Retained secretions		
Aspiration		
After Extubation		
Hoarseness		
Dysphagia		
Laryngeal motor dysfunction		
Laryngeal synechiae		
Laryngeal granuloma		
Subglottic stenosis		
Tracheal stenosis		
Tracheal granuloma		
Tracheal dilatation		
Tracheomalacia		

bation.[21,85–90] In one such study of 226 intubations in critically ill adults, we found an overall complication rate of 62 percent.[21] In a prospective study of 100 critically ill children, Orlowski and co-workers[90] noted major complications in 10 percent and 11 percent of patients with oral and nasal intubation, respectively. Mortality due to endotracheal intubation is extremely rare, in contrast to the mean 3 percent (range 0 to 5.3 percent) mortality with tracheotomy.[91,92] The risk of complications can undoubtedly be reduced by: (1) proper training and experience in intubation; (2) a confident and assured approach by the intubator; (3) intubation in as controlled a setting as possible, with good lighting and support facilities; (4) the assembly of necessary equipment and checking for its proper function before intubation; and (5) full preparation of the patient.

A minimum of force is necessary to pass a tube through the mouth or nose, and excessive force should be avoided. Only soft-cuff endotracheal tubes approved by the Z-79 Committee should be used. Motion, traction, and leverage applied to the tube should be minimized. Self-extubation, noted in 13 percent of intubations in the critical-care setting,[21] probably cannot be prevented, but can be reduced with skilled nursing and respiratory care. Right mainstem bronchus intubation, which occurs in 9 percent of intubations in critically ill adults,[21,93] can be prevented by resisting the urge to thrust the endotracheal tube deep into the airway after its successful placement through the glottis. If right mainstem bronchus intubation does occur, the tube should be pulled back at once because of the risk of right pneumothorax and left lung atelectasis.[93] If epistaxis occurs during nasal intubation, the tube should be temporarily left in place to tamponade major bleeding. If esophageal intubation occurs, the patient should be placed in the Trendelenburg position and the airway protected so as to avoid aspiration.

Complications of Esophageal Obturator Airway

Major complications of use of the EOA are rare; Gordon noted 95 percent success in its proper placement.[94] Experience with the EOA in 29,000 cardiac resuscitation cases in Los Angeles revealed only a handful of complications, including two cases of esophageal rupture and three cases of tracheal intubation.[33,43] Among the complications that have been reported are esophageal perforation and rupture,[43,46,95–99] pharyngeal-esophageal laceration,[97] supraglottic obstruction,[100] failure to achieve an adequate seal on the face,[45] tracheal intubation,[101] post-extraction vomiting, and inability to intubate the esophagus. Esophageal perforation and rupture are the most common complications of EOA use, with at least 19 cases having been reported by 1980.[43] The mechanism of this complication is not entirely clear,[95] but high intraluminal esophageal pressure during forced vomiting against the inflated cuff of the device is the likely cause. Subcutaneous emphysema and pneumomediastinum are found in 75 percent of cases of esophageal perforation,[43] with the diagnosis being confirmed by an esophagram with water-soluble contrast medium. The esophageal gastric-tube airway, which allows decompression of the esophagus, may prevent this complication.[43]

Complications of Cricothyroidotomy and Tracheotomy

The complication rates in emergency cricothyroidotomy and emergency tracheotomy are unknown because of the absence of reliable data. The complication rate of elective cricothyroidotomy was 6.1 percent in one retrospective analysis.[52] Complications of emergency tracheotomy are two to five times more common than complications of elective tracheotomy.[54,102–106] The overall complication rate in tracheotomy varies widely, from 13 percent[107] to 66 percent[21] in reported series. It is expected that emergency cricothyroidotomy would have fewer complications than emergency tracheotomy because of reduced risks of bleeding, trauma to adjacent structures, and pneumothorax, but this is conjectural in the absence of data.

Although tracheotomy is not the preferred method for emergency surgical access to the trachea, critical-care personnel should still be aware of its complications. Numerous reviews on this subject have appeared in the literature.[91,108–115] Complications during tracheotomy include hemorrhage, injury to the thyroid gland, location of the stoma at a level that is too high or too low, subcutaneous emphysema, mediastinal emphysema, pneumothorax, pneumomediastinum, pneumopericardium, prolonged hypoxemia, placement of the tube in the pretracheal space, inadequate ventilation due to malposition of the distal end of the tube, recurrent laryngeal nerve injury, esophageal penetration, cuff laceration during tube placement, hypotension, prolonged hypoxemia, and cardiac arrest. Early postoperative complications include discomfort, wound infection, hemorrhage, pulmonary infection, tube obstruction, pneumothorax, pneumomediastinum, pneumopericardium, subcutaneous emphysema, accidental decannulation, malfunction of the tube or cuff, aspiration, malposition or dislocation of the tube, tracheal injury (ulceration, inflammation, tracheomalacia, and dilatation), pseudomembrane formation, tracheoesophageal fistula, mediastinitis, sepsis, tracheal granuloma, various mechanical problems with the tube, reduction in mucociliary transport, epithelial squamous metaplasia, and ineffective cough. Decannulation may be painful or difficult for a variety of reasons, including a tight stoma. Late sequelae of tracheotomy include dysphagia, scarring, keloid formation, a persistent open stoma, tracheal stenosis, tracheomalacia, tracheal granuloma, and tracheoesophageal fistula. Some of these adverse outcomes are also potential complications of cricothyroidotomy.

Complications of Translaryngeal and Transtracheal Jet Ventilation

Because of limited experience, there are few reports of complications of transcricothyroid and transtracheal jet ventilation. Among the complications that have been reported are subcutaneous and mediastinal emphysema,[60] pneumothorax,[65] coughing,[65] transient hemoptysis,[63] and tracheitis.[63] Other complications and potential complications include hemorrhage, perforation of the esophagus, laceration of the thyroid, perforation of the subclavian artery or innominate vein,[116] broken needle, and hypercapnia. No deaths have been reported.[60]

EARLY POSTINTUBATION MANAGEMENT

The intubated, critically ill patient depends totally upon the critical-care staff to maintain his or her airway and to meet many physical and psychologic needs. Only the general principles of care of the patient with an artificial airway will be reviewed here; the reader is referred to other sources for additional information.[15,20,117]

The intubated patient is managed in an intensive care unit, where diligent and skilled respiratory care is available around the clock. In this setting, nurses and respiratory therapists are immediately available to serve the patient, to care for the airway, and to manage any complications. The patient is examined at every nursing shift or more often, with particular attention being given to the nose, mouth, neck, chest, and artificial airway. The endotracheal tube is always connected to a source that warms and humidifies inspired gas. Inhalation of dry, cold air depresses mucociliary transport, increasing the risk of infection and atelectasis. Tracheobronchial secretions are suctioned with a meticulous, gloved technique and sterile disposable catheters as often as necessary to keep the airway clear. Excessive and routine suctioning are avoided. The risk of pulmonary aspiration is minimized by preventing gastric distention, avoiding the use of large nasogastric tubes which impair the competence of the esophageal sphincters, keeping the soft cuff of the endotracheal tube inflated at all times, and elevating the head of the bed.

Pulmonary infection is a constant threat to the patient with an artificial airway. The risk of tracheitis, pneumonia, and lung abscess may be reduced if particular care is taken to use sterile suctioning technique, to follow infection control guidelines, to use only humidified and warmed inspired gases, and to change ventilator tubing and humidifiers frequently. Nevertheless, Gram staining of the sputum is frequently necessary for the detection of organisms that may appear in the tracheobronchial tree, particularly Gram-negative bacilli. Leverage and traction on the endotracheal tube are minimized by the use of two-way swivel adaptors, elastic connectors, and tubing support arms. Both coughing and motion between the endotracheal tube and the patient are controlled in order to reduce the raking action of the tube across the mucosa of the larynx and trachea. The oral endotracheal tube is repositioned from one side of the mouth to the other every day, and a new oral airway is inserted if necessary. Mouth care is given at least once a day at the time of repositioning of the oral tube. The ears and sinuses are examined regularly for infection if a nasogastric or nasotracheal tube is being used.[21] The simultaneous use of large nasogastric and nasal endotracheal tubes is avoided. The patient's arms and hands are restrained to avoid self-extubation, although this can occur even without use of the hands.[118] Cuff pressure requirements are determined at least twice a day, and the lowest effective cuff pressure, usually less than 20 mmHg, is used as long as the endotracheal tube is in place. With this precaution, serious complications, such as tracheomalacia, tracheal stenosis, and tracheal dilatation are less likely to occur.

The complications of artificial airways should be sought diligently and routinely, since most may be treated effectively if they are detected early. An endotracheal tube should not be changed routinely unless mechanical problems or complications develop. Whenever an endotracheal or tracheostomy tube is removed, the physician must be ready to re-establish the airway immediately. If severe stridor develops after extubation, it usually can be managed with topical phenylephrine or epinephrine.

The patient should always be extubated or decannulated as early as possible, consistent with optimal respiratory care and improvement or resolution of the underlying disease process. Attending staff members should ask themselves each day, "Is the artificial airway still necessary?" How long an endotracheal tube may safely be left in place is a matter of considerable debate, but in many centers it is now possible to continue endotracheal intubation for as long as 3 weeks.[21] In considering elective tracheotomy for a patient with the long-term need for an artificial airway, the clinician should consider the following factors: (1) the estimated duration of need for an airway; (2) the patient's tolerance of endotracheal intubation, including nutritional status; (3) any observed complications of endotracheal intubation; (4) the likelihood of improved airway management with tracheotomy; and (5) the morbidity, mortality, and expense of tracheotomy in relation to the patient's underlying disease and prognosis.

REFERENCES

1. McLaughlin AJ, Scott W: Training and evaluation of respiratory therapists in emergency intubation. Respiratory Care 26: 333, 1981.
2. Conley JM, Smith DJ: Emergency endotracheal intubation by respiratory care personnel in a community hospital. Respiratory Care 26: 336, 1981.
3. Sladen A: Emergency endotracheal intubation: Who can—Who should? Chest 75: 535, 1979.
4. Downs JB: Who should intubate? Respiratory Care 26: 331, 1981.
5. Emergency Care Research Institute: Artificial airways. Health Devices 7: 67, 1978.
6. Way WW, Sooy FA: Histological changes produced by endotracheal intubation. Ann Otol Rhinol Laryngol 24: 799, 1965.
7. Dripps RD, Eckenhoff JE, Vandam LD: Introduction to Anesthesia: The Principles of Safe Practice. 5th Ed. WB Saunders, Philadelphia, 1977.
8. Loeser EA, Hodges M, Gliedman J, et al: Tracheal pathology following short-term intubation with low- and high-pressure endotracheal tube cuffs. Anesth Analg (Cleve) 57: 577, 1978.
9. Lewis FR Jr, Schlobohm RM, Thomas AN: Prevention of complications from prolonged tracheal intubation. Am J Surg 135: 452, 1978.
10. Gregory GA: Respiratory care of the child. Crit Care Med 8: 582, 1980.
11. Kamen JM, Wilkinson CJ: A new low-pressure cuff for endotracheal tubes. Anesthesiology 34: 482, 1971.
12. Emergency Care Research Institute: Suction catheters. Health Devices 6: 132, 1977.
13. Sackner MA, Landa JF, Greeneltch N, Robinson MJ: Pathogenesis and prevention of tracheobronchial damage with suction catheters. Chest 64: 284, 1973.

14. Venus B: Five year experience with Kistner tracheostomy tube. Crit Care Med 8: 106, 1980.
15. Smith RB, Safar P: Emergency airway control and long-term airway care. p. 1587. In Pulmonary Diseases and Disorders, ed Fishman AP, McGraw Hill Book Company, New York, 1980.
16. Shapter RK, Katz HJ, Cobb LA, et al: Cardiopulmonary resuscitation: basic life support. Clin Symp 26: 4, 1974.
17. Hoff BH, Flemming DC, Sasse F: Use of positive airway pressure without endotracheal intubation. Crit Care Med 7: 559, 1979.
18. Kopman AF, Wollman SB, Ross K, Surks SN: Awake endotracheal intubation: A review of 267 cases. Anesth Analg (Cleve) 54: 323, 1975.
19. Newsum JK, Smith RM, Crocker D: Intubation for acute respiratory failure in Guillain-Barré syndrome. JAMA 242: 1650, 1979.
20. Orringer MB: Endotracheal intubation and tracheostomy: Indications, techniques and complications. Surg Clin North Am 60: 1447, 1980.
21. Stauffer JL, Olson DE, Petty TL: Complications and consequences of endotracheal intubation and tracheotomy: A prospective study of 150 critically ill adult patients. Am J Med 70: 65, 1981.
22. Dubick MN, Wright BD: Comparison of laryngeal pathology following long-term oral and nasal endotracheal intubations. Anesth Analg (Cleve) 57: 663, 1978.
23. Danzyl DF, Thomas DM: Nasotracheal intubations in the emergency department. Crit Care Med 8: 677, 1980.
24. Magill IW: Technique in endotracheal anaesthesia. Br Med J 2: 817, 1930.
25. Pedersen B: Blind nasotracheal intubation: a review and a new guided technique. Acta Anaesthesiol Scand 15: 107, 1971.
26. Gold MI, Buechel DR: A method of blind nasal intubation for the conscious patient. Anesth Analg (Cleve) 39: 257, 1960.
27. Gold MI, Buechel DR: Translaryngeal anesthesia: A review. Anesthesiology 20: 181, 1959.
28. Thomas JL: Awake intubation: Indications, techniques and a review of 25 patients. Anaesthesia 24: 28, 1969.
29. Brown EM, Krishnaprasad D, Smiler BG: Pancuronium for rapid induction technique for tracheal intubation. Can Anaesth Soc J 26: 489, 1979.
30. Churchill-Davidson HC: A Practice of Anaesthesia. WB Saunders, Philadelphia, 1978.
31. Goodman LR, Conrardy PA, Laing F, Singer MM: Radiographic evaluation of endotracheal tube position. Am J Roentgenol 127: 433, 1976
32. Conrardy PA, Goodman LR, Lainge F, Singer MM: Alteration of endotracheal tube position: flexion and extension of the neck. Crit Care Med 4: 8, 1976.
33. Don Michael TA, Gordon A, Schofferman J: Esophageal obturator airway—A new adjunct in emergency airway management. Am J Cardiol 39 (a): 259, 1977.
34. Don Michael TA: Esophageal obturator airway. Med Instrum 11: 331, 1977.
35. Schofferman J, Oill P, Lewis AJ: The esophageal obturator airway: A clinical evaluation. Chest 69: 67, 1976.
36. Don Michael TA, Gordon AS: Esophageal obturator airway: a new adjunct for artificial ventilation. Presented at the National Conference on Standards for Cardiopulmonary Resuscitation and Emergency Cardiac Care. Washington DC, May 16, 1973.

37. Meislin HW: The esophageal obturator airway: A study of respiratory effectiveness. Ann Emerg Med 9: 54, 1980.
38. Don Michael TA, Lambert EH, Mehran A: "Mouth-to-lung airway" for cardiac resuscitation. Lancet 2: 1329, 1968.
39. American Heart Association: Standards for cardiopulmonary resuscitation (CPR) and emergency cardiac care (ECC). JAMA, 244: 453, 1980.
40. Gordon AS: Improved esophageal obturator airway (EOA) and new esophageal gastric tube airway (EGTA). p. 58. In Advances in Cardiopulmonary Resuscitation, ed Safar P, Springer-Verlag, New York, 1977.
41. Farley M: The esophageal obturator airway. Respir Ther 3: 95, 1973.
42. Smock SN: Esophageal obturator airway: preferred CPR technique. JACEP 4: 232, 1975.
43. Harrison EE, Nord HJ, Beeman RW: Esophageal perforation following use of the esophageal obturator airway. Ann Emerg Med 9: 21, 1980.
44. Meislin HW: The esophageal obturator airway: it works, but. . . . Ann Emerg Med 9: 171, 1980.
45. Cameron AE: The oesophageal obturator airway. Br Med J 282: 316, 1981.
46. Pilcher DB, DeMeules JE: Esophageal perforation following use of esophageal airway. Chest 69: 377, 1976.
47. Eisenberg RS: A new airway for tracheal or esophageal insertion: description and field experience. Ann Emerg Med 9: 270, 1980.
48. Nicholas TH, Rumer GF: Emergency airway—A plan of action. JAMA 174: 1930, 1960.
49. Safar P, Penninckx J: Cricothyroid membrane puncture with special cannula. Anesthesiology 28: 943, 1967.
50. Gann DS: Emergency management of the obstructed airway. JAMA 243: 1141, 1980.
51. Brantigan CO, Grow JB Sr: Cricothyroidotomy revisited again. Ear Nose Throat J 59: 26, 1980.
52. Brantigan CO, Grow JB Sr: Cricothyroidotomy: elective use in respiratory problems requiring tracheotomy. J Thorac Cardiovasc Surg 71: 72, 1976.
53. Caparoza RJ, Zavatsky AR: Practical aspects of the cricothyroid space. Laryngoscope 67: 577, 1957.
54. Carlton DM, Zide MF: An easily constructed cricothyroidotomy device for emergency airway management. J Oral Surg 38: 623, 1980.
55. Jacoby JJ, Hamelberg W, Ziegler CH et al: Transtracheal resuscitation. JAMA 162: 625, 1956.
56. Jacobs HB: Needle catheter brings oxygen to the trachea. JAMA 222: 1231, 1972.
57. Jacobs HB: Emergency percutaneous transtracheal catheter and ventilator. J Trauma 12: 50, 1972.
58. Klain M, Smith RB: High frequency percutaneous transtracheal jet ventilation. Crit Care Med 5: 280, 1977.
59. Rock JJ, Pfaeffle H, Smith RB et al: High pressure jet insufflation used to prevent aspiration and its effect on the tracheal mucosal wall. Crit Care Med 4: 135, 1976.
60. Smith RB, Schaer WB, Pfaeffle H: Percutaneous transtracheal ventilation for anaesthesia and resuscitation: A review and report of complications. Can Anaesth Soc J 22: 607, 1975.

61. Dobbinson TL, Whalen J, Pelton DA, et al: Needle tracheostomy: a laboratory study. Anaesth Intensive Care 8: 72, 1980.
62. Bougas TP, Cook CD: Pressure-flow characteristics of needles suggested for transtracheal resuscitation. N Engl J Med 262: 511, 1960.
63. Spoerel WE, Narayanan PS, Singh NP: Transtracheal ventilation. Br J Anaesth 43: 932, 1971.
64. Smith RB: Transtracheal ventilation during anesthesia. Anesth Analg (Cleve) 53: 225, 1974.
65. Spoerel WE, Greenway RE: Technique of ventilation during endolaryngeal surgery under general anesthesia. Can Anaesth Soc J 20: 369, 1973.
66. Smith RB, Babinski M, Pfaeffle H: Percutaneous transtracheal ventilation in emergency medicine. Crit Care Med 4: 135 (a), 1976.
67. Smith RB, Cutaia F, Hoff BH, et al: Long-term transtracheal high frequency ventilation in dogs. Crit Care Med 9: 311, 1981.
68. Attia RR, Battit GE, Murphy JD: Transtracheal ventilation. JAMA, 234: 1152, 1975.
69. Payne KA: Difficult tracheal intubation. Anaesth Intensive Care 8: 84, 1980.
70. Salem MR, Mathrubhutham M, Bennett EJ: Difficult intubation. N Engl J Med 295: 879, 1976.
71. Duncan JAT: Intubation of the trachea in the conscious patient. Br J Anaesth 49: 619, 1977.
72. Moller CT: Use of a suction catheter to change a nasotracheal tube. Anaesth Intensive Care 7: 192, 1979.
73. Rucker RW, Silva WJ, Worcester CC: Fiberoptic bronchoscopic nasotracheal intubation in children. Chest 76: 56, 1979.
74. Taylor PA, Towey RM: The broncho-fiberscope as an aid to endotracheal intubation. Br J Anaesth 44: 611, 1972.
75. Messeter KH, Pettersson KI: Endotracheal intubation with the fibre-optic bronchoscope. Anaesthesia 35: 294, 1980.
76. Whitehouse AC, Klock LE: Evaluation of endotracheal tube position with the fiberoptic intubation laryngoscope. Chest 68: 848, 1975.
77. Ducrow M: Throwing light on blind intubation. Anaesthesia 33: 827, 1978.
78. Sleeman KW: An introducer to facilitate nasotracheal intubation. Anaesth Intensive Care 7: 381, 1979.
79. Akinyemi OO: Complications of guided blind endotracheal intubation. Anaesthesia 34: 590, 1979.
80. Waters DJ: Guided endotracheal intubation for patients with deformities of the upper airway. Anaesthesia 18: 158, 1963.
81. Taryle DA, Chandler JE, Good JT Jr, et al: Emergency room intubations—Complications and survival. Chest 75: 541, 1979.
82. Lewis RN, Swerdlow M: Hazards of endotracheal anaesthesia. Br J Anaesth 36: 504, 1964.
83. McGovern FH, Fitz-Hugh GS, Edgemon LJ: The hazards of endotracheal intubation. Ann Otol 80: 556, 1971.
84. Blanc VF, Tremblay NAG: The complications of tracheal intubation: A new classification with a review of the literature. Anesth Analg (Cleve) 53: 202, 1974.
85. Deane RS, Mills EL: Prolonged nasotracheal intubation in adults: a successor and adjunct to tracheostomy. Anesth Analg (Cleve) 49: 89, 1970.

86. Lindholm C-E: Prolonged endotracheal intubation. Acta Anaesthesiol Scand 33 (Suppl): 1, 1969.
87. Lake KB, Van Dyke JJ: Prolonged nasotracheal intubation. Heart Lung 9: 93, 1980.
88. El-Naggar M, Sadagopan S, Levine H, et al: Factors influencing choice between tracheostomy and prolonged translaryngeal intubation in acute respiratory failure. Anesth Analg (Cleve) 55: 195, 1976.
89. Burns HP, Dayal VS, Scott A, et al: Laryngotracheal trauma: observations on its pathogenesis and its prevention following prolonged orotracheal intubation in the adult. Laryngoscope 89: 1316, 1979.
90. Orlowski JP, Ellis NG, Amin NP, Crumrine RS: Complications of airway intrusion in 100 consecutive cases in a pediatric ICU. Crit Care Med 8: 324, 1980.
91. Meade JW: Tracheotomy—Its complications and their management: a study of 212 cases. N Engl J Med 265: 519, 1961.
92. Kuner J, Goldman A: Prolonged nasotracheal intubation in adults versus tracheostomy. Dis Chest 51: 270, 1967.
93. Zwillich CW, Pierson DJ, Creagh CE, et al: Complications of assisted ventilation: a prospective study of 354 consecutive episodes. Am J Med 57: 161, 1974.
94. Melker RJ, Gordon AS: The esophageal obturator airway. Chest 76: 611, 1979.
95. Kassels SJ, Robinson WA, O'Bara KJ: Esophageal perforation associated with the esophageal obturator airway. Crit Care Med 8: 386, 1980.
96. Scholl DG, Tsai SH: Esophageal perforation following the use of the esophageal obturator airway. Radiology 122: 315, 1977.
97. Johnson KR, Genovesi MG, Lassar KH: Esophageal obturator airway: use and complications. JACEP 5: 36, 1976.
98. Strate RG, Fischer RP: Midesophageal perforations by esophageal obturator airways. J Trauma 16: 503, 1976.
99. Carlson WJ, Hunter SW, Bonnabeau RC: Esophageal perforation with obturator airway. JAMA 241: 1154, 1979.
100. Bryson TK, Benumof JL, Ward CF: The esophageal obturator airway: a clinical comparison to ventilation with a mask and oropharyngeal airway. Chest 74: 537, 1978.
101. Yancey W, Wears R, Kamajian G, Derovanesian J: Unrecognized tracheal intubation: A complication of the esophageal obturator airway. Ann Emerg Med 9: 18, 1980.
102. Davis HS, Kretchmer HE, Bryce-Smith R: Advantages and complications of tracheostomy. JAMA 153: 1156, 1953.
103. Eiseman B, Spencer FC: Tracheostomy: An underated surgical procedure. JAMA 184: 683, 1963.
104. Greene DA: Tracheostomy or not? JAMA 234: 1150, 1975.
105. Glas W, King OJ, Liu A: Complications of tracheostomy. Arch Surg 85: 56, 1962.
106. King OJ Jr, Glas WW: Complication of tracheostomy. Rocky Mt Med J 57: 36, 1960.
107. Figi FA: Tracheotomy: A study of 200 consecutive cases. Ann Otol 43: 178, 1934.
108. Kirchner JA: Tracheotomy and its problems. Surg Clin North Am 60: 1093, 1980.
109. Stemmer EA, Oliver C, Carey JP, Connolly JE: Fatal complications of tracheotomy. Am J Surg 131: 288, 1976.
110. Andrews MJ, Pearson FG: Incidence and pathogenesis of tracheal injury following cuffed tube tracheostomy with assisted ventilation: analysis of a two-year prospective study. Ann Surg 173: 249, 1971.

111. Timmis HH: Tracheostomy: an overview of implications, management and morbidity. Adv Surg 7: 199, 1973.
112. McClelland RMA: Complications of tracheostomy. Br Med J 2: 567, 1965.
113. McClelland RMA: Tracheostomy: Its management and alternatives. Proc R Soc Med 65: 401, 1972.
114. Kenan PD: Complications associated with tracheostomy: prevention and treatment. Otolaryngol Clin North Am 12: 807, 1979.
115. El-Kilany SM: Complications of tracheostomy. Ear Nose Throat J 59: 59, 1980.
116. Toy FJ, Weinstein JD: A percutaneous tracheostomy device. Surgery 65: 384, 1969.
117. Stauffer JL: Establishment and care of the airway. In Intensive and Rehabilitative Respiratory Care, 3rd Ed, ed. Petty TL, Lea & Febiger, Philadelphia, (In press).
118. Ripoll I, Lindholm C-E, Carroll R, Grenvik A: Spontaneous dislocation of endotracheal tubes. Anesthesiology 49: 50, 1978.

3

Upper Airway Obstruction

John G. Brooks, M.D.

INTRODUCTION

The upper airway includes the larynx, pharynx, nose, and mouth, and can be obstructed by a wide variety of acute or chronic disease processes.[1] The obstruction may be fixed, variable (dynamic), or a combination of the two. An upper airway obstruction may also be persistent or intermittent as, for example, in the syndrome of obstructive sleep apnea. Upper airway obstruction can cause severe dyspnea, respiratory failure, and death.

Viral laryngotracheobronchitis in infants and young children is the most common clinically important form of upper airway obstruction (Table 3–1). Other infectious causes of upper airway obstruction in children include epiglottitis or bacterial croup, diphtheria and measles croup (both relatively rare today), and bacterial tracheitis. Retropharyngeal abscesses and epiglottitis can occur in adults as well as children. Noninfectious potential causes of upper airway obstruction in the pediatric population include unilateral or bilateral vocal cord paralysis (congenital or acquired), congenital laryngeal stridor (laryngomalacia), and a congenital laryngeal or tracheal web or stenosis. Laryngeal or subglottic cysts and subglottic tumors such as hemangioma may produce upper airway obstruction at birth or during infancy. Laryngeal polyps may present at any age. Most aberrant vessels or vascular rings cause a tracheal obstruction that is primarily intrathoracic. Aspirated foreign bodies usually lodge in the intrathoracic airways, but on rare occasions may lodge in the larynx or subglottic area, particularly at the level of the cricoid cartilage, and may present as acute upper airway obstructions. Occasionally, enlarged tonsils or adenoids may cause enough chronic airway obstruction to result in cor pulmonale. A similar problem may develop if the tongue is relatively large for the oral cavity, owing to macroglossia or micrognathia. Clinically important upper airway obstruction is much less common in the adult than in the child. The most common causes of upper airway obstruction in adults include blunt trauma to the neck and throat, complications from endotracheal intubation or tracheostomy, and malignancies.

Table 3–1. Differential Diagnosis of Acute Onset of Inspiratory Stridor

Common	Viral croup
Less common	Bacterial tracheitis Epiglottitis Foreign body aspiration Retropharyngeal abscess Vocal cord paralysis Malignancy Trauma Tonsillar/adenoidal hypertrophy

PATHOPHYSIOLOGY

The patency of the upper airways is normally maintained by a variety of anatomic and reflex mechanisms.[2] While the infant is an obligate nose breather for the first several weeks or months of life, most other patients who develop significant nasal or nasopharyngeal obstruction will switch to mouth breathing to bypass an obstruction. The pharyngeal and laryngeal airways are normally larger during inspiration than expiration, due to the phasic activity of the genioglossus (which pulls the tongue forward, out of the pharyngeal airway) and the posterior cricoarytenoid (which is the main abductor of the vocal cords) muscles, in phase with respiration. With sedation or decreased levels of consciousness (such as those due to anesthesia, head injury, or alcohol ingestion), these protective reflexes, particularly that of the genioglossus, may be less effective.

Extrathoracic airway obstruction is usually characterized by inspiratory stridor—that is, greater inspiratory obstruction than expiratory obstruction. The reverse is true with intrathoracic obstruction, such as asthma. This clinically useful distinction results from the different transmural pressure gradients which develop across the airway wall during inspiration and expiration and cause dynamic narrowing when the intraluminal pressure is more negative than the extraluminal pressure. This dynamic compression can narrow the airway to one-half or less of its resting cross-sectional area. With extrathoracic airway obstruction, a more vigorous than usual inspiratory effort is generated, with the effect that the intraluminal airway pressure on the lung side of the point of greatest obstruction becomes very negative. If this negative airway pressure occurs in a segment of the extrathoracic airway, this segment will undergo dynamic compression. The more compliant the airway, the more marked the dynamic compression. During expiration in a patient with extrathoracic airway obstruction, there will be minimal dynamic compression of the airways, and inspiratory stridor will therefore be much worse than expiratory stridor. In patients old enough to perform a forced expiratory and inspiratory maneuver for spirometry, dynamic compression due to extrathoracic airway obstruction is manifested as a much greater limitation of maximal inspiratory than of maximal expiratory flow rates. If the lesion is fixed and involves the airway at the level of the thoracic inlet, there may be inspiratory and expiratory obstruction of relatively similar magnitude.

There are several important differences between the upper airway of the infant and the adult, some of which contribute to the infant's greater susceptibility and vulnerability to upper airway obstruction. The small diameter of the infant airway, particularly at the external naris, where the diameter may be less than 1 mm, and in the subglottic trachea, puts the infant at a disproportionate disadvantage, since any slight further narrowing of the airway will critically increase the airway resistance; by Poiseuille's law, the resistance in an airway is inversely proportional to the fourth power of the radius. Additionally, the infant has a relatively longer soft palate, relatively more posterior pharyngeal tissue between the pharyngeal airway and the spine, and a more mobile temporomandibular joint than the adult; all of these characteristics contribute to a greater tendency toward partial or complete pharyngeal airway obstruction by soft tissue. Moreover, since the larynx is from one to two cervical vertebrae higher in the infant than in the adult, the epiglottis, which like the larynx is more compliant than in the adult, owing to incomplete cartilaginous development, is another upper airway structure that can contribute to airway obstruction in the infant. Until the age of 3 to 6 years, the extrathoracic trachea at the level of the cricoid cartilage is the narrowest part of the airway; it is also the only part of the airway in which there is a complete cartilaginous ring restricting any outward expansion, thus making the infant particularly likely to develop symptoms from subglottic inflammation. The trachea also is more compliant in the infant than in the adult, due to the incomplete development of tracheal cartilage.

VIRAL CROUP

Viral croup (laryngotracheobronchitis) is a common cause of airway obstruction in infants and children between 3 months and 3 years of age. It occurs particularly in the late fall or early winter, is more common in boys than in girls, and produces symptoms resulting from subglottic narrowing due to mucosal edema, inflammation, and possibly exudate. Approximately 85 percent of laryngotracheobronchitis is of viral etiology, and most of this is due to parainfluenza virus type I. Croup may also be due to parainfluenza types II and III and to respiratory syncytial, influenza, rubeola, and adenovirus.

A major clinical concern when dealing with a patient who has the croup syndrome is to rule out bacterial epiglottitis. The typical clinical presentation of viral croup is quite different from that of epiglottitis; the two are contrasted in Table 3–2. The symptoms of upper airway obstruction in a patient with viral croup are usually preceded by several days of symptoms of upper respiratory tract infection, such as coryza and cough. The temperature is usually normal or slightly elevated. The entire clinical picture is typical of a viral infection, with a normal or slightly elevated white blood cell count and a normal differential count. Blood cultures are negative. Over a 1- to 3-day period there is gradual development of a "brassy" cough which sounds like the bark of a seal or dog, and in some patients there is progression to intermittent and then persistent inspiratory stridor. There

Table 3–2. Clinical Characteristics of Epiglottitis and Viral Croup

	Epiglottitis (Bacterial Croup)	Viral Croup (Laryngotracheobronchitis)
Usual cause	*Hemophilus influenzae*	Parainfluenza virus type I
Usual age range	3–7 years	3 months–3 years
Seasonal occurrence	None	Late fall, early winter
Clinical onset	Rapidly (<24 hours), acutely ill	Preceded by rhinitis and cough for several days
Dysphagia	Marked; may be drooling	None
Fever	>39.4°C (103°F)	Variable, usually <39.4°C (103°F)
White blood count	High (>15,000/μl) with neutrophilia	Usually normal
Blood culture	Positive	Negative
Neck radiograph	Supraglottic swelling	Subglottic narrowing
Criteria for diagnosis	"Cherry-red" epiglottis on direct visualization	Clinical presentation and exclusion of other diagnoses
Treatment	Intravenous chloramphenicol; artificial airway	Cool mist; racemic epinephrine
Complications	Pneumonia Cervical lymphadenitis Exudative tonsillitis Otitis media Pulmonary edema Respiratory failure	Pneumonia Pulmonary edema Respiratory failure Cardiac failure

is usually no sore throat, but the voice may be hoarse. The signs of upper airway obstruction usually resolve over 2 to 7 days, but marked obstruction may develop before resolution begins. In addition to the brassy cough and inspiratory stridor, the child with croup may demonstrate varying degrees of chest wall retraction, tachypnea, tachycardia and, if the obstruction is severe, cyanosis, decreased air entry, lethargy, coma, or respiratory arrest. The chest radiograph is usually normal, although some patients may have associated pneumonia, and pulmonary edema and cardiomegaly are occasionally seen.[3]

The diagnosis is usually established on the basis of the typical clinical presentation and by the exclusion of other diagnoses, particularly epiglottitis. The lateral radiograph of the soft tissues of the neck is helpful for establishing or excluding the diagnosis of epiglottitis but is less helpful for the diagnosis of croup.[4,5]

Therapy for viral croup is based on symptomatic treatment of the upper airway obstruction and careful observation to permit the use of an artificial airway at the correct time if severe obstruction and respiratory failure are imminent. All patients who, while at rest, manifest a persistent inspiratory stridor due to acute viral croup should be hospitalized. Most croup patients do not reach this degree of severity and can be appropriately managed as outpatients. When patients are to be cared for at home, it is important that the parents or other caretakers understand that they must watch closely for signs of increasing airway obstruction, such as an increased respiratory rate, respiratory distress, cyanosis, or chest wall retraction. Often, an acute exacerbation of upper airway obstruction can be relieved by having the home-treated patient sit in a bathroom with the doors closed, and generating heavy steam by running the shower. Sometimes, taking a child into the cool night air will provide relief of upper airway obstruction, presumably by causing local subglottic mucosal cooling and vasoconstriction and by decreasing swelling of the airway lining. If there are questions about the parents' ability to closely observe the child or to return the child to a medical facility if the airway obstruction should increase, it may be appropriate to observe the child in the hospital even if there is no persistent stridor during rest. This is particularly true for infants under 6 to 12 months of age.

Close observation and the use of a continuous cool mist (bland aerosol) are the cornerstones of in-hospital therapy for the patient with viral croup. The mist can be delivered in a steam room, a mist tent, a head hood (for young infants only) or occasionally, by mist mask (for older patients). On admission, patients with croup may be somewhat dehydrated if their dyspnea has interfered with their oral fluid intake. The goal should be to restore and maintain a normal hydration status (urine specific gravity = 1.010 to 1.020); this often may require giving intravenous fluid. Overhydration could theoretically potentiate a tendency to pulmonary edema.[3]

It is important to minimize patient anxiety, since agitation will increase oxygen consumption which, in the face of limited oxygen availability, is likely to increase the hypoxemia in viral croup. Anxiety will also be associated with more vigorous inspiratory efforts, which will exaggerate the dynamic compression of the extrathoracic trachea, thus further increasing the work required for inspiration. The child's anxiety often can be minimized by the close presence of a parent or sympathetic staff member. Pharmacologic sedation almost always is contraindicated, since any effective sedation may be associated with a decrease in the patient's respiratory drive.

Any patient meeting the criteria for hospitalization for viral croup will be hypoxemic, most likely due to the associated lower airway involvement, which interferes with normal ventilation-perfusion relationships.[6] For this reason, it is often appropriate to administer low-flow, humidified oxygen (usually at an FIO_2 of 0.24 to 0.28). The child should be observed closely when the oxygen is first administered, since an occasional child with moderate or severe obstruction will hypoventilate when given oxygen as a result of removal of the hypoxic stimulus to breathing. The use of arterial or "arterialized" capillary blood gas measurements for monitoring the course of a patient with viral croup is controversial. The rationale for their use is that they provide a quantitative assessment of the adequacy of oxygenation and alveolar ventilation. However, except when the blood samples are drawn from an indwelling arterial catheter, the measurements are not likely to represent the patient's steady state. The agitation and anxiety associated with the drawing of the blood will change the PO_2 and PCO_2 in unpredictable ways. Additionally, the agitation will contribute to increased functional airway obstruction by increasing the dynamic airway compression. The best solution, which hopefully will be available in the near future, is either continuous transcutaneous monitoring of carbon dioxide and oxygen tensions or end-tidal CO_2 monitoring. An indirect reflection of oxygenation can be obtained by counting the resting respiratory rate, since there is a significant inverse correlation between the arterial PO_2 and the respiratory rate.[6] This is not true for the arterial PCO_2, and there is no significant relationship between blood gas results and other clinical findings such as the heart rate, chest wall retractions, or air entry.

Mist therapy alone will provide substantial relief of upper airway obstruction in about 50 percent of viral croup patients who exhibit stridor while at rest.[7,8] When mist therapy fails to provide adequate relief of the symptoms of upper airway obstruction, the inhalation of nebulized racemic epinephrine (0.5 cc of a 2.25 percent racemic epinephrine solution in 3.5 cc of preservative-free sterile water) usually will provide marked, although transient, improvement. Nebulized racemic epinephrine solution delivered by IPPB has also been proven effective[7,9]; but in most if not all patients, this nebulized solution is equally effective when delivered by face mask with active inhalation. The benefit from this treatment may last no longer than 1 to 2 hours,[7] but there is no definite evidence of a "rebound" phenomenon after the inhalation of racemic epinephrine. The symptoms of upper airway obstruction may be worse 2 hours after the administration of the racemic epinephrine than they were prior to the treatment, but this may be due to the progression of the underlying disease itself. However, because there is a real potential for the recurrence of severe symptoms after a treatment, racemic epinephrine should not be administered to outpatients. The treatments can be repeated on hospitalized patients at 1- to 2-hour intervals if upper airway obstruction and stridor have recurred. There is no evidence for any benefit from the prophylactic use of racemic epinephrine in less severely affected croup patients.

Since the therapeutic effect of inhaled racemic epinephrine solution is most likely due to localized vasoconstriction in the subglottic tracheal mucosa, with a subsequent decrease in edema and swelling, an alpha-adrenergic agent might be equally or more effective. The administration of 2 cc of an 0.25 percent phenylephrine solution by nebulization has been shown to cause a transient decrease in total respiratory resistance in viral croup patients, but the benefit lasted only about 30 minutes.[10]

Despite numerous studies of their efficacy, the role of corticosteroids in the treatment of croup remains unclear.[11–13] A reasonable approach to the use of these agents in the viral croup patient is to administer a short course of dexamethasone (0.5 to 2 mg/kg/day parenterally or by mouth, either as a single dose or for a 48-hour period) to patients with severe or moderately severe upper airway obstruction, particularly if the airway narrowing has become unresponsive to nebulized racemic epinephrine.

The goal of the treatment and monitoring which have been reviewed thus far is to avoid respiratory failure from severe upper airway obstruction. This is achieved by the appropriate use of medical measures to reverse the upper airway obstruction and by careful observation and monitoring so that an artificial airway may be introduced if respiratory failure is imminent. Certain complications, such as underlying fixed airway narrowing, pneumonia, or heart failure may increase the

Table 3–3. Recommended Endotracheal Tube Sizes (Internal Diameter)

Age	Normal (mm)	Croup or Epiglottitis (mm)
Premature (<1 kg)	2.5	2.5
Premature (1–2.5 kg)	3.0	3.0
Newborn (2.5–4 kg)	3.5	3.0
1–12 months	4.0	3.0–3.5
1–3 years	4.5	3.5–4.0
3–10 years	5.0–5.5	4.0–5.0

likelihood that an artificial airway will be required. The indications for tracheal intubation are marked chest wall retractions, cyanosis, markedly decreased air entry, severe agitation, and loss of consciousness. When there is uncertainty about the adequacy of alveolar ventilation, an arterial blood gas sample to document hypercarbia may be helpful. If tracheal intubation is necessary, it should preferably be done by the nasotracheal route. The intubation should be performed under controlled circumstances by the most experienced person available. A tracheostomy is not necessary, since the artificial airway is likely to be in place for only 2 to 7 days. The size of the endotracheal tube should be 0.5 to 1 mm smaller in diameter than that which would usually be used for a patient of the size being treated (Table 3–3).

Although complete symptomatic recovery from croup is the rule, there is some recent evidence that children who have had croup are at increased risk of demonstrating bronchial hyperreactivity when tested during the mid-childhood years.[14,15]

"Spasmodic croup" is a common but poorly understood variant of the typical presentation of croup; it is characterized by the sudden onset of inspiratory stridor and a barking cough, usually in the middle of the night, in a child who has been completely well or is suffering from only a very mild upper respiratory infection. "Spasmodic croup" tends to respond particularly well to mist therapy. This type of airway obstruction may recur on several consecutive nights. Like recurrent croup,[16] "spasmodic croup" may be a manifestation of airway hyperreactivity or atopy.

BACTERIAL TRACHEITIS

Bacterial tracheitis, a recently re-described respiratory tract disease which is usually caused by *Staphylococcus aureus*, usually presents with inspiratory stridor and a brassy cough, but with a higher temperature and more of a left shift in a differential white blood count than is seen in viral croup.[17] Bacterial tracheitis is probably most common during the winter months and in children less than 3 years old. Its precise incidence is unknown, although it may be slightly more comman than bacterial epiglottitis. While the presentation is quite similar to that of viral croup, patients with bacterial tracheitis will fail to respond to the usual croup therapy. They require anti-staphylococcal antibiotic therapy and often tracheal intubation for the removal of profuse, thick, purulent tracheal secretions. The incidence of long-term tracheal scarring in bacterial tracheitis is unknown.

EPIGLOTTITIS

Epiglottitis (bacterial croup or bacterial supraglottitis) is the most serious infectious cause of the croup syndrome. It is usually caused by *Hemophilus influenzae* type B, and consists of a bacterial cellulitis of the epiglottis, sometimes involving other supraglottic structures such as the arytenoid cartilages and aryepiglottic folds. Epiglottitis represents a medical emergency since there is a real possibility of sudden, complete upper airway obstruction. The mortality in untreated epiglottitis is greater than 50 percent. With currently available forms of therapy, the mortality is 2 to 5 percent, with upper airway obstruction being the cause of death. While epiglottitis is most common in children between the ages of 2 and 7 years, it can occur at any age and has been reported in a 2-month-old infant and a 66-year-old adult.[18] There is no consistent seasonal pattern to the occurrence of epiglottitis, but there is a slight male predominance.

In contrast to viral croup, epiglottitis has a very rapid onset, often over a few hours, with high fever, toxicity, an extreme sore throat, muffled voice, inability to swallow, and signs and symptoms of upper airway obstruction including inspiratory stridor and respiratory distress (see Table 3–2). There is no brassy cough. Patients with severe upper airway obstruction due to epiglottitis often assume a characteristic posture, sitting forward with the mouth open and the tongue protruding. There often is drooling of excessive secretions, pallor, tachycardia, restlessness, and in more severe cases, cyanosis and even confusion and loss of consciousness.

The white blood cell count is usually elevated to greater than 15,000 per μl, with a marked neutrophilia. Moltini[19] reported that 85 percent of his series of 72 patients presented with more than 500 bands per μl. In approximately 80 percent of patients with acute epiglottitis, *Hemophilus influenzae* type B can be grown from the blood. There is a slightly higher percentage of positive culture for *H. influenzae* from the pharynx. Because of the possibility of precipitating a marked increase in upper airway obstruction, it is not safe to obtain pharyngeal cultures until an artificial airway has been introduced.

The diagnosis of epiglottitis is most definitively established by direct visualization of an epiglottis that is "cherry-red," enlarged, edematous, and markedly inflamed and friable. Optimal visualization of the epiglottis and adjacent supraglottic structures that may be involved by an *H. influenza* infection is achieved by direct laryngoscopy. Since this may cause discomfort to the patient, it is sometimes appropriate to attempt to visualize the epiglottis by cautiously advancing a tongue depressor toward the posterior part of the tongue until the epiglottis rises above the base of the tongue as the patient gags. Since this procedure, like any

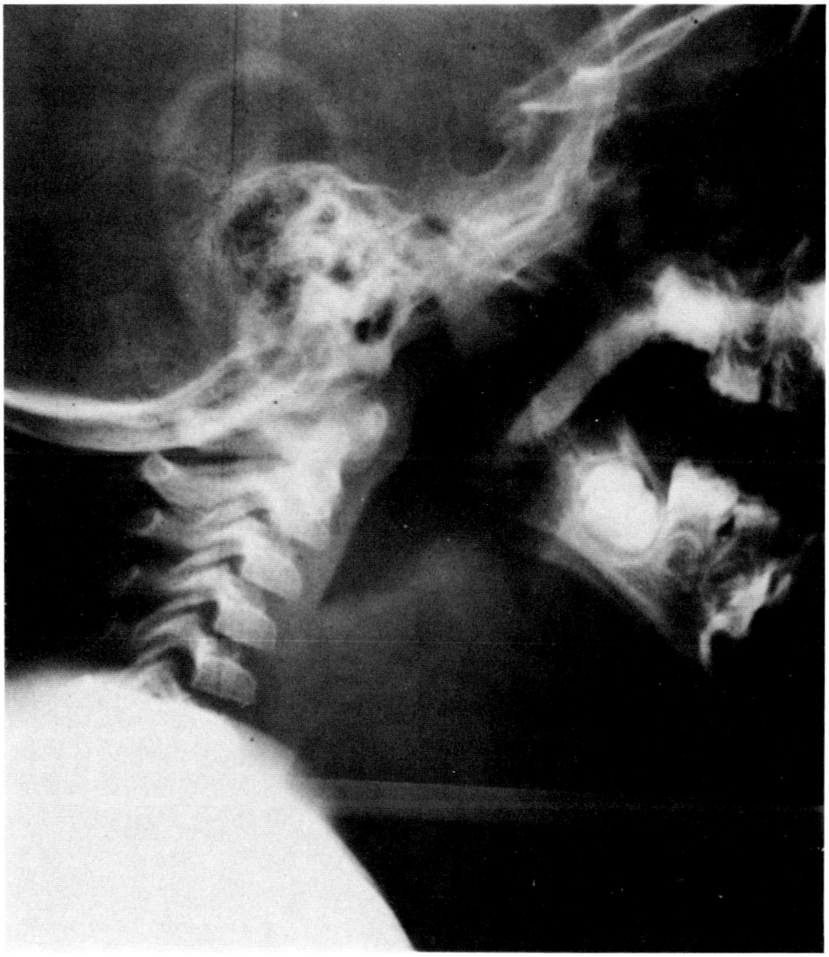

Figure 3–1. Soft-tissue lateral neck roentgenogram of a 5-year-old boy with epiglottitis. Note enlarged epiglottis and aryepiglottic folds, partial obliteration of the vallecula, pharyngeal distension, and normal subglottic airway caliber.

other instrumentation of the oropharynx, may precipitate a marked increase in airway obstruction, it is important that all appropriate precautions be taken, including pre-oxygenating the patient, having the equipment and personnel for pharyngeal suctioning and introduction of an artificial airway immediately available. The equipment for assisted positive pressure ventilation by bag and mask should also be immediately available.

Lateral roentgenography of the soft tissues of the neck is an alternative, noninvasive method which is quite useful in establishing or ruling out the diagnosis of epiglottitis.[4] In the patient with epiglottitis, the epiglottis is swollen, and the aryepiglottic folds may also be swollen (Fig. 3–1). There is likely to be pharyngeal "ballooning" (distension) if the film is taken during inspiration, but this is a nonspecific indication of airway obstruction in the glottic or subglottic area. A patient with suspected epiglottitis who is to have an x-ray must be accompanied to the radiology department by a physician with the skills and equipment for providing assisted ventilation or an artificial airway should there be an increase in airway obstruction. The supine position should be avoided in patients with suspected epiglottitis until an artificial airway has been introduced, since it may precipitate total airway obstruction by the enlarged epiglottis.

The goals of treatment of epiglottitis are to ensure an adequate airway and to eradicate the bacterial infection. There is great urgency in initiating steps toward both of these goals as soon as the diagnosis is established. The diagnosis of epiglottitis is considered to be the indication for an artificial airway, and this should be established on an emergency basis. The key to successful treatment of patients with epiglottitis is a good understanding and acute awareness among primary care physicians and especially emergency room doctors so as to facilitate an early diagnosis. In order to ensure rapid and optimal in-hospital therapy when the diagnosis is suspected, there must be systematic, expeditious, multidisciplinary collaboration among pediatricians, anesthesiologists, surgeons, and radiologists. Based on the specific facilities and personnel available, each medical center must devise its own protocol for the optimal handling of every patient suspected of having epiglottitis. Each center's protocol will differ slightly, depending upon the particular hospital or medical setting.

Once the diagnosis of epiglottitis has been established by direct visualization or by lateral neck roentgenogram, the standardized protocol for the medical center treating each particular case should be activated immediately, so as to ensure rapid and expert introduction of an artificial airway. An intravenous line should be inserted, a blood culture and complete blood count done, and the first dose of chloramephenicol administered intravenously (100 mg/kg/day in four divided doses). The patient should never be left alone because of the possible development of total airway obstruction. If the patient is having severe respiratory difficulty, humidified oxygen should be delivered by face mask. If the patient's status should deteriorate suddenly, assisted ventilation by bag and mask should be attempted, using 100 percent oxygen. Rapid, short, hard compressions of the ventilation bag should be used to maximize gas delivery to the lungs and to minimize the gas transmitted by the esophagus to the stomach. With these techniques and a tight mask-to-face seal, sufficient alveolar ventilation usually can be achieved, at least for a short period of time, to prevent serious respiratory acidosis. It is almost never necessary to perform an emergency, uncontrolled tracheotomy.

As soon as possible after the diagnosis is established (optimally, the initial direct visualization of the epiglottis will have been performed in the operating room), the patient should be taken directly to the operating room. After thorough preoxygenation of the patient, a nasotracheal tube should be inserted by someone who is particularly skilled in this procedure.[20] This is likely to be one of the most difficult of all intubations. Orotracheal intubation can be used if the person performing the intubation is more comfortable with this procedure. A surgeon should be present to perform an emergency tracheotomy in the unusual circumstance in which it may become necessary. Some medical personnel are experienced in performing intubations on patients who are in the sitting position. This has the advantage of obviating the need for the patient to lie supine, risking the possibility of increased airway obstruction. The endotracheal tube used for the intubation should be approximately 1 mm smaller than that which would normally be used (Table 3–3); the tube must be carefully stabilized to minimize the risk of accidental extubation. For this same purpose, the intubated patient should be cared for in an intensive care unit under close observation. Elbow splints are helpful for preventing young children from getting their hands to the endotracheal tube. In infants, 2 cmH_2O of continuous positive airway pressure may help prevent alveolar collapse.

Unless a patient has had central nervous system damage from an hypoxemic episode associated with severe airway obstruction, assisted ventilation is not necessary once an artificial airway is established. In some cases, mild sedation may be necessary when an endotracheal tube is in place, to prevent the patient from becoming too agitated. The epiglottis can be visualized daily in the intensive care unit by direct laryngoscopy. The endotracheal tube should be removed when the epiglottic swelling has subsided and the patient can handle oral secretions and breathe around the tube; this usually occurs from 1 to 3 days after antibiotic therapy has been initiated. After a definite clinical response, the 10-day course of antibiotics can be completed using oral preparations if adequate serum drug levels are maintained. Dexamethasone (0.4 mg/kg/q. 4–6 h. for a total of two to four doses) has been advocated by some, but its value is unproven and it generally is not used.

More extensive involvement of the respiratory tract can occur in patients with epiglottitis. There is a 25 percent incidence of coexistent pneumonia which may be either lobar or bronchopneumonia. Other associated complications include cervical lymphadenitis, exudative tonsillitis, otitis media, and cervical cellulitis.[21]

EXTERNAL TRAUMA TO THE UPPER AIRWAY

Severe upper airway obstruction can result from external blows and penetrating wounds of the neck. The immediate cause of the obstruction may be the dislocation of the cricoarytenoid cartilages, or airway narrowing due to hematoma or edema of the airway mucosa or surrounding soft tissues. In such cases, bronchoscopic examination of the upper airway is necessary for determining the extent of the injury and whether or not there is substantial hemorrhage. It may be necessary to perform a tracheostomy or tracheal intubation to ensure an adequate airway, or prophylactically in anticipation of airway surgery.

FOREIGN BODIES

Foreign body aspiration is most common in the 6-month to 4-year age range, and the foreign body usually lodges in the intrathoracic airway. In one pediatric series, 4 percent of aspirated foreign bodies were located in the larynx.[22] This is usually associated with severe respiratory distress with a striking cough, dyspnea, and inspiratory stridor. The foreign body is usually (95 percent of the time) radiolucent, and when the foreign body is in the upper airway, the chest radiograph is normal. The removal of a laryngeal or tracheal foreign body is an emergency procedure. In infants and young children the foreign body may become lodged at the level of the cricoid cartilage, since the tracheal lumen is narrower at this point than at the level of the vocal cords.

The aspiration of foreign bodies by adults usually occurs during meals.[23] The typical victim is middle-aged or elderly, often is wearing dentures, and has ingested alcohol which may have decreased some of the normal protective laryngeal reflexes. "Café coronary" refers to a situation in which a bolus of food, usually steak, becomes lodged in the hypopharynx and upper larynx, causing complete airway obstruction and aphonia. This occurrence often has been mistaken for myocardial infarction. The aphonia and normal state of alertness are key points in the differential diagnosis. Emergency treatment should be directed toward removing the meat or obstructing material from the posterior pharynx with the back blow, manual thrust (Heimlich maneuver), or finger sweep (see Chapter 1). It is estimated that the "café coronary" is responsible for 1000 to 2500 adult fatalities annually in the United States.

REFERENCES

1. Maze A, Bloch E: Stridor in pediatric patients. Anesthesiology 50:132, 1979.
2. Proctor DF: The upper airways. II. The larynx and trachea. Am Rev Resp Dis 115:315, 1977.
3. Travis KW, Todres ID, Shannon, DC: Pulmonary edema associated with croup and epiglottitis. Pediatrics 59:695, 1977.
4. Rapkin RH: Simplicity and reliability of radiograph of the neck in the differential diagnosis of the croup syndrome. J Pediatr 80:96, 1972.
5. Mills JL, Spackman J, Borns P, et al: The usefulness of lateral neck roentgenogram in laryngotracheobronchitis. Am J Dis Child 133:1140, 1979.
6. Newth CJL, Levison H, Bryan AC: The respiratory status of children with croup. J Pediatr 81:1068, 1972.
7. Westley CR, Cotton EK, Brooks JG: Neubulized racemic epinephrine by IPPB for croup: A double blind study. Am J Dis Child 132:484, 1978.
8. Gardner HG, Powell KR, Roden VJ, Cherry JD: The evaluation of racemic epinephrine in the treatment of infectious croup. Pediatrics 52:52, 1973.
9. Taussig LM, Castro O, Beaudry PH, et al: Treatment of laryngotracheal bronchitis (croup). Am J Dis Child 129:790, 1975.
10. Lenney W, Milner AD: Treatment of acute viral croup. Arch Dis Child 53:704, 1978.

11. Leipzig B, Oski FA, Cummings CW, et al: A prospective randomized study to determine the efficacy of steroids in treatment of croup. J Pediatr 94:194, 1979.
12. Cherry JD: The treatment of croup: continued controversy due to failure of recognition of historic, ecologic, etiologic and clinical perspectives. J Pediatr 94:352, 1979.
13. Tunnessen WW Jr, Feinstein AR: The steroid-croup controversy: An analytic review of methodologic problems. J Pediatr 96:751, 1980.
14. Loughlin GM, Taussig LM: Pulmonary function in children with a history of laryngotracheobronchitis. J Pediatr 94:365, 1979.
15. Gurwitz D, Corey M, Levison H: Pulmonary function and bronchial reactivity in children after croup. Am Rev Resp Dis 122:95, 1980.
16. Zach MS, Schnall RP, Landau LI: Upper and lower airway hyperreactivity in recurrent croup. Am Rev Resp Dis 121:979, 1980.
17. Jones R, Santos, JI, Overall JC Jr: Bacterial tracheitis. JAMA 242:721, 1979.
18. Lazoritz S, Saunders BS, Bason WM: Management of acute epiglottitis. Crit Care Med 7:285, 1979.
19. Moltini RA: Epiglottitis: Incidence of extra epiglottic infection: Report of 72 cases and review of the literature. Pediatrics 58:526, 1976.
20. Oh RH, Motoyama EK: Comparison of nasotracheal intubation and tracheostomy in management of acute epiglottitis. Anesthesiology 46:214, 1977.
21. Faden HS: Treatment of *Hemophilus influenzae* type B epiglottitis. Pediatrics 63:402, 1979.
22. Blazer S, Naveh Y, Friedman A: Foreign body in the airway. A review of 200 cases. Am J Dis Child 134:68, 1980.
23. Eller WC, Haugen RK: Current concepts. Food asphyxiation—Restaurant rescue. N Engl J Med 289:81, 1973.

4

Acute Respiratory Failure

David J. Pierson, M.D.

INTRODUCTION

Acute respiratory failure (ARF) is any acute impairment of oxygen uptake, carbon dioxide elimination, or both that is severe enough to be a threat to life. Its key elements are acuteness and degree. As such, ARF is not a disease but rather a physiologically defined situation which may result from a wide variety of disease processes. Disruption of any aspect of respiratory or circulatory function which is severe enough to produce the risk of death within hours may be thought of as ARF. Oxygenation, ventilation, or both may be affected primarily. Confirmation of the existence of ARF requires the measurement of arterial blood gas (ABG) tensions and pH, yet no rigid PO_2 and PCO_2 criteria can be given that would apply to all patients. This is because ARF develops when there is a sudden change in cardiorespiratory function, whatever the baseline state.

It is convenient both conceptually and for purposes of therapy to separate ARF into *hypoxemic* and *hypercapnic* forms, in which there is failure of oxygenation and failure of ventilation, respectively. Both processes may be present in a given patient, but one usually is primary. With few exceptions the following ABG criteria indicate the existence of ARF:

Oxygenation: an acute decrease in arterial PO_2 to 50 mmHg or below.

Ventilation: an acute increase in arterial PCO_2 such that the pH drops below 7.30.

Acute hypoxemia with a PO_2 of around 50 mmHg implies that hemoglobin desaturation to an extent that the normal tissue oxygen supply cannot be maintained, and that cardiac arrhythmias and other serious organ dysfunction are likely. Unless there is good evidence that this degree of hypoxemia has existed for many days, the finding of a PO_2 below 50 mmHg warrants the immediate institution of supplemental oxygen therapy and a repeat ABG measurement within 30 minutes.

In an otherwise normal individual, an acute increase in PCO_2 to 50 mmHg or higher will result in a pH decrease to 7.30 or below. However, when chronic alveolar hypoventilation is present, as may be the case in chronic obstructive pulmonary disease (COPD) and other conditions, a PCO_2 of 50 mmHg may be "normal" in that compensation has occurred through renal bicarbonate retention, and the arterial pH will be normal or near normal. Although both patients in the following sets of ABG results have a PCO_2 of 55, only one is in ARF:

Patient A	*Patient B*
Acute hypoventilation	Chronic hypoventilation
pH 7.27	pH 7.39
PCO_2 55	PCO_2 55
PO_2 58	PO_2 58

Patient A's baseline serum bicarbonate concentration was normal (no base excess or deficit); a sudden rise in PCO_2 from 40 to 55 has produced life-threatening acidemia (acute hypercapnic respiratory failure). Patient B, however, presumably has been chronically hypercapnic, with an increased serum bicarbonate concentration (a positive base excess) providing a compensatory metabolic alkalosis, with the result that the pH is normal. This is a stable state that may be termed "chronic ventilatory insufficiency," and the high PCO_2 requires no emergency intervention.

Since ARF is defined by an acute change in ABG values, it is important to recognize the limitations of these values in reflecting tissue oxygenation. Most clinical laboratories measure pH, PCO_2, and PO_2, and from these values the serum bicarbonate concentration and hemoglobin saturation are calculated. If the patient's hemoglobin is functionally abnormal, as in carbon monoxide poisoning, this will not be detected by routine ABG measurement, and the reported saturation will be wrong. Nor do blood gas measurements measure the blood's oxygen content, which may be severely deficient despite a normal PO_2 if the hemoglobin is abnormal in quantity, as in anemia. Finally, ABGs do not necessarily reflect tissue oxygen delivery, the determination of which requires the assessment of cardiac output as well as of blood oxygen content.

Causes of Acute Respiratory Failure

Many specific disease entities can lead to ARF, through pathophysiologic mechanisms discussed later. A convenient step-by-step approach to differential diagnosis in hypoxemic ARF, first devised by Dr. Paul Stevens of the University of Texas, makes use of the general appearance of the lung fields on the frontal chest radiograph at initial presentation. The main diagnositc possibilities can be divided into those that produce "white" (radio-opaque) lung fields and those in which the lungs are "black" (normal or hyperlucent), and can be further classified according to whether there is alveolar hypoventilation as shown by an elevated arterial PCO_2. Table 4–1 demonstrates this "black-and-white" schema for differential

Table 4–1. "Black and White" Differential Diagnosis of Hypoxemic Acute Respiratory Failure[a]

	$PO_2 < 50$ mmHg			
	$PCO_2 < 40$ mmHg		$PCO_2 > 40$ mmHg	
Lung Fields on Chest Radiograph	Black	White	Black	White
Most likely diagnosis	Acute pulmonary embolism Other vascular obstruction Circulatory failure Anatomic right-to-left shunt	If diffuse ARDS (any cause) Cardiac pulmonary edema Pulmonary fibrosis with acute insult If localized Pneumonia Acute atelectasis Infarction	COPD Status asthmaticus Alveolar hypoventilation Drug overdose Neuromuscular weakness/paralysis	If diffuse ARDS or cardiac pulmonary edema with superimposed respiratory depression Pulmonary fibrosis End-stage (irreversible) With airways disease (some reversibility) If localized Pneumonia plus: COPD Respiratory depression (drugs, O_2)

[a]A modification of the differential system devised and popularized by Dr. Paul Stevens.

diagnosis. As will be discussed later, ARF has several immediate therapeutic implications regardless of the disease process responsible for its development. Thus, although identification and management of the specific etiology is important, the distinction between respiratory failure that is primarily due to a failure in oxygenation from that which is primarily due to ventilation failure, and the appropriate initial treatment of these, is of greater urgency.

Diagnosis

Acute respiratory failure is defined by ABG abnormalities in an appropriate clinical setting. ABG measurement is also the only reliable way in which to make the diagnosis, because the symptoms and signs of ARF are notoriously nonspecific and misleading. Respiratory symptoms and abnormalities may be present in a chest physical examination, but may simply reflect the underlying disease, and do not help in deciding whether ARF is present. The findings in ARF reflect *tissue hypoxia* and *acidosis*, and are cardiovascular and neurologic, not respiratory. The usual symptoms include restlessness, confusion, and a disturbance of consciousness, ranging from mild lethargy to coma. Headache, tremor, and asterixis may be present. The cardiovascular findings include tachycardia, cardiac arrhythmias, diaphoresis, and either hypotension or elevated blood pressure.

Moreover, the bedside assessment of either oxygenation or ventilation is so unreliable as to be clinically useless in the diagnosis of ARF. Thus, although cyanosis accurately reflects an arterial oxygen desaturation (of at least 5 gm of hemoglobin per 100 ml blood) in some patients, it is often present without ARF, and is sometimes absent in profound hypoxemia; consequently, relying upon the presence or absence of cyanosis is misleading and dangerous.[1] Likewise, the bedside prediction of effective alveolar ventilation and arterial PCO_2 has been shown to be haphazard, even by experienced clinicians.[2] Thus, in the absence of clinically reliable noninvasive measures of PO_2 and acid-base status in critically ill patients, the ABG is the only available way to diagnose ARF.

Because the nonspecific clinical signs noted above are often present in patients who are critically ill from any cause, the ready availability of ABG measurements and a high index of suspicion are necessary if the diagnosis of ARF is not to be missed. Four clear indications for drawing ABGs are: (1) symptoms or signs, in an initial assessment, that are consistent with ARF; (2) an acute clinical change in the critically ill patient; (3) monitoring of the effects of therapy; and (4) assessment of the progression of or recovery from ARF over time. Repeat ABG assessment after initiating supplemental oxygen therapy has dual importance: it allows the immediate adjustment of therapy and, as discussed next, it indicates the main physiologic mechanism for the hypoxemia.

Hypoxemic ARF: Pathophysiology and Etiologies

Failure to adequately oxygenate the arterial blood (hypoxemia) can be caused by alveolar hypoventilation, the mismatching of ventilation and perfusion ($\dot{V}/\dot{Q}$) in the lung, a right-to-left shunt, diffusion limitation, or a low inspired oxygen fraction

(FIO_2). Hypoxia at the tissue level also can result from inadequate tissue perfusion, or from insufficient or chemically abnormal hemoglobin. Of primary clinical concern in patients with ARF are the first three of these seven pathophysiologic mechanisms. Among the others, poor perfusion is usually clinically apparent because of other signs of shock or because of a diminished cardiac output. Diffusion limitation, once taught as a major cause of hypoxemia, now is not believed to be a factor of clinical importance in ARF at sea level or moderate altitude. Low FIO_2 as a cause of severe hypoxemia occasionally occurs through the inadvertent interruption of supplemental oxygen therapy, and thus should be kept in mind; it is not otherwise a factor in the hospital setting.

Finally, it is important to realize that fatal hypoxia may occur with an adequate arterial PO_2 in carbon monoxide poisoning. The partial pressure of oxygen measured in a blood sample is unaffected by the quantity of hemoglobin present. Thus, replacement of normal hemoglobin with carboxyhemoglobin, which is unavailable for the carriage of oxygen, will not lower the PO_2, but will profoundly reduce the oxygen content of arterial blood. The saturation figure provided with ABG results is calculated using the PO_2, pH, and temperature, and assumes the hemoglobin to be chemically normal. Whenever CO poisoning is a possibility, measurement of the carboxyhemoglobin concentration of the blood, or *direct* colorimetric measurement of the O_2 saturation should be made.

Identification of the main physiologic cause of hypoxemia is of great importance both in understanding the pathophysiology of ARF in the individual patient and in planning treatment. Of the major mechanisms of hypoxemia—hypoventilation, $\dot{V}/\dot{Q}$ mismatch, and shunt—the first is evident on the initial ABG specimen, and the others can be differentiated for clinical purposes by the response to supplemental O_2.

Hypoventilation is defined as an arterial PCO_2 value above normal (40 ± 2 mmHg at sea level, 36 ± 2 mmHg at 5280 feet). When hypercapnic ARF is present (elevated PCO_2, pH below 7.30), hypoventilation is identified by definition. The etiologies for hypercapnic ARF (ventilatory failure) are discussed in the next section. Hypoventilation may be accompanied by hypoxemia from either a $\dot{V}/\dot{Q}$ mismatch or a shunt.

Figure 4–1 shows in a diagrammatic form the mechanism of the essential clinical difference between a $\dot{V}/\dot{Q}$ mismatch and a shunt: in $\dot{V}/\dot{Q}$ problems, the PO_2 increases substantially with supplemental O_2; in a shunt, it does not. The figure illustrates only oxygen exchange, since CO_2 passes more readily out of the lung, and its elimination is not ordinarily a clinical problem so long as overall ventilation is provided. In Figure 4–1A, a representative lung unit (two alveoli or two adjacent areas of lung) is shown under normal conditions. Ventilation ($\dot{V}$) is evenly matched with perfusion ($\dot{Q}$), so that the oxygen entering from the airway and the venous blood in the capillaries are exposed to one another uniformly enough so that essentially all of the hemoglobin in the capillary blood becomes saturated. The blood enters 75 percent saturated and leaves about 97 percent saturated, increasing the O_2 content by approximately 5 gm/100 ml.

Figure 4–1B, depicts, on the right, an area of impaired ventilation as the result of a constriction: this produces a low $\dot{V}/\dot{Q}$ ratio in that lung unit. The desaturated

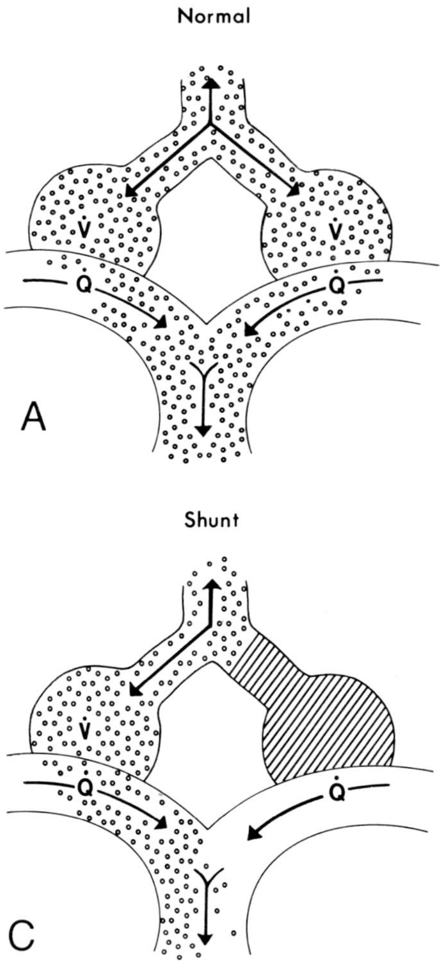

Figure 4–1. Diagrammatic illustration of the physiologic differences between (A) normal gas exchange, (B) ventilation:perfusion ($\dot{V}/\dot{Q}$) mismatch, and (C) right-to-left pulmonary shunt. These figures correspond to the ABG findings and responses to supplemental O_2 shown in Table 4–2. (For explanation see text.)

blood passing the unit in normal quantity removes all of the O_2 molecules that are presented to it; but since they are present in greatly reduced number, it does not become fully saturated. It passes away from the affected unit and mixes with the fully saturated blood from the left side, where $\dot{V}/\dot{Q}$ matching is normal, with the result that the mixed effluent from the two lung units is incompletely saturated and, thus, hypoxemic. Note that the PO_2 in the mixed effluent (and thus the arterial PO_2 drawn at the wrist) is determined by the mean oxygen *contents* of its component streams, not their partial pressures. Since the blood O_2 content is mainly determined by hemoglobin saturation, it is clear that desaturated blood coming from the low-$\dot{V}/\dot{Q}$ unit will lower the mixed arterial PO_2.

To correct the hypoxemia caused by the low $\dot{V}/\dot{Q}$ unit shown in Figure 4–1B, it is necessary only to increase the number of O_2 molecules reaching the unit through the constricted airway. This is accomplished by raising the "driving pressure" of O_2 in the inspired gas—increasing the FIO_2 that the patient breathes. In the clinical disorders in which $\dot{V}/\dot{Q}$ mismatching most often accounts for hypoxemia—COPD and asthma—the disturbance is almost always such that it can be corrected with only a modest increase in FIO_2.

The lung area depicted in Figure 4–1C is very different from that in Figure 4–1B, in that there is *no* ventilation of the lung unit on the right. Ventilation and perfusion are evenly matched on the left, as before, but the desaturated blood entering on the right "sees" no O_2 at all, and leaves the affected unit completely desaturated, to mix with the oxygenated blood. This situation might occur when the adjacent airspace is collapsed or completely filled with fluid, as in atelectasis or pulmonary edema. If widespread, such a process can result in profound hypoxemia.

In the case of a shunt, increasing the FIO_2 alleviates the hypoxemia very little. This is because, as can be seen in Figure 4–1C, the right-hand unit remains unventilated regardless of the composition of the ventilating gas, and is perfused by blood that does not come into contact with O_2. Blood leaving the normally-ventilated lung unit is already 97 percent saturated; and although increasing the FIO_2 will greatly increase the PO_2 of this blood, its O_2 content will increase very little because even at a high PO_2, most of the oxygen in the blood is carried by saturating the hemoglobin. Once the latter is 100 percent saturated, little additional O_2 can be carried. When the high- and low-saturation effluents, with their very different O_2 contents, are mixed, the result will be blood that is still partially desaturated, with a correspondingly low PO_2. This is why supplemental O_2 alone usually is not sufficient in hypoxemic ARF caused primarily by a shunt.

Direct measurements of $\dot{V}/\dot{Q}$ ratios in the lungs of patients with hypoxemic ARF have shown that what has been thought to be shunt is often a case of lung units having a very low $\dot{V}/\dot{Q}$, with or without a true right-to-left shunt ($\dot{V}/\dot{Q} = 0$).[3] For clinical purposes, this distinction usually is unimportant, since the therapeutic maneuvers used for a "shunt" are effective for very low $\dot{V}/\dot{Q}$ units as well. Hypoxemia in patients with such low $\dot{V}/\dot{Q}$ units behaves as described above, and it is very helpful therapeutically to distinguish between the "$\dot{V}/\dot{Q}$ effect"—a good PO_2 response to low-flow O_2—and the "shunt effect." For the rest of this chapter, however, "shunt" as defined clinically will be placed in quotation marks to acknowledge a possible technical discrepancy with what actually might be measurable in the lung.

Table 4–2 illustrates the clinical distinction between $\dot{V}/\dot{Q}$ mismatch and "shunt," as shown by the initial response to supplemental O_2. No exact FIO_2 figures have been included because the pertinent result is assessed by ABG measurement, and the important difference is between "low" FIO_2 and "high" FIO_2. Thus, modest concentrations of O_2—24 to 40 percent—which are safe when given acutely and are easy to administer, sufficiently alleviate the hypoxemia as seen in COPD or status asthmaticus, conditions characterized by widespread $\dot{V}/\dot{Q}$ mismatching, to provide an acceptable clinical response. Conversely, hypoxemia as seen in ARDS or acute lobar atelectasis, characterized by a "shunt," is improved very little even by 100 percent O_2. Furthermore, such O_2 concentrations

Table 4–2. Hypoxemia: $\dot{V}/\dot{Q}$ Mismatch or "Shunt"? (Clinical Distinction According to Initial Response to Supplemental O_2)

Setting	ABG Breathing Room Air		ABG Breathing "Low" Supplemental O_2 (2 L/min by Nasal Prongs)		ABG Breathing "High" Supplemental O_2 (70–80% by Mask)	
Normal	PO_2	90	PO_2	152	PO_2	362
	PCO_2	40	PCO_2	40	PCO_2	40
	pH	7.40	pH	7.40	pH	7.40
Mainly $\dot{V}/\dot{Q}$ mismatch (example: COPD)	PO_2	48	PO_2	60	PO_2	244
	PCO_2	55	PCO_2	58	PCO_2	78
	pH	7.36	pH	7.34	pH	7.23
Mainly "shunt" (example: ARDS)	PO_2	42	PO_2	45	PO_2	58
	PCO_2	34	PCO_2	34	PCO_2	36
	pH	7.44	pH	7.44	pH	7.42

are hazardous and difficult to administer without endotracheal intubation. Making the clinical distinction between a $\dot{V}/\dot{Q}$ mismatch and a "shunt" in the initial hour of assessment and management, as shown in the examples in Table 4–2, is important in planning subsequent therapy for hypoxemic ARF.

Hypoxemic ARF with the characteristic "shunt" response to supplemental O_2 can result from either localized or generalized processes in the chest. Figure 4–2 shows the chest radiographs of two patients with profound hypoxemia unresponsive to the breathring of a high FIO_2. The patient in Figure 4–2A had heroin-induced pulmonary edema and the clinical features of ARDS, while the patient in Figure 4–2B presented with right upper-lobe pneumococcal pneumonia which spared the other lobes radiographically. The responses of these two patients to therapy directed at reversing the "shunt" were dramatically different, as will be discussed later.

Hypercapnic ARF: Pathophysiology and Etiologies

Hypoventilation occurs whenever alveolar ventilation fails to keep up with the body's CO_2 production. A reduction in overall ventilation, an enlargement of anatomic or physiologic dead space, or an increased CO_2 production, or all three, may lead to hypercapnic ARF. The mechanisms responsible for diminished ventilation may be any or all of the following: (1) central—depression of normal respiratory drives; (2) neuromuscular—interference with neural transmission or muscular translation of the drive message; (3) chest cage—disruption of the bony thorax as a bellows; and (4) lungs and airways—proximal or distal airflow limitation. The first three of these mechanisms are causes of ARF in individuals with normal lungs; drug overdosage, head trauma, cerebrovascular accident, drug-induced or infectious neuromuscular paralysis, cervical cord or phrenic nerve injury, and massive flail chest injury are the most commonly responsible sources.

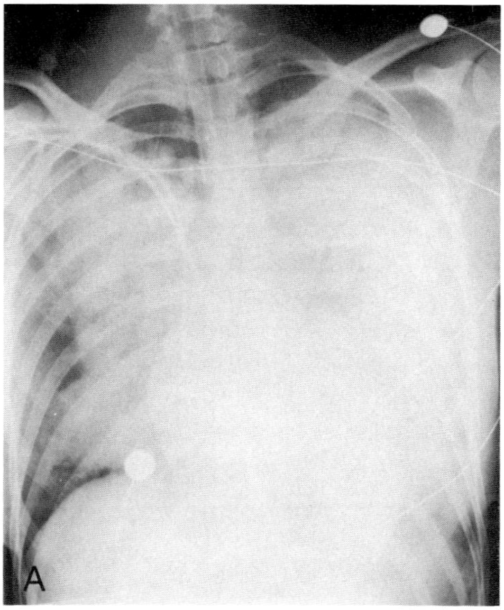

Figure 4–2. Chest radiographs of two patients with similar ABG findings (severe "shunt") who presented to the same emergency room 10 days apart. (A) ARDS secondary to heroin-induced pulmonary edema. This patient improved dramatically with PEEP and recovered. (B) Pneumococcal pneumonia in a debilitated chronic alcoholic. This patient developed cardiovascular collapse during a PEEP trial and expired within 24 hours of admission.

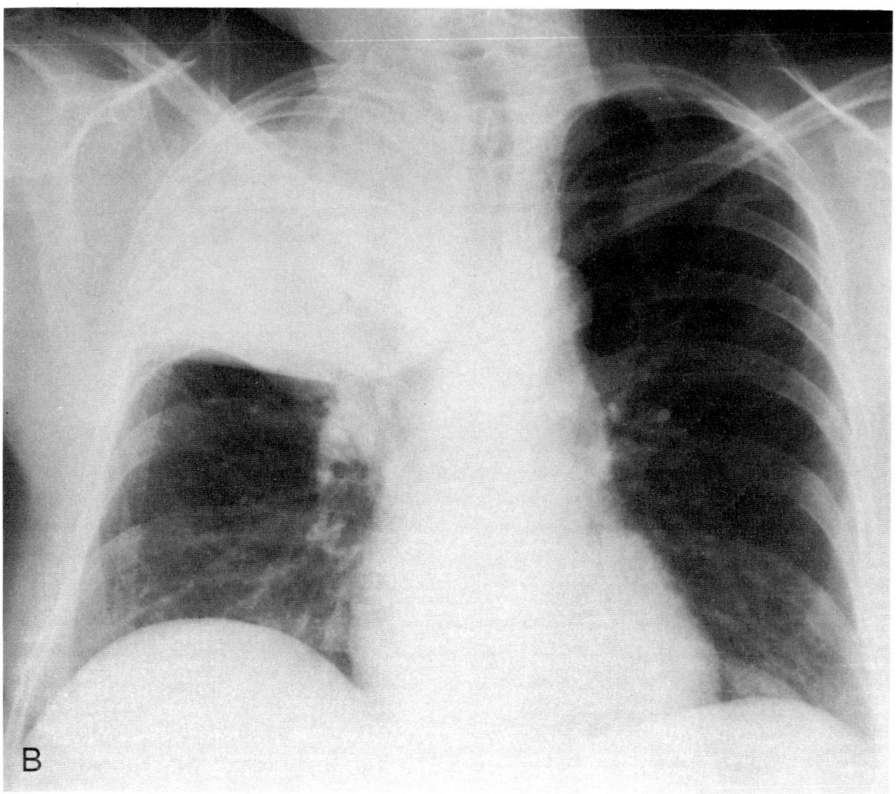

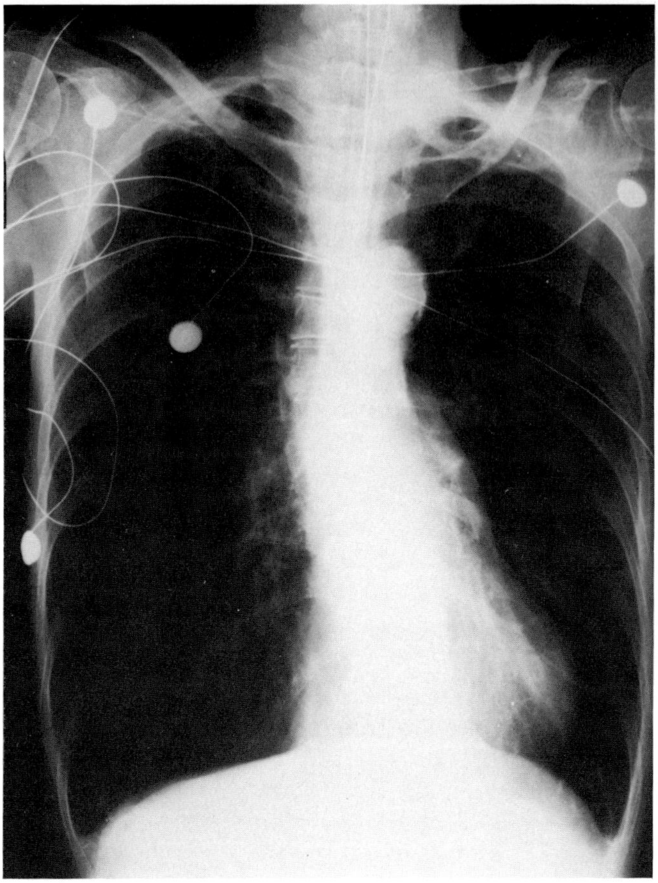

Figure 4–3. Acute respiratory failure in a patient with severe COPD. The lung fields are "black." This 67-year-old woman presented semicomatose with a several-day history of increased cough and sputum production. Admission ABG values breathing room air: pH = 7.20, $PCO_2 = 77$, $PO_2 = 36$. After 4 days of mechanical ventilation she was successfully weaned and extubated and later returned to her previous functional level.

Acute upper airway obstruction can also occur in persons with normal underlying lung function.

Chronic obstructive pulmonary disease with superimposed exacerbation, and status asthmaticus, are the pulmonary conditions most often responsible for hypercapnic ARF. In these conditions, acute respiratory acidosis occurs because of mechanical limitation of the patient's ability to excrete CO_2, with or without superimposed depression of the respiratory drive. Increased CO_2 retention, from an acute exacerbation of COPD, is usually a result of several factors, including increased airways resistance from edema, bronchospasm, and secretions, and elevated CO_2 production both from the presence of acute inflammation and from a greater work of breathing. In COPD the dead space: tidal volume ratio (V_D/V_T) is abnormally high, and alveolar ventilation may be insufficient despite a normal or even elevated overall minute ventilation.

Patients with hypercapnic ARF constitute most cases of "black" lung fields, as described in Table 4–1. An example is shown in Figure 4–3—the admission chest radiograph of a COPD patient with profound hypercapnia and acidemia secondary to an acute respiratory infection. Such patients typically have hypoxemia due to hypoventilation and $\dot{V}/\dot{Q}$ mismatch rather than "shunt." When pulmonary infiltrates producing "white" lung fields, whether diffuse or localized, occur in combination with hypercapnia, more than one process is usually present. Examples of such processes are pulmonary edema with a superimposed respiratory drive depression and pneumonia in patients with COPD or asthma. Physiologically, such patients may demonstrate either a $\dot{V}/\dot{Q}$ or a "shunt" effect in response to supplemental O_2.

MANAGEMENT OF ACUTE RESPIRATORY FAILURE

Because of the life-threatening nature of ARF, its management must begin as soon as the diagnosis is suspected. Several processes must occur simultaneously—assessment, nonspecific general measures to combat the physiologic effects of ARF, and specific treatment of the precipitating event or disease process. Patient assessment continues throughout the management process and includes the early differentiation between a $\dot{V}/\dot{Q}$ mismatch and a "shunt" as the dominating cause of hypoxemia. Some form of oxygen therapy should begin immediately when hypoxemia is present; a repeat of the ABG measurement after the first 20 minutes of oxygen therapy will allow the differentiation of $\dot{V}/\dot{Q}$ mismatch from "shunt", as discussed earlier, and reveal the need for further oxygen therapy manipulation.

Nonspecific supportive management in ARF is directed at physiologic derangement, as revealed by ABGs plus the patient's history, a physical examination, and other laboratory results. This supportive management consists of measures to relieve hypoxemia, the use of mechanical ventilation, and airway care to maintain patency, prevent aspiration, and remove secretions.

MEASURES TO RELIEVE HYPOXEMIA

Oxygen therapy in ARF is based upon the hemoglobin-oxygen dissociation curve (Fig. 4–4). In the curve, the "S" shaped relationship between PO_2, hemoglobin saturation, and oxygen content illustrates why PO_2 values below about 50 mmHg are life-threatening, and why raising the PO_2 above this level is the first goal of therapy. It should be kept in mind, however, that supplemental O_2 is administered to patients in order to increase the O_2 delivery to their tissues, which depends upon an adequate cardiac output and hemoglobin concentration as well

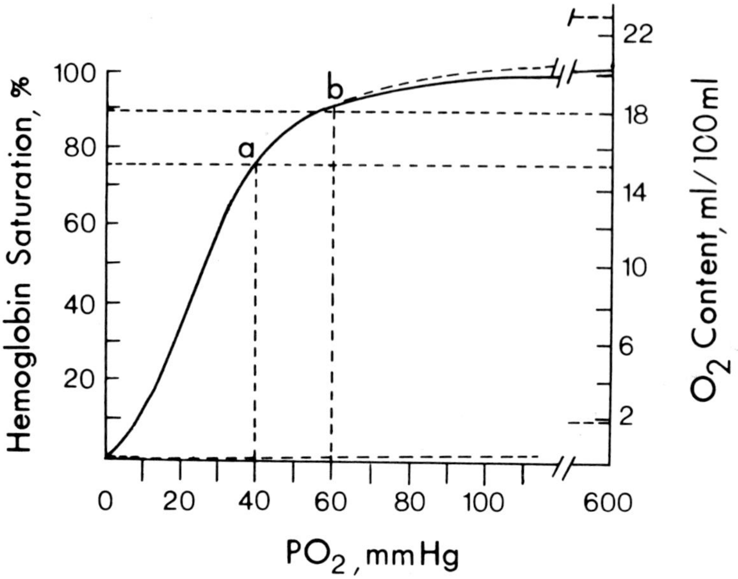

Figure 4–4. The hemoglobin-oxygen dissociation curve. The solid line represents oxygen carrying by hemoglobin; saturation and O_2 content are determined by the "S" shape of the curve. The curve is steep below PO_2 values of about 50 mmHg, indicating severely reduced O_2 carrying by hemoglobin below this PO_2 and suggesting the physiologic definition for ARF used in this chapter. The lower dashed line represents oxygen in solution in the blood, and the upper dashed line shows total oxygen (dissolved O_2 plus O_2 bound to hemoglobin). Note that dissolved O_2 contributes little to blood O_2 content, even at very high PO_2 values. The points a and b illustrate the increase in O_2 saturation and content when the PO_2 is raised from 40 to 60 mmHg: the saturation increases from 75 to 89 percent and the O_2 content increases from 15 to 17.8 ml/100 ml blood. (Adapted from West, JB: Respiratory Physiology: The Essentials. p. 75. © 1974, The Williams & Wilkins Co., Baltimore.)

as on the arterial PO_2. Thus, although PO_2 is the major indicator of therapeutic effect in most cases of ARF, it is important to remember the other determinants of oxygen delivery, especially when severe hypoxemia persists despite therapy.

Except for a small amount in physical solution, oxygen in the blood is carried by hemoglobin. As shown in Figure 4–4, once all of the available hemoglobin is fully saturated with O_2, little additional O_2 carriage is achieved even by raising the PO_2 to very high values. In the "normal" example in Table 4–2, raising the PO_2 from 152 to 362 mmHg would result in an increase in the O_2 *content* of not more than 1 ml/100 ml of blood, or less than 5 percent.

The "S" shape of the hemoglobin-oxygen dissociation curve is the key not only to understanding blood oxygenation, but also to the proper goals of O_2 therapy. The curve is steep at PO_2 values below 50 mm Hg, and hemoglobin loses O_2 rapidly as the PO_2 drops further. Therefore, in this range, raising the PO_2 by even a few millimeters of mercury results in substantial increases in O_2 carrying. The curve "humps" at 50 to 60 mmHg, and above 60 mmHg the increases in O_2 content with increasing PO_2 become less and less. At PO_2 values above 80 mmHg, normal hemoglobin, at neutral pH and 37° C, is essentially completely saturated. There is, thus, little to be gained by increasing the FIO_2 in order to raise the PO_2 above about 80 mmHg.

In any patient, regardless of the techniques used to deliver supplemental O_2, the goals of therapy should be:

1. To raise the PO_2 above the steepest part of the curve—to at least 50 mmHg.
2. To avoid raising the PO_2 above about 80 mmHg, since doing so does not appreciably increase the carriage of O_2, and may require toxic O_2 concentrations.

An exception to the second rule is carbon monoxide poisoning, in which an FIO_2 equal to 1.0 or even hyperbaric oxygen may be indicated for short periods.[4] For patients with COPD or other chronic respiratory insufficiency, the goal of O_2 therapy is a PO_2 between about 55 and 65 mmHg, avoiding higher partial pressures because of the risk of depressing ventilation by reducing the hypoxic drive. For all other patients a reasonable goal is a PO_2 between 60 and 80 mmHg.

Low-FIO_2 versus High-FIO_2 Supplemental Oxygen

As discussed under pathophysiology, hypoxemia due to a $\dot{V}/\dot{Q}$ mismatch or hypoventilation usually is correctable with low concentrations of supplemental O_2, while a "shunt" produces hypoxemia often refractory even to a very high FIO_2. Although the FIO_2 above which oxygen toxicity is a hazard to hypoxemic patients is uncertain,[5] fractions of 0.50 or less appear to be safe for extended periods.[6] Supplemental O_2 can be considered in two basic dose ranges: an FIO_2 of below 0.50, which is safe and adequate for reversing hypoxemia due to $\dot{V}/\dot{Q}$ mismatching and hypoventilation; and an FIO_2 above 0.50, which is potentially hazardous, more difficult to administer, and typically required when a large "shunt" effect is present.

Aside from the knowledge of whether the FIO_2 is in the potentially toxic range, its actual value as delivered to the patient is relatively unimportant. In every case of ARF, the effects of supplemental O_2 must be checked by measuring ABG values 15 to 30 minutes after oxygen therapy is begun or changed. The "bottom line" in O_2 therapy is its effect on the arterial blood PO_2, rather than the exact FIO_2 delivered.

Low-FIO_2 supplemental oxygen may be given either by mask or by nasal prongs (see Fig. 4–5). Venturi masks (Fig. 4–5A) rely upon air entrainment around an O_2 stream, producing a fixed FIO_2 of 0.24, 0.28, 0.35, or 0.40, depending upon the jet orifice. However, this precisely accurate FIO_2 actually is present only in the mask itself, and not necessarily in the patient's airway. If the patient is tachypneic or can generate high peak inspiratory flow rates, room air will be entrained around the mask, and the delivered FIO_2 will be lower. Thus, the fact that the FIO_2 with

(Text continues on p. 91.)

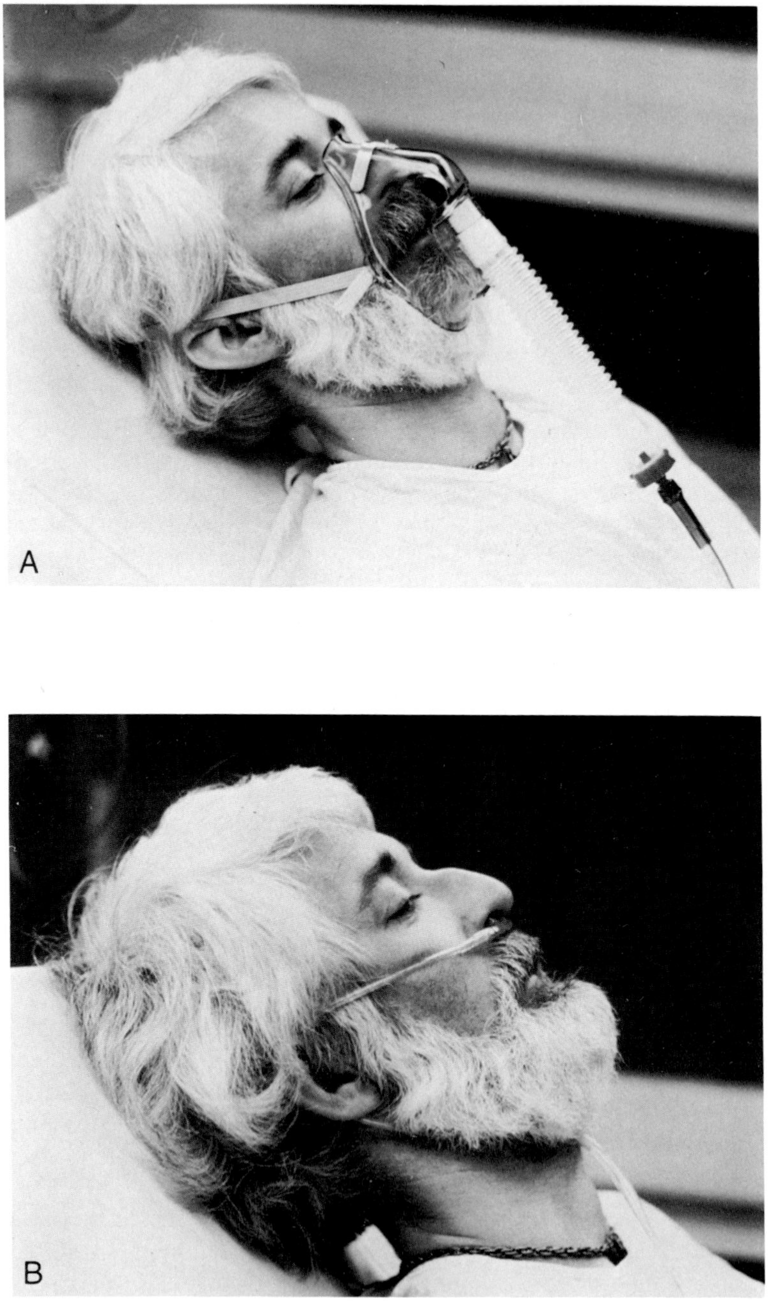

Figure 4–5. Low-FIO_2 supplemental O_2 therapy. Venturi masks (A and C) and nasal prongs (B and D) deliver similar tracheal FIO_2 and are appropriate for hypoventilation and $\dot{V}/\dot{Q}$ mismatch. Therapy must be monitored by ABG values in both cases.

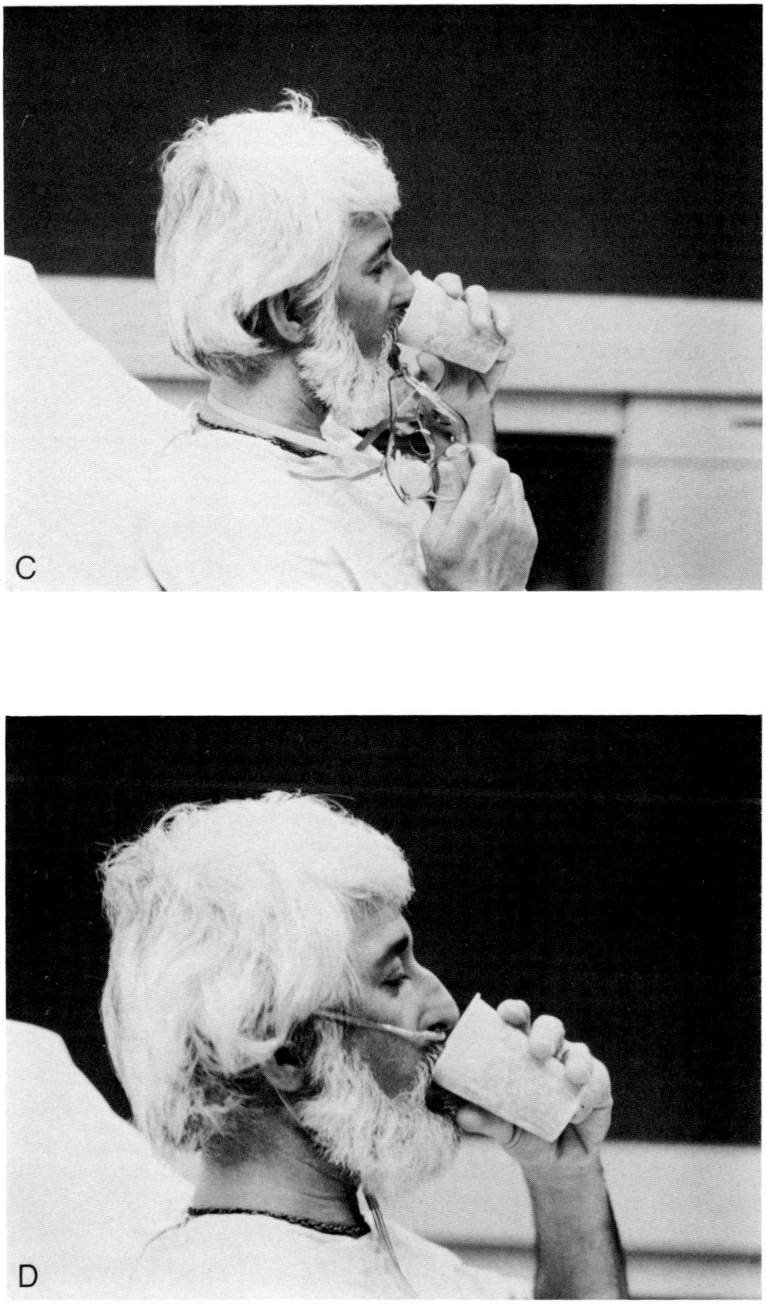

Figure 4–5 (continued). Patients must remove masks when coughing, eating, or drinking (see C); nasal prongs allow continuous O_2 delivery during all patient activities (D).

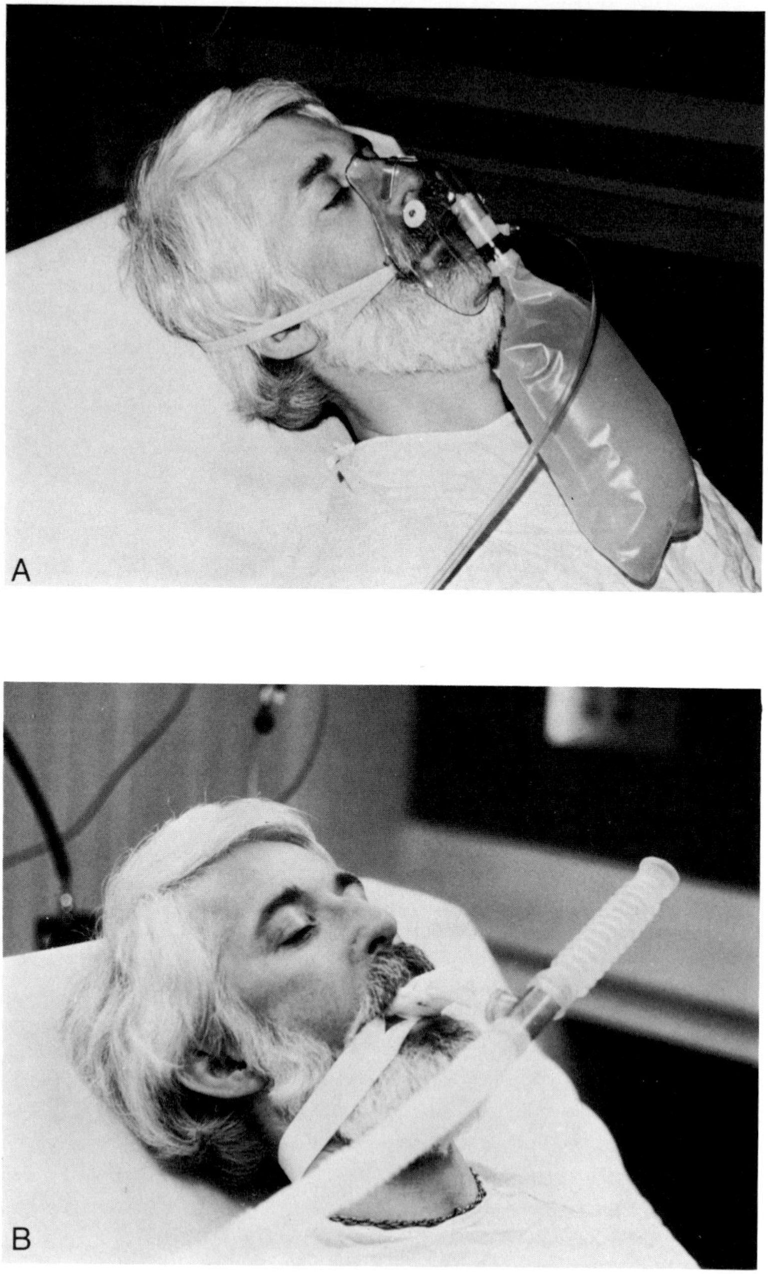

Figure 4–6. (A) High-FIO_2 supplemental O_2 by non-rebreathing mask. FIO_2 in mask is up to 1.0, but air entrainment during inspiration almost always reduces this in trachea. (B) Supplemental O_2 via T-piece and endotracheal tube. With sufficient extension tubing to prevent air entrainment during inspiration, any FIO_2 from 0.21 to 1.0 can be delivered.

a Venturi mask is "known" is misleading. This is especially true if the mask becomes dislodged or is taken off while the patient coughs, eats, or drinks (Fig. 4–5C).

Nasal prongs (Fig. 4–5B) deliver humidified O_2 at rates of 0.5 to 10 or 12 liters per minute, although most patients cannot tolerate flows above 5 or 6 liters per minute. The FIO_2 attainable with nasal prongs is in the same range as with Venturi masks. As with the masks, the therapy must be empirical, in that the exact FIO_2 is unknown, and oxygen administration must be guided by the PO_2. The chief advantages of nasal prongs are that most patients tolerate them better than masks for long periods, and that they may be left on the patient at all times (Fig. 4–5D). Nasal prongs are effective whether the patient breathes through the nose or the mouth. During exhalation through the mouth, the nasopharynx collects O_2, which is inhaled by entrainment with the next breath. Nasally administered O_2 should be humidified, since many patients otherwise experience uncomfortable drying of the nasopharynx.

In contrast to the ease of delivery of O_2 fractions below 0.50 with low-FIO_2 therapy, supplemental O_2 fractions above 0.50 are difficult to deliver accurately for more than a short time without endotracheal intubation. Nonrebreathing (reservoir) masks (Fig. 4–6A) deliver FIO_2 levels up to 1.0; however, because the maximum flow through narrow tubing from a wall- or tank outlet is limited, and less and less air is entrained into the breathing mixture as the FIO_2 increases, the bulk flow from such masks grows progressively smaller. At an FIO_2 of 1.0, the flow is limited to that available from the O_2 source, usually 12 to 15 L/min. Depending on how tightly the mask fits, how cooperative the patient is, and how vigorously he or she inhales, air is virtually always entrained around the mask, with a consequent reduction in the tracheal FIO_2. One-hundred percent oxygen can seldom be delivered effectively by mask to patients with ARF.

These mask-related difficulties increase with time and with increasing patient distress. Many dyspneic patients find tight-fitting masks "smothering," and most cannot keep them on correctly for hours or days. An examination of 10 patients being treated with high-FIO_2 masks will show that in at least 5 of them the device will be off the face or otherwise ineffective at any given moment, unless a nurse or therapist is providing constant supervision; this is a reflection on the mask, not the patient.

Most patients with hypoxemic ARF who need high-FIO_2 therapy for more than a few hours will require endotracheal intubation (see Chapter 2). With this, supplemental O_2, given via a T-piece as illustrated in Figure 4–6B, can be adjusted to any FIO_2 between 0.21 (the oxygen fraction in room air) and 1.0. However, room air entrainment will still occur if the peak flow through the endotracheal tube during spontaneous inhalation exceeds the bulk flow rate from the O_2 source. This is usually the case, and may lower the effective FIO_2 substantially in patients with high minute volumes. Extending the expiratory side of the T-piece with a section of large-bore tubing will correct this problem. Since mist coming from the expiratory side should be visible at all times to make sure that humidification and bulk flow are adequate, the extension tube should be long enough to prevent the momentary interruption in mist production that occurs when air is entrained from the room. Furthermore, because a continuous flow is provided during exhalation to wash away expired gas, extending the expiratory side of the T-piece circuit does not add external dead space (as would be the case if tubing were added between the T-piece and the endotracheal tube), and substantial CO_2 retention does not occur.

Positive End-Expiratory Pressure (PEEP) and Continuous Positive Airway Pressure (CPAP)

Both of these techniques are mechanical means for correcting hypoxemia by increasing the lung volume. Both PEEP and CPAP impose an expiratory "threshold" pressure of anywhere from 1 to 20 cmH_2O or more, with the effect that the pressure in the apparatus and in the patient's airway is not allowed to fall below that level during the respiratory cycle. With this continuous expiratory threshold pressure, the volume of gas in the patient's chest at the end of each exhalation increases over what it was before the pressure was applied. This end-expiratory volume, the position of rest at which the lung elastic recoil is most nearly balanced by that of the chest wall, is the functional residual capacity (FRC). Both PEEP and CPAP act by increasing the FRC.

By convention, a continuous expiratory pressure threshold that is imposed during mechanical breathing from a ventilator is called positive end-expiratory pressure, whereas the pressure threshold that accompanies spontaneous breathing is properly called continuous positive airway pressure (see Fig. 4–7). Both PEEP and CPAP therapy are intended for the treatment of severe hypoxemia, and are not part of the management of alveolar hypoventilation. CPAP may be provided with or without a ventilator and, in carefully selected patients, even without endotracheal intubation.[7–9] Because PEEP/CPAP therapy works by increasing the FRC, such therapy would be expected to improve hypoxemia due to a diffuse restrictive process. In such a process, typified by ARDS, the hypoxemia results from generalized alveolar collapse, filling, or both, which produces decreased lung compliance and a "shunt" effect (see Chapter 6). In ARDS, the appropriate application of PEEP/CPAP increases lung compliance and improves oxygenation.[3,10,11]

As PEEP/CPAP therapy has become commonplace, there has occasionally been a tendency to use it routinely in any critically ill patient with hypoxemia. This can be disastrous, as is outlined in Table 4–3 and illustrated with the patient in Figure 4–2B. While PEEP/CPAP is appropriate in a generalized restrictive ventilatory process, its application in cases of localized disease causing a "shunt" is likely to produce preferential expansion of uninvolved areas of lung. In such areas, volume increases above normal raise the pulmonary vascular resistance, and may well *increase* the shunt by diverting more perfusion to the involved area. Also, whenever the FRC is raised substantially above normal, positive pressure breaths increase the risk of barotrauma through overdistension of individual alveoli. In a disease process such as COPD or status asthmaticus, in which hyperinflation

Table 4–3. Expected Effects of PEEP/CPAP in Different Forms of Acute Respiratory Failure

Setting	Effect on Lung Volume (FRC)	Effect on Lung Compliance	Risk of Barotrauma	Effect on Pulmonary Blood flow	Effect on Gas Exchange	Effect on PaO_2
Diffuse infiltrates (lungs "white") Hypoxemia (shunt effect) FRC: low Example: ARDS (any cause) (see Fig. 4–2A)	↑ Toward normal*	↑ Toward normal (more open alveoli)	+	No overall effect better matching of $\dot{Q}$ to $\dot{V}$	↓ Shunt effect	↑
	↑ Above normal†	↓	+ +	No effect	↑ Dead-space	0 or ↓
Localized infiltrate Hypoxemia (shunt effect) FRC: low in involved area; nl or ↑ in uninvolved lung Examples: lobar pneumonia (see Fig. 4–2B)	Involved area— No change	No effect	No effect	↑ Vascular resistance in uninvolved lung	No effect	No effect
acute lobar atelectasis (see Fig. 4–8)	Surrounding uninvolved lung: ↑ above normal	↓	+ +	↑ Blood flow to involved areas	↑ Shunt effect	↓
Diffuse hyperinflation (lungs "black") Hypoxemia (mainly $\dot{V}/\dot{Q}$) FRC: high Examples: COPD; status asthmaticus (see Fig. 4–3)	↑ To further above normal	↓	+ + +	↑ Vascular resistance	↑ Dead-space ventilation; ↑ $\dot{V}/\dot{Q}$ mismatching	↓

*Desirable effect of PEEP used optimally.
†Undesirable effect of excessive PEEP.

Table 4–4. Indications for a Trial of PEEP or CPAP

Severe hypoxemia
"Shunt effect" as demonstrated by response to initial O_2 therapy
High FIO_2 requirement (example: $PO_2 < 60$ mmHg on $FIO_2 > 0.40$)
Acute diffuse process
Clinically compatible with ARDS
Cardiac pulmonary edema unlikely
Effect restrictive rather than obstructive (lung volumes low)

already exists, the application of PEEP/CPAP could not be expected to improve gas exchange by further increasing the FRC.

From the foregoing discussion it is apparent that PEEP/CPAP therapy would be expected to improve oxygenation in clinical situations characterized by acute, diffuse lung injury with a restrictive rather than obstructive effect, and in which hypoxemia is due to a "shunt" rather than a $\dot{V}/\dot{Q}$ mismatch. Table 4–4 outlines the indications for a therapeutic trail of PEEP/CPAP which are consistent with this pathophysiologic approach. The practical applications, monitoring, and complications of PEEP/CPAP therapy are discussed in Chapter 6.

Extracorporeal membrane oxygenation (ECMO) has received attention as a possible treatment modality for severe hypoxemic ARF refractory to other therapy. However, a recent multi-center study of ECMO in carefully selected patients has demonstrated that although this invasive therapy can support gas exchange in severe ARF, it does not appear to improve overall survival.[12] These findings imply that the high mortality in such patients is due to the severity of the underlying disease process rather than to the therapy applied. Most clinicians also think that ECMO is not indicated in less severe ARF, since adequate support of oxygenation usually is attainable by conventional therapy.

MANAGEMENT OF HYPOVENTILATION

With few exceptions, the acute failure of adequate alveolar ventilation requires immediate mechanical ventilation. The primary goals of mechanical ventilation are to maintain adequate alveolar ventilation and provide proper lung inflation. Occasionally, mechanical ventilation is also used to reduce the oxygen consumption that results from excessive work of breathing, in which case it fulfills the other two goals as well. Deciding when to initiate mechanical ventilation in a given patient requires experience in the management of ARF, although a number of guidelines can be given to aid in this decision. Table 4–5 outlines several indications for mechanical ventilation, based upon the etiology of ARF.

Indications for Mechanical Ventilation

Apnea requires the immediate institution of ventilatory assistance in any patient. This may consist of temporary ventilation via mouth-to-mouth resuscitation or a manual resuscitation bag, or long-term ventilator therapy via an endotracheal or

Table 4–5. Indications for Mechanical Ventilation

In any patient:
Apnea
Acute respiratory acidosis: ↑ PCO_2; pH < 7.25
In hypoxemic ARF:
Need for larger tidal volumes (with or without PEEP/CPAP—See Table 4–4): spontaneous tidal volume < 5 ml/kg
Excessive work of breathing: minute ventilation > 15 L for PCO_2 40 (or equivalent)
In head trauma:
Apneic episodes or acutely unstable breathing pattern
Need for hyperventilation to reduce brain swelling in first 24–48 hours
In chest trauma: See Chapter 11
In chronic obstructive pulmonary disease:
Inability to cooperate with care: decreased consciousness; uncontrollable agitation
Worsening acidosis: PCO_2 < 7.30 despite vigorous bronchodilator and respiratory therapy
In status asthmaticus: See Chapter 5
In neuromuscular weakness or sedative overdose:
Progressive hypoventilation with pH < 7.30
Vital capacity < 15 ml/kg
Tidal volume < 5 ml/kg
Inspiratory force < −20 cmH_2O

tracheostomy tube. Acute failure of ventilation, with a CO_2 elevation that reduces the pH to below 7.25 to 7.30, should be corrected with mechanical ventilation regardless of the cause because of the acute threat to life from arrhythmias and the other adverse effects of acidosis and hypoxemia.

Whether or not to initiate mechanical ventilation in hypoxemic ARF in the presence of normal alveolar ventilation (a normal or low PCO_2) is a clinical decision. However, because spontaneous breathing at low tidal volumes is associated with hypoxemia that can be corrected by providing periodic deep breaths,[13] regular lung inflation in such patients is reasonable, whether done manually or with a ventilator. Early mechanical ventilation is especially important when progressive hypoxemia complicates severe trauma or an acute inhalation injury (drowning, smoke inhalation).[14,15] In such cases, and in postoperative sepsis and severe burns, high CO_2 production may result in an excessive ventilatory demand. Mechanical ventilation may be indicated because of the very high work of breathing required to maintain a normal PCO_2 when the minute volume exceeds 2 to 3 times normal, and especially if the critical illness is likely to be prolonged.

In comatose patients with severe head injuries, mechanical ventilation has two potential indications. If periodic apnea occurs in a setting of changing neurologic status, "prophylactic" ventilation may be indicated until the patient stabilizes. Additionally, hyperventilation in severely head-injured patients reduces cerebral blood flow via both hypocapnia and alkalemia, and two groups of investigators have reported better survival rates in such cases with intensive regimens including mechanical hyperventilation to a PCO_2 of 25 to 30 mmHg.[16,17] The clinical benefit from hyperventilation appears to diminish after 24 to 48 hours. In a study of patients with cerebrovascular accidents, no differences in outcome were found when patients were mechanically hyperventilated to PCO_2 values of about 25 mmHg, were mechanically ventilated to a PCO_2 of 40 mmHg, or were allowed to breathe spontaneously.[18]

Patients with COPD who develop ARF because of an acute exacerbation of this condition seldom require intubation and mechanical ventilation.[19,20] The need for intubation increases with worsening hypoxemia and a falling pH,[21] and becomes unavoidable if the patient is unresponsive or unable to follow commands.

Inability to fully inflate the lungs is the major indication for mechanical ventilation in patients with neuromuscular disease.[22] This is assessed by the same criteria used for ventilator weaning (see Table 4–7), which are the vital capacity and maximum inspiratory effort, in addition to the tidal volume. In such patients, as well as in cases of sedative drug overdose, progressive respiratory acidosis indicates the need for institution of mechanical ventilation.

Choice of Ventilator Settings

Although pressure-cycled ventilators were used regularly for continuous ventilation in the past, they have been superseded by volume-preset machines. In addition to allowing adjustment of the tidal volume, currently available ventilators allow adjustment of the peak inspiratory flow rate and inspiratory waveform. During anesthesia, ventilation with constant, "normal" tidal volumes (5 ml/kg) results in hypoxemia and a decreasing lung compliance, which are corrected when periodic hyperinflations are provided.[23,24] For this reason, currently available ventilators have "sigh" features which enable patients to receive larger breaths intermittently. However, constant ventilation with large tidal volumes (10 to 15 ml/kg) without "sighs" also prevents hypoxemia[25], and because large volumes have become the popular standard for mechanical ventilation, "sigh" features are seldom used today. Whether constant large-tidal-volume ventilation is superior to physiologic tidal volumes with periodic hyperinflation has not been demonstrated.

Although some ventilators are equipped to adjust inspiratory waveforms, which include square-wave, sinusoidal, and decelerating flow patterns, it is doubtful that such adjustment affects gas exchange in any clinically significant way.[26] More important is adjustment of the ventilator settings according to individual patient comfort. In this regard many alert patients prefer higher (70 to 90 L/min) over lower (40 to 60 L/min) peak inspiratory flow rates. When high cycling rates are used, or there is expiratory airflow limitation from COPD or asthma, rapid inspiratory flows are necessary to allow sufficient time for exhalation before the next breath begins. Whatever the tidal volume, frequency, or flow settings employed when a patient is begun on mechanical ventilation, it is imperative that an ABG measurement be obtained within 30 minutes and that appropriate adjustments be made as guided by the results.

Monitoring Mechanical Ventilation

Because mechanical ventilation and the disorders necessitating it are associated with numerous complications,[27] careful and continuous monitoring of all patients receiving such therapy is mandatory. The mechanical ventilation of patients with ARF should not be attempted outside an intensive care unit (ICU) unless ICU-level nursing and respiratory therapy personnel and equipment are available on a one-to-one basis. Appropriate physiologic monitoring depends upon the type and severity of physiologic abnormalities present in the individual patient. Some aspects of respiratory monitoring are discussed later in this section, under "Weaning"; however, a general review of available critical-care monitoring techniques is beyond the scope of this chapter, and the reader is directed to sources dealing with this subject in detail.[28,29]

Available Modes of Mechanical Ventilation

Figure 4–7 illustrates schematically the differences between intermittent mandatory ventilation (IMV) and assisted mechanical ventilation (AMV), the two main ventilator modes in current use, along with the largely outdated controlled mechanical ventilation (CMV) and spontaneous breathing. With CMV, the first volume-cycled ventilator mode to become available, the respiratory rate is set and cannot be increased by patient efforts to take more breaths. AMV allows the patient to set his or her own cycling rate, but each breath is delivered by the ventilator. The ventilator is set to deliver a certain number of breaths per minute: if the patient makes no inspiratory efforts this set value is the actual rate of breath delivery, but the patient can trigger additional breaths at will. Once a patient-triggered breathing rate is established with AMV, the machine backup rate should be set to just below the frequency set by the patient, so that if the patient stops triggering, ventilation will not decrease substantially.

IMV is presently the most popular ventilator mode in many areas. Originally popularized as a weaning technique,[30,31] it has found widespread use as a means of providing continuous ventilatory support. It is a mode which effectively combines CMV with spontaneous breathing in that the machine cycling rate is fixed, but the patient can also breathe independently from a reservoir system between machine breaths. This ordinarily results in a few large breaths (10 to 15 ml/kg) interspersed with a variable number of smaller ones. The primary purpose of this combined pattern is to allow (or force) the patient to provide a substantial part of the necessary minute ventilation.

Considerable controversy has accompanied the rise of IMV as a continuous ventilator mode, with outspoken advocates and opponents both in practice and in the literature.[32] Although a number of its theoretical advantages are as yet unsupported by objective data, IMV appears to be preferable to AMV for patients with respiratory alkalosis who are unresponsive to ventilator adjustment or sedation,

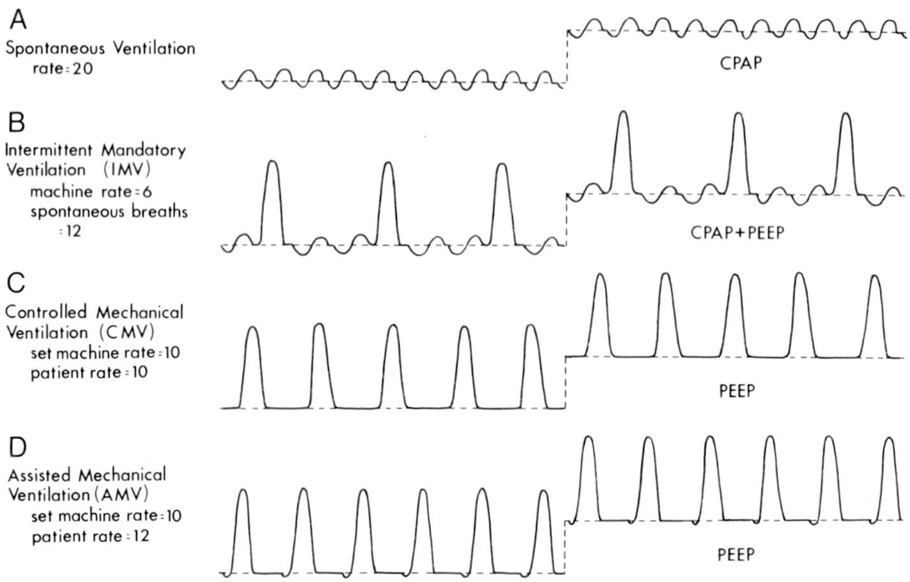

Figure 4–7. The three ventilator modes in current use, shown schematically in comparison with spontaneous ventilation. Changes in airway pressure are shown as deflections above and below the "zero" level of atmospheric pressure. Ventilation is depicted for one full minute, half before and half after the addition of PEEP (ventilator breaths) and/or CPAP (spontaneous breaths). (A) *Spontaneous breathing.* The pressure deflection is negative during inspiration and becomes positive with expiration. (B) *IMV.* The patient is effectively connected to two breathing circuits at once. Six mandatory breaths from the ventilator (as in C) are interspersed with 12 spontaneous breaths (as in A), which do not necessarily bear any temporal relationship to the mandatory breaths. The ventilator rate is fixed and additional breaths cannot be initiated by the patient. The mandatory rate should be slow enough that the patient contributes a significant fraction of the total ventilation. (C) *CMV.* The machine rate of 10 breaths per minute cannot be increased by the patient's attempts to trigger. All pressure deflections are positive. (D) *AMV.* The machine rate of 10 breaths per minute can be increased by patient effort. In this example all 12 breaths are "assist" breaths, or patient-initiated, as shown by the small negative deflections preceeding each one. Once the patient establishes a stable assist rate, the machine rate should be set to within 3 to 5 breaths per minute of it to prevent hypoventilation if the patient ceases to trigger.

for those who continue to fight the ventilator despite these measures, and when cardiovascular instability is exacerbated by the higher mean intrathoracic pressures attained with AMV. The use of IMV is inadvisable when paralytic agents such as pancuronium bromide are employed to control muscular activity or agitation, and when there is apnea or a changing neurologic status. Patients with small-diameter endotracheal tubes may experience excessive work of breathing if their ventilatory demand is high and the mandatory IMV rate is low. Relatively few patients fall into these groups, however, and in most instances of mechanical ventilation either IMV or AMV may be used, depending upon the experience and expertise of the attending personnel and the equipment available.

Table 4–6 provides guidelines for the use of IMV, AMV, and CMV, and summarizes relative advantages and disadvantages of each.

The Respiratory Muscles and Mechanical Ventilation

One area of persistent controversy in mechanical ventilation concerns its effects on the respiratory muscles.[32,33] Respiratory muscle discoordination is common in patients with ARF,[28] and weakness of the respiratory muscles may result from—or at least be worsened by—disuse, malnutrition, electrolyte imbalance, and the catabolic effects of the illness leading to ARF.[34] In severe COPD, some ambulatory patients have respiratory muscle asynchrony, and evidence suggests that this subgroup of patients is more likely to develop ARF than those with more normal breathing patterns.[35,36] Among COPD patients with ARF, those with respiratory muscle asynchrony are more likely to require intubation and mechanical ventilation, especially if hypercapnia is also present.[37] The importance of these findings with regard to patients without severe COPD is unclear.

The mechanical ventilation–muscle controversy is complicated by uncertainty about whether the respiratory muscles should be exercised or rested in ARF.[32,33] IMV is said to strengthen the respiratory muscles and is recommended by some for its role in exercising them,[38] although few data have appeared to support this recommendation.[32] In contrast, resting the diaphragm through ventilation in a negative pressure tank has been shown to improve dyspnea and may slow or halt clinical deterioration in patients with chronic ventilatory insufficiency and hypercapnia.[39] While it is reasonable to conclude from the available data that respiratory muscle dysfunction may cause or predispose to ARF, the role of mechanical ventilation, and of different ventilator modes, in worsening or improving the function of the respiratory muscles must be regarded as unknown. In the majority of patients with ARF, the mode of ventilation used appears to make little difference, so long as it is properly used.

"Fighting the Respirator"

Agitation and distress during mechanical ventilation develop in four main circumstances:

1. An incorrect ventilator setup for the patient's needs.
2. An acute change in the patient's status.
3. An obstructed airway.
4. Ventilator malfunction.

Regardless of which one or more of these general problems is the cause, "fighting the respirator" must always be regarded as a potentially life-threatening situation.

The statement that a given patient "can't adjust to the respirator" after being placed on mechanical ventilation reveals a basic mistake in thinking with regard to ventilator management. By varying the cycling frequency, tidal volume, trigger-

(Text continues on p. 102.)

Table 4–6. Choice of Ventilator Mode in Acute Respiratory Failure

Mode	Use Appropriate	Advantages	Disadvantages	Use Inappropriate
Intermittent mandatory ventilation (IMV)	Any patient requiring mechanical ventilation (see Table 4–5) if: No contraindication to IMV is present (see "use inappropriate") Ventilator requires no additional apparatus or expense to deliver IMV Patients who "fight the ventilator" in whom sedation is ineffective or contraindicated Patients with hemodynamic instability To decrease mean intrathoracic pressure (compared with AMV) To decrease oxygen consumption from work of breathing (compared with spontaneous ventilation) Hypoxemic ARF with low spontaneous tidal volume (< 5 ml/kg) ? Refractory respiratory alkalosis on AMV ? To preserve respiratory muscle function in patients requiring ventilation for > 4–5 days	Prevents asynchrony with ventilator Decreased mean intrathoracic pressure may reduce cardiovascular effects of PEEP/CPAP Provides periodic deep breath to prevent atelectasis in patients with low tidal volume ? Prevents hyperventilation by allowing patients to "set their own PCO_2" ?? Maintains tone and coordination of respiratory muscles	Cannot respond to increased patient demand with increased ventilator minute volume Increased work of breathing as compared with AMV if: High patient minute ventilation requirement Small diameter endotracheal tube Longer total ventilator time if weaning with IMV not done as intended Increased cost to patient and complexity of apparatus if ventilator does not have built-in IMV mode ? Danger of barotrauma from "stacking" mandatory breath on top of spontaneous breath	Apnea Use of paralytic agents Severe respiratory depression Drug overdose, head trauma, etc. Large or increasing doses of sedatives Unstable neurologic or metabolic status Use of high mandatory rates such that patient's contribution is nil or negligible (effectively CMV) Small-diameter endotracheal tube (7 mm or less for average size adult)

Table 4–6 (continued). Choice of Ventilator Mode in Acute Respiratory Failure

Mode	Use Appropriate	Advantages	Disadvantages	Use Inappropriate
Controlled mechanical ventilation (CMV) (patient does not trigger ventilator)	Use of paralytic agents or heavy sedation *if* sensitivity control set to allow possible triggering by patient Chronic ventilatory support in the home (high cervical cord injury, bilateral diaphragmatic paralysis, etc)	Decreased oxygen consumption in patients with high spontaneous breathing work ? Rests respiratory muscles Least expensive, simplest available mode for ventilation at home or during transport	Cannot respond with increased minute ventilation to increased patient demand Patient distress if alert and dyspneic Usually requires paralysis or heavy sedation ?Respiratory muscle dysfunction from disuse	Any patient capable of triggering a ventilator breath: turning sensitivity down to prevent triggering is clinically unacceptable
Assisted mechanical ventilation (AMV) (patient triggers some or all ventilator breaths)	Any patient requiring mechanical ventilation (see Table 4–5), unless: Respiratory alkalosis is refractory to machine adjustment and sedation ? Prolonged ventilation (> 4–5 days) will be required Increased work of breathing in patients with high minute ventilation requirement or small (≤ 7 mm) endotracheal tubes Patients with unstable neurologic or metabolic status whose respiratory drive may fluctuate	Can respond to increased patient demand with higher minute ventilation Decreased oxygen consumption in patients with high work of breathing as compared to IMV or spontaneous ventilation Less cost to patient than IMV if ventilator does not have built-in IMV mode	Respiratory alkalosis in patients with dyspnea, COPD, or brainstem dysfunction Increased mean intrathoracic pressure in comparison with IMV Possible cardiovascular compromise, especially with PEEP/CPAP ? Increased risk of barotrauma ?? Respiratory muscle dysfunction in comparison with IMV	Respiratory alkalosis unresponsive to ventilator adjustment and sedation (increased ventilatory drive uncorrectable except by paralysis) Patients with cardiovascular instability whose cardiac outputs are compromised more by AMV than by IMV when used with PEEP/CPAP ? Prolonged ventilation (> 4–5 days) because of possible effects on tone and coordination of respiratory muscles

ing sensitivity, and inspiratory flow rate, the ventilator can usually be matched to the patient's requirements, rather than vice versa. This requires some experimentation at the bedside, since no fixed combination of settings is appropriate for all patients. Calm reassurance first, and moderate sedation second, in addition to the above measures, will allow successful matching of the patient and ventilator in most instances.

The sudden onset of agitation and "fighting the respirator" in a patient previously tolerating mechanical ventilation signifies either an abrupt worsening of clinical status or malfunction of the ventilator or artificial airway. As is the case in making an original diagnosis of ARF, there are few specific physical findings to aid in discovering the source of the problem. However, a rapid bedside check is vital in assessment of this medical emergency.[40] The following steps should be taken:

1. Disconnect the patient from the ventilator and provide manual ventilation via a self-inflating resuscitator or anesthesia bag.
2. Make a quick check of the vital signs, chest, other physical factors (are both lungs being ventilated? Is there diffuse wheezing? Is the patient suddenly hypotensive?), and bedside monitoring equipment.
3. Suction the airway and make sure the endotracheal or tracheostomy tube is patent.
4. Run an ABG and make a more thorough general check of the patient (is a process in another organ system primarily causing respiratory distress?).

Many potentially fatal complications occur during mechanical ventilation.[27,40] Pneumothorax, fluid overload with acute pulmonary edema, pulmonary embolism, ICU-acquired bacterial pneumonia, and other intercurrent processes can complicate ARF and demand prompt attention. It is crucial that "fighting the ventilator" be viewed as a sign of acute clinical change rather than as an annoyance, and that it be a signal for urgent evaluation and intervention rather than for the routine administration of sedatives or paralytic agents.

Sedation and Paralysis

Although there are occasional settings in which paralytic agents such as pancuronium bromide are indicated in ARF[41]—including tetanus, manic behavior uncontrollable with sedation, and when high CO_2 production increases the work of breathing in a harmful way—muscle paralysis must be regarded as a "last resort" in ventilator management. It renders the patient incapable of manifesting distress, which takes away an important indicator of clinical status. Furthermore, although paralyzing the patient may remove the overt expression of distress, it does nothing to reveal or reverse its cause, and introduces the added problem of immobility and its complications. Additionally, because paralytic agents do not affect consciousness, sedatives such as diazepam must be given concomitantly.

Drugs that produce sedation rather than paralysis are usually preferable to agents such as curare and pancuronium in patients with ARF. If used in doses sufficient to calm the patient but not to induce unconsciousness, they allow some preservation of responsiveness as an indicator of clinical status. Sedation, whether with benzodiazepines (diazepam, chlordiazepoxide) or with narcotic analgesics (morphine, demerol) is best administered with small, frequent intravenous doses rather than intermittent, larger boluses, since the latter are more likely to cause hypotension. It is advisable to stay with a single agent and give progressively larger doses rather than adding different pharmacologic agents to the regimen. Morphine has the advantage of ready reversibility with naloxone if overdosage is suspected; however, this drug should be avoided in patients with asthma because of its potential for triggering bronchospasm.[42] Diazepam's major side effect of hypotension can be prevented if small incremental doses (2 to 5 mg i.v., q. 5 to 20 min.) are used, and although not acutely reversible like morphine, it has the added advantage of being a good amnesic agent. The most important concept in sedating patients with ARF is that this never be done simply to render them "easier to handle," but rather as therapy for a process that is both fully understood and unmanageable by other means.

Intermittent Positive Pressure Breathing (IPPB)

IPPB—frequent 10-to-15-minute pressure-ventilator treatments administered via a mouthpiece or mask—has no place in the treatment of acute ventilatory failure. The idea that IPPB treatment can temporarily assist patients and preclude the need for endotracheal intubation and mechanical ventilation is both incorrect and dangerous. If alveolar ventilation is acutely insufficient because of central nervous system depression or airway obstruction, it is unlikely that the cause can be reversed during the course of a single IPPB treatment. After the IPPB treatment, the need for ventilatory assistance will still exist, and the patient's ability to meet this need may be diminished if the treatment temporarily lowers the PCO_2, thus decreasing the ventilatory drive. Patients who are comatose or otherwise unable to insure airway protection should not be treated with IPPB because of the risk of gastric distension, vomiting, and aspiration.

IPPB *can* increase alveolar ventilation and, thus, lower the PCO_2 acutely.[43] The effect is limited to the duration of the treatment itself, however, and is lost almost immediately thereafter. In addition, one study of COPD patients with ARF showed that the PCO_2 actually increased in more than half, due to increased dead space ventilation, increased work of breathing, or both.[44]

Properly delivered IPPB occasionally can provide larger breaths than the patient can generate spontaneously.[45] This can be important in preventing postoperative atelectasis and pneumonia, rather than in supporting alveolar ventilation. IPPB and spontaneous deep breathing can be compared using a beside spirometer to see which produces the larger inspiration. If IPPB results in a deeper breath than a properly coached spontaneous effort, its use in a patient at risk for postoperative atelectasis or pneumonia is reasonable as part of a complete postoperative respiratory therapy regimen. Experience shows that if it is to be effective in this way, the IPPB treatment must be supervised directly by a respiratory therapist or nurse familiar with the physiologic objectives of the procedure; acutely ill patients can seldom do this correctly by themselves.

Respiratory Stimulants

The quest for a pharmacologic substitute for mechanical ventilation has been largely unsuccessful.[46] Currently, there are several "respiratory stimulant" drugs—doxapram, nikethamide, and methylphenidate are the most frequently used—which act by stimulating the central nervous system, including, with varying degrees of specificity, the centers controlling ventilation. These analeptic agents, along with the xanthines, carbonic anhydrase inhibitors, progesterone, and strychnine, do stimulate ventilation.[46] Doxapram, the analeptic with widest current use, increases the minute ventilation, tidal volume, and respiratory frequency, and may result in an acute lowering of arterial PCO_2. However, these effects, which have been demonstrated in patients with ARF,[47–49] are accomplished through an increase in energy expenditure and breathing work. This may not have adverse effects if the patient's respiratory mechanics are not severely impaired and the primary problem is an acute, reversible depression of respiratory center function, as is seen in postanesthesia hypoventilation.[50,51] On the other hand, if acute respiratory acidosis occurs because of mechanical limitation of the patient's ability to eliminate CO_2, as in COPD with acute exacerbation or in status asthmaticus, further stimulation of the central ventilatory drive would be ineffective in lowering the PCO_2, and might well increase it by increasing the work of breathing.[46]

A carefully done multi-center comparison of doxapram and placebo in preventing the progression of respiratory acidosis among patients with ARF found statistically significant increases in pH and decreases in PCO_2 during the 2 hours the analeptic agent was used.[49] However, the clinical course of ARF was unaffected: 38 percent of the doxapram-treated patients eventually required intubation and mechanical ventilation, as compared to 32 percent of those in the control group. Thus, doxapram temporarily improved the laboratory manifestations of ARF, but did not affect the outcome.

Doxapram and other analeptics have a very brief duration of action. Because the respiratory stimulant effect of doxapram is lost in 5 to 10 minutes, it must be given by continuous intravenous infusion. It must also be administered under continuous supervision, in the same manner as with dopamine, nitroprusside, and other potent intravenous agents. Respiratory stimulants must not be considered an alternative to ICU care, since patients receiving these drugs have to be monitored as closely as those on mechanical ventilators.

Although not used in most centers, respiratory stimulants still are considered by some to be potentially useful adjuncts to other therapy. Bone[52] considers the administration of analeptics a useful temporizing measure while instituting definitive management in ARF complicating COPD, and others[53] have reported occasional apparent benefit from this approach. Most authors, however, do not include respiratory stimulants in their treatment of ARF.[19,28,54–56] These drugs should not be considered a substitute for any of the aspects of ARF management discussed in this chapter.

High-Frequency Positive-Pressure Ventilation (HFPPV)

For the last decade and a half, a Swedish group has been studying HFPPV, a radically different means of supporting gas exchange, in which small tidal volumes (usually about equal to the calculated dead space) are delivered using respiratory frequencies of 60 to 120 cycles per minute.[57] Variations in the technique, utilizing as many as 5,000 oscillations per minute, have been tried. Although the mechanism by which HFPPV supports gas exchange is yet unknown, this technique has been effective not only in experimental animals but also in humans.[58] Its recent successful use in an adult patient with bronchopleural fistula[59] has stimulated interest in HFPPV in the United States,[60] and the technique is sure to "catch on" in this country for trials in other clinical settings. Whether HFPPV will prove to be a safe, effective alternative to currently available modes of mechanical ventilation is very much in doubt at present, although it may find limited application in situations in which large tidal volumes are lost via air leaks, or cause severe cardiovascular compromise.

WEANING FROM MECHANICAL VENTILATION

General Considerations

In most cases of ARF, once the underlying disease process has resolved or improved, and the indications for ventilatory support (Table 4–5) are no longer present, the patient may simply be removed from the ventilator. This is not "weaning" in the sense of gradual withdrawal over a period of time, but rather a discontinuation of a therapeutic modality that is no longer indicated. However, the discontinuation of mechanical ventilation by whatever means has come to be known as weaning, and this section will conform to this common usage.

Numerous bedside and laboratory predictors of successful ventilatory weaning have been proposed.[15,28,61,62] Some combination of the following parameters indicative of "weanability" is usually implied:

1. Ventilatory requirement for a normal PCO_2 and pH = 10 L/min or less.
2. A maximum voluntary ventilation (MVV) of at least 2 × ventilatory requirement.
3. A spontaneous tidal volume (V_T) greater than 5 ml/kg body weight.
4. A vital capacity (VC) greater than 10 ml/kg body weight.
5. A maximum inspiratory force greater than −20 cm H_2O.
6. An alveolar-arterial oxygen gradient ($P(A\text{-}a)O_2$) of less than 350 mmHg on FIO_2 of 1.0.
7. A dead space:tidal volume ratio (V_D/V_T) of less than 0.6.

The foregoing parameters are indices for assessing as quantitatively as possible: (1) the patient's resting metabolic demand; (2) the patient's ability to meet this demand on a continuing basis, taking into account both lung and neuromuscular function; and (3) the patient's ventilatory reserve: the ability to increase ventilation in response to a further increase in demand.

The minute volume required for normal alveolar ventilation (a PCO_2 of 40 mmHg) reflects both CO_2 production and dead-space ventilation. Substantial increases in either or both put added stress on the patient's ventilatory apparatus. Measurements of the VC and V_T help to predict the adequacy of spontaneous lung inflation and the avoidance of atelectasis once the ventilator is removed. A criterion for efficiency of oxygenation, whether formal calculation of the $P(A\text{-}a)O_2$ or a rule of thumb such as a PO_2 of greater than 80 mmHg at an FIO_2 equal to or less than 0.40, helps to assure that adequate oxygen delivery can be maintained even if the PO_2 falls initially when the ventilator is removed. The patient's ability to generate an inspiratory force exceeding 20 cmH_2O below atmospheric pressure is a good indicator of adequate muscle strength and neuromuscular coordination for spontaneous ventilation. Finally, although many patients with ARF are unable to cooperate for measurement of the MVV, the ability to double the required resting minute ventilation suggests adequate ventilatory reserve should additional demand for CO_2 removal occur.

Traditional Weaning

Removal of a patient from continuous ventilatory support is a major step in the management of ARF and should be approached as such. The protocol given in Table 4–7 emphasizes the importance of choosing the appropriate time to initiate weaning. The patient's overall condition should be such that those factors indicating the need for mechanical ventilation (Table 4–5) are substantially improved and no new or complicating process has appeared to increase the ventilatory demand. The physiologic parameters shown are those most readily available at the bedside, and are the ones primarily relied upon at Harborview Medical Center. Clinical experience and the existing literature indicate that fulfilling some preset objective criteria, whether those shown in Table 4–5 or others, improves the rate of weaning success in comparison with a "seat-of-the-pants" approach based upon how the patient looks in general.[61]

Just as patient distress, vital signs, and the chest physical examination are unreliable guides to the diagnosis of ARF prior to instituting mechanical ventilation, these signs cannot accurately gauge success in weaning. Gilbert and his associates studied patients being weaned to a T-piece after 3 to 80 days of AMV and found that acute changes in the V_T, respiratory rate, heart rate, and dyspnea did not correlate with weaning success.[63] The arterial PCO_2 tended to rise and the PO_2 to fall commensurate with an increased V_D/V_T as the V_T fell and the frequency of respiration increased, although these changes were not severe enough to produce significant acidemia or hypoxemia. The results of this study suggest that ABG values, rather than bedside parameters and clinical impression, should be

Table 4–7. Weaning from Continuous Mechanical Ventilation

Appropriate time:
Underlying cause of ARF has resolved or improved
Oxygenation adequate on $FIO_2 \leq 0.50$
Patient otherwise stable
Physiologic parameters:
Spontaneous VC > 10 ml/kg
Inspiratory force > $-20-25$ cmH_2O
Minute ventilation required for normal PCO_2 < 10 L
Technique:
Satisfy some preselected physiologic criteria (above parameters or others)
Pick the right time: early in day, adequate available staff, patient emotionally appropriate
Withhold sedatives and depressant analgesics
Suction and position appropriately
Switch patient to spontaneous breathing (T-piece with same FIO_2 and humidification)
Observe and reassure patient
Check ABG in 20–30 minutes

used in assessing weaning success. While it is advisable to return the patient to the ventilator if respiratory distress develops, an arterial blood specimen should be drawn first if possible and another weaning attempt made if the results fail to show acute deterioration. Calm reassurance of the patient and the presence of members of the respiratory care team at the bedside during weaning can greatly reduce agitation and distress caused by apprehension about being taken off the ventilator.

Weaning with IMV

IMV initially was popularized as a method of weaning from mechanical ventilation.[30–32] Whether the initial mode of mechanical ventilation is AMV or IMV, the rationale for IMV during weaning is that mechanical assistance is withdrawn gradually and smoothly, rather than abruptly, allowing the patient to increase his or her own ventilatory contribution in a progressive manner.[31] Weaning with IMV is accomplished by reducing the frequency of mandatory (ventilator) breaths, in decrements of 1 to 3 breaths per minute, such that the arterial pH does not fall below a given value, usually 7.35. As originally intended, this technique employs short intervals between setting changes, with ABG measurements after each change and the completion of weaning within a few hours in most instances.

Although it has been claimed that ventilator weaning time is shorter when IMV is used than with traditional weaning,[31,38] this has been difficult to demonstrate.[32] Milbern and co-workers[64] studied 33 patients during recovery from anesthesia. They measured spontaneous ventilatory parameters during a protocol of rapid IMV weaning and found that the time required before the patients could maintain an arterial pH of greater than 7.35 during spontaneous breathing averaged 1.4 hours less than that necessary to satisfy the "conventional" weaning criteria of a VC greater than 15 ml/kg and an inspiratory force greater than -20 cmH_2O. Whether a difference of 1.4 hours weaning time in postanesthesia patients without intrinsic lung disease implies a clinically important difference between IMV and conventional weaning after ARF is uncertain.

In order to minimize the duration of ventilation when IMV is used, it is important to decrease the mandatory breathing rate frequently, as originally intended with this method.[31,38,64] Unfortunately, the adoption of IMV as the standard mode of both continuous ventilatory support and weaning has led to longer, rather than shorter, ventilator time in some institutions.[32,65] This is because of a tendency to reduce the mandatory ventilation rate only once or twice per day. When high mandatory rates (12 to 16 per minute) are used initially, a weaning process that could be accomplished in a few hours may take several days.

Traditional weaning consists of waiting until the patient meets certain preset physiologic criteria and then discontinuing ventilatory support, either abruptly or in a series of progressively longer periods of spontaneous ventilation.[61] Weaning with IMV consists of empirically withdrawing ventilatory support using ABG results as the main physiologic guidelines. Both methods require close monitoring, and which of the two accomplishes total weaning faster depends mainly on how they are used. In the majority of patients recovering from ARF, the difference in weaning time is probably a few hours at most if both methods are employed correctly. Because weaning with IMV requires re-checking the patient's status repeatedly during a series of mandatory rate reductions, this technique probably requires more ABG measurements than traditional weaning. In other respects and in most clinical situations, there appears to be little to recommend either method over the other.

The Patient Who Cannot Be Weaned

Application of the basic principles of weaning (Table 4–7) will lead to the successful discontinuation of ventilatory assistance in most patients. When the usual criteria for traditional weaning are not met, an orderly approach to assessment, as is shown in Table 4–8, can be helpful.

If the patient had no symptoms of muscle weakness prior to the onset of ARF, and has not sustained an irreversible neurologic injury, failure to meet the inspiratory force and vital capacity criteria should be assumed to be due to some reversible process. Paralytic agents should be discontinued if weaning is being attempted, sedation and narcotic analgesics should be given at the lowest possible dosages, and consideration should be given to switching from aminoglycosides to other antibiotics, especially if the patient's weakness occurred soon after the suspect drugs were started. Hypophosphatemia can cause neuromuscular weakness in patients with ARF,[66] and measurement of the serum phosphorus as well as magnesium and potassium concentration should be part of the evaluation of patients who cannot be weaned because of weakness.

Weakness and discoordination of the respiratory muscles can hamper or prevent weaning, especially in patients who have been critically ill for a period of weeks.[28,34] When evaluation fails to reveal a specific cause for weakness, a period of hyperalimentation, either via the gastrointestinal tract or parenterally, may eventually enable the patient to be weaned when all other methods have failed. The maintenance of a proper caloric intake and nitrogen balance in critically ill patients

Table 4–8. Failure to Meet Weaning Criteria

Weakness: (VC < 10 ml/kg, inspiratory force <–20 cmH_2O)		
	Problem:	Patient is not strong enough to keep up with ventilatory needs
	Causes:	Primary neuromuscular disease
		Drugs: paralytic agents (pancuronium, curare); aminoglycosides (rare)
		Metabolic disorders: hypophosphatemia, hypomagnesemia, hypokalemia
		Malnutrition
Low respiratory drive: (apnea or ↓ spontaneous ventilation off ventilator)		
	Problem:	Patient is not stimulated to breathe
	Causes:	Respiratory alkalosis (overventilation)
		Metabolic alkalosis (diuresis; gastric suction)
		Drugs: sedatives and depressant analgesics
		(Malnutrition)
		(Myxedema)
Excessive breathing effort: (high frequency, low tidal volume)		
	Problem:	Work of breathing exceeds patient's capacity
	Causes:	Endotracheal tube too small (usually 7 mm or less)
		Obstruction of tube or airway (secretions, foreign body, kinking, tube defect)
		Chest restriction (bandages, positioning, restraints)
		Pain
		Anxiety (check ABG; try calming patient)
High ventilation requirement: (V_E > 10 L/min to maintain PCO_2 = 40)		
	Problem:	Required minute ventilation for normal CO_2 elimination exceeds patient's capacity
	Causes:	High CO_2 production (sepsis; inflammation; excessive hyperalimentation)
		High dead-space (ARDS: airways disease; pulmonary emboli)

has received increasing attention in recent years.[67] This has special importance in ventilator weaning because of the recognition that even short periods of semistarvation cause a marked depression of ventilatory drives.[68]

The most common cause of an insufficient drive to breathe during mechanical ventilation is alkalosis, often a combination of both respiratory and metabolic processes. If the arterial pH is much above 7.45, many patients will not start breathing within the first minute or two when taken off the ventilator. As is the case for initial adjustment of a ventilator, a safe physiologic pH rather than any specific PCO_2 value should be the goal in weaning, even if hypercapnia occurs. If metabolic alkalosis is severe, it should be corrected over a day or two, and weaning should be reattempted. When hypocapnia has been longstanding, it may be necessary to raise the PCO_2 gradually so as to avoid acidemia; IMV may be useful in this situation.

Narcotic analgesics and other sedating drugs depress the ventilatory drive and may contribute to difficulty in weaning. Intercostal nerve blocks or epidural anesthesia may enable postoperative patients to ventilate adequately and to cough without the use of systemic agents.[69] In other patients, it is necessary to balance the assumed degree of respiratory depression against the need for sedation and analgesia. Frequently, weaning and extubation will reduce patient agitation and the need for sedation.

Excessive work of breathing through a small-diameter endotracheal tube can prevent successful weaning. The resistance to flow through a tube and the work required to overcome it vary with the length of the tube and inversely with the fourth power of the tube radius (Poiseuille's law). The following resistances to flow through endotracheal tubes at 1 L/sec illustrate the importance of this point[61]:

9 mm inside diameter: 0.6 cm H_2O/L/sec
8 mm inside diameter: 1.9 cm H_2O/L/sec
7 mm inside diameter: 4.0 cm H_2O/L/sec
6 mm inside diameter: 4.8 cm H_2O/L/sec

Prolonged spontaneous ventilation through a 6- or 7-mm-diameter endotracheal tube may be beyond the capability of the patient, particularly if the patient's resting minute ventilation is greater than 10 L. If maintenance of a patent airway and secretion removal are not a problem, such patients can sometimes be weaned and extubated at the same time. Otherwise it may be necessary to change the tube to a larger size, preferably of 8-mm inside diameter or greater.

Measurement of CO_2 production and calculation of the V_D/V_T are simple procedures which can help to gauge the relative contributions of metabolic demand and dead space to a high minute ventilation requirement. They are most useful when attempting to wean patients with surgical sepsis, burns, or resolving, severe ARDS, in that they identify the major barrier to weaning and provide an objective parameter to follow during therapy. A high CO_2 production can potentially be reduced by controlling fever, sepsis, and muscular activity. Hyperalimentation increases O_2 consumption, although in most cases its associated increase in CO_2 production does not interfere with weaning, and its benefit greatly outweighs this side effect. A high dead-space ventilation in a patient with acute severe lung injury suggests that improvement can be expected as the injury resolves.[3]

Although meeting the physiologic criteria for weaning listed in Table 4–7 means that a patient almost certainly can be weaned,[61,70] patients who "fail" these criteria often can also be weaned successfully. Weaning with the use of IMV relies upon ABG results after each mandatory respiratory rate reduction rather than prospective measurements, and experience with this technique shows that the conventional weaning criteria may be too strict for some patients.

Attention to the overall status of the patient is important in weaning the difficult patient. Fluid overload, the presence of fever or untreated infection in other systems, and insufficient attention to nutritional support are frequent findings in such patients.[62] On most occasions when consultation is requested because of ventilator weaning problems, the problem is found to be in these areas and in insufficient adherence to the basic guidelines for weaning (Table 4–7).

AIRWAY AND SECRETION MANAGEMENT

Acute respiratory failure usually leads to the need to protect or maintain the airway (see Chapter 2) and to impairment of normal secretion clearance. The main indications for tracheal intubation in ARF are, first, the need for mechanical ventilation or a controlled, high FIO_2; second, inability of the patient to maintain airway patency or protection from aspiration; and third, failure to adequately remove respiratory secretions spontaneously or by catheter suction. Once an endotracheal tube is in place it must be managed carefully and monitored for malfunction.[27] Nasotracheal tubes must be examined frequently for excessive pressure on the external nares from tape or other equipment attached to the tube.[71]

Objective predictors of success are not currently available for extubation, as they are for weaning from mechanical ventilation. If intubation was done because of the need for mechanical ventilation, spontaneous ventilation must obviously be adequate and stable before a tracheal tube can be removed. Upper airway obstruction must be resolved or markedly reduced if this was the reason for intubation. The patient must be judged capable of adequately eliminating secretions, a factor that may be hard to assess but which involves a combination of secretion volume and viscocity and the patient's predicted ability to cough. Finally, the patient must be capable of protecting his or her airway so as to prevent the aspiration of gastric or oral contents. This last assessment is the most difficult to make, especially in patients with depressed consciousness.

Deglutition and glottic function are usually impaired immediately following extubation, even when this is done after brief anesthesia. How well the gag reflex and stimulated cough predict the ability to prevent aspiration is unknown. Extubation remains largely an empirical experiment based upon clinical judgment.

Adequate secretion clearance is a major problem in many patients with ARF. Among the factors that impair mucociliary clearance mechanisms in such patients are the following[72,73]:

Abnormal secretion volume and viscocity.

Central nervous system depression (depression of the cough reflex; abolition of the normal sighing mechanism).

Endotracheal intubation (loss of glottic function; airway drying; interruption of the mucociliary escalator).

Supine position (gravitational secretion pooling).

Although the contribution of each of these factors varies in a given patient, attention to the adequacy of secretion clearance is an important part of ARF management. Available methods for increasing secretion clearance include hydration, the facilitation of coughing, chest physiotherapy, and catheter suction.

Both local airway drying and systemic dehydration impair mucociliary clearance.[72,74] Replacing depleted total-body fluids can restore clearance rates to normal,[74] and this aspect of general ICU care can be important in secretion management, particularly if the secretions are abnormally viscous. Breathing incompletely humidified gases, whether by mouth or via an endotracheal tube, can cause severe airway drying which is not fully reversed until a relative humidity of at least 75 percent is achieved in the trachea.[75] Whether the addition of moisture to the respiratory tract beyond that necessary to maintain 100 percent relative humidity is clinically useful in managing ARF is doubtful.[73,76]

The purposes of chest physiotherapy (chest percussion and postural drainage) in ARF are to reduce the work of breathing by removing obstructing secretions and improving airflow, and to improve gas exchange.[73] In addition, in postoperative patients, chest physiotherapy is intended to prevent atelectasis, pneumonia, and other sequelae of poor lung expansion and secretion clearance.[77] Several clinical studies have documented its effectiveness in the latter situation,[77–79] and it is reasonable to assume that the same effectiveness could be expected in ARF. Unfortunately, this has been difficult to show in clinically relevant studies.[73,80] Chest physiotherapy was shown in one study to have no effect on the acute course of pneumonia in patients who could cough spontaneously.[81] Other investigators found no clinical benefit from chest physiotherapy in COPD patients with acute exacerbations,[82] while yet another group reported decreases in FEV_1 after physiotherapy in such patients, presumably because of aggravation of bronchospasm.[83]

There are few data pertaining to the question of how chest physiotherapy should most effectively be done in ARF. Studies to date have not shown any advantage of mechanical percussors over traditional manual techniques.[84,85] Because of the effort and time involved on the part of the nurse or respiratory therapist in properly performing chest percussion and postural drainage, this treatment probably should be reserved for patients with demonstrable difficulty in raising their own secretions, or in whom a test treatment results in a substantial increase in the expectoration of sputum. Suitable patients for chest physiotherapy would be those with large sputum volumes[80] or thick, tenacious secretions which are difficult to clear.

Chest physiotherapy should be directed at a particular lung segment or area. The frequency of treatments should be dictated by the sputum volume and viscosity; fewer than two treatments per 24 hours would seem insufficient in ARF, while giving treatment more often than every 3 or 4 hours may be logistically prohibitive.

Chest physiotherapy is not innocuous. In addition to the possibility of inducing bronchospasm,[83] it may worsen hypoxemia if the patient has predominately unilateral lung disease and is positioned with the abnormal lung down.[86,87] The latter may result in increased perfusion to already non- or hypoventilated lung areas, worsening a "shunt" effect.[88] On the other hand, positioning patients so that the more abnormal lung tissue is uppermost can improve $\dot{V}/\dot{Q}$ matching and increase the PO_2.[86,89] Patients with hypoxemia and severe unilateral lung disease, such as major atelectasis or lobar pneumonia, should be monitored closely during chest physiotherapy, and should not be positioned with the affected side down.

Although it is less effective than spontaneous coughing, catheter suction via the endotracheal or nasotracheal route is often necessary when patients cannot clear secretions spontaneously. Standard-size suction catheters can reach farther down the respiratory tract through a tracheostomy tube than through oral- or nasotracheal tubes, but at best they do not extend far beyond the mainstem bronchi. Attempts to devise catheters and suctioning techniques that can predictably allow cannulation of a particular bronchus have had little success.

In addition to mucosal bleeding from catheter-induced local trauma, suctioning procedures can occasionally produce life-threatening complications. Despite preoxygenation procedures, hypoxemia can worsen acutely during both endotracheal[90] and nasotracheal[91] suctioning. Additionally, cardiac arrhythmias have been observed during suctioning via both routes,[92] possibly due to hypoxemia in combination with vagal stimulation; and fatal cardiac arrest has occurred during nasotracheal suctioning.[93] The latter procedure has also been shown to be associated with transient bacteremia.[94]

Considering the potential hazards and relative efficacy of both catheter suctioning procedures and chest physiotherapy, in comparison with spontaneous coughing and expectoration, every effort should be made to induce patient cooperation and effort so that these procedures will be unnecessary. Extra time spent with the patient by the physician, nurse, and respiratory therapist can help a great deal in this regard.

ARF IN THE COPD PATIENT

Because of several unique features of ARF in an acute exacerbation of COPD, the approach to its management differs in certain respects from that in other conditions. The most important of these differences are a greater concern for the precision of oxygen therapy, and the avoidance of endotracheal intubation and mechanical ventilation if at all possible.

The natural course of severe COPD is one of gradual deterioration, sometimes punctuated by acute exacerbations that markedly compromise lung function.[95,96] Such exacerbations seldom result in marked permanent pulmonary-function loss.[20] Thus, when ARF occurs during an exacerbation of COPD, the physician, in the absence of personal knowledge that the patient's underlying lung function and course over a period of months or years have demonstrated otherwise, must assume the acute process to be reversible. In the emergency room or ICU setting, it is seldom possible to know the patient well enough to be able to withhold lifesaving therapy acutely.

In ARF, the pathophysiology of COPD remains, but is exaggerated; airflow limitation by bronchospasm, mucosal edema, and airway secretions is worsened acutely, resulting in increased breathing work, elevated CO_2 production, and often, acute respiratory acidosis. Consequently, in the absence of a specific intercurrent process (such as congestive heart failure, pneumothorax, or bacterial pneumonia), the management of ARF in COPD is essentially an intensification of outpatient comprehensive care.[95,97] Measures for relieving hypoxemia, bronchospasm, and retained secretions are the keystones of this management.

The first goal of oxygen therapy in acute exacerbations of COPD is the same as in other forms of ARF: to relieve life-threatening hypoxemia. Once severe hypoxemia is detected, the PO_2 should immediately be raised above the steepest part of the oxygen-hemoglobin dissociation curve (Fig. 4–4). Thereafter, the goal of oxygen therapy is somewhat different from that in other ARF situations in that the PO_2 should not rise above 65 mmHg. The reason for this is that patients with chronic hypercapnia are often driven to breathe primarily by their hypoxic ventilatory drive, unlike normal individuals, and if the PO_2 is raised above a point at which input from the peripheral chemoreceptor largely stops, the patient will hypoventilate further and become more acidemic. Clinical experience shows that in most COPD patients, the hypoxic drive is preserved at PO_2 values below 60 to 65 mmHg. Thus, the initial goal of supplemental oxygen administration should be a PO_2 between 50 and 65 mmHg (ideally between 55 and 60 mmHg to allow a margin for error and steady-state variability.)

In order to avoid an excessively high PO_2, oxygen should be given to COPD patients at precisely controlled rates. As described earlier, the exact FIO_2 is unknown during oxygen therapy unless it is measured directly in the trachea, regardless of whether a Venturi mask or nasal prongs are used. What is important is that the oxygen delivery be constant and that the results be determined by ABG analysis. The major problem with Venturi masks is keeping them on the patient (Fig. 4–5); with nasal prongs it is accurate delivery of often very low flows of oxygen. A pediatric-style flowmeter is useful for the precise delivery of flow rates of less than 2 L/min.

Even when the PO_2 is kept below 60 to 65 mmHg in patients with acute exacerbations of COPD, the PCO_2 often rises once oxygen therapy is begun. It is important that the arterial pH, rather than PCO_2, be used as the gauge of severity when this happens. So long as the pH remains above 7.30, and if the patient remains alert and cooperative, a modest further increase in the PCO_2 is acceptable in order to relieve severe hypoxemia.

Intubation and mechanical ventilation should be avoided in COPD patients for four reasons[52]: (1) intubation impairs their clearance of secretions; (2) they frequently develop complications from intubation and mechanical ventilation; (3) prolonged ventilation often becomes necessary because of difficult weaning; and, perhaps most important (4) they usually can be managed successfully without intubation and mechanical ventilation.[20] Patients who are awake and can follow instructions seldom need to be intubated. If the patient is comatose or uncontrollably agitated, if general anesthesia becomes necessary, or if respiratory acidemia worsens despite vigorous therapy, mechanical ventilation may be unavoidable. Patients in the last category were found in one study to be those most profoundly hypoxemic and acidemic when first seen.[21] These two parameters, and not the actual PCO_2 value, were the best predictors of the need for intubation; 11 of 15 patients with both a pH below 7.30 and a PO_2 below 40 mmHg (on admission FIO_2) required this intervention.[21]

When COPD patients are mechanically ventilated, the goal of support should be their "normal" ABG values. Thus, the PO_2 should be between 50 and 65 mmHg and the pH between about 7.35 and 7.40. Since the patient's usual PCO_2 is frequently unknown, and may have risen over a period of several days prior to admission, use of the pH as a guide to ventilator settings will help to avoid acute alkalosis. The duration of mechanical ventilation, whether AMV or IMV, should be kept as short as possible. PEEP/CPAP should be avoided in COPD patients because of the likelihood of cardiovascular compromise and barotrauma (see Table

4–3). While sedation is appropriate when agitation persists despite ventilator adjustment, all respiratory depressant drugs should be stopped, if possible, prior to a weaning attempt.

Bronchodilator Therapy

All patients with ARF complicating severe COPD should be assumed to be bronchodilator-responsive. The reasons for this statement are twofold: underlying reversibility of the COPD may be obscured during the acute episode, and may thus not be demonstrable, and presently available bronchodilating agents can be given and monitored safely enough to make empirical treatment justifiable. The pharmacology and clinical use of bronchodilators have recently been reviewed.[98,99] Both intravenous aminophylline and an inhaled beta-adrenergic agent should be used.

As theophylline pharmacokinetics have become more fully understood, and clinical experience with previous dosage guidelines has accumulated, it has become apparent that regimens published from 1973 to 1977 for the use of this drug resulted in overdosage in some acutely ill patients.[52,100,101] The following intravenous aminophylline dosage schedule should result in serum theophylline levels within but not exceeding the therapeutic range of 10 to 20 μg/ml. Theophylline as measured in the serum is the active agent, whether theophylline or aminophylline is given. To convert the dosage of the two drugs, 1.0 mg theophylline = 1.2 mg aminophylline)

Loading doses (all patients):
- No theophylline-containing drugs within the last 24 hours: 6 mg/kg, given i.v. over 20 minutes.
- Theophylline-containing drugs taken within the last 24 hours but at a clinically subtherapeutic level: 3 mg/kg, given i.v. over 20 minutes.
- Theophylline-containing drugs taken within the last 24 hours and level clinically in or above therapeutic range: no loading dose.

Maintenance infusion (via continuous infusion pump):
- COPD without overt liver disease or congestive heart failure: 0.4 mg/kg/hr
- Evidence of liver disease or congestive heart failure present: 0.2 mg/kg/hr

A 3 mg/kg loading dose of aminophylline should result in an increase in serum theophylline concentration of about 5 μg/ml. This half-loading dose can be given with reasonable confidence to patients not considered clinically to have theophylline serum levels above 20 μg/ml, since serious toxicity seldom occurs at levels below 25 to 30 μg/ml. A serum theophylline-level specimen should be drawn 6 to 12 hours after the maintenance infusion is begun, and dosage adjustment should be made accordingly. As patients improve, their theophylline clearance may change, and occasional monitoring of the serum theophylline level throughout the acute episode is therefore necessary even if the level is initially appropriate.

In addition to aminophylline, all patients should be given a trial of inhaled beta-agonists. The following are appropriate beginning doses for patients of average size:

Metaproterenol, 0.2 ml of a 5 percent solution
(10 mg) in 2 to 3 ml total volume, every 4 to 6 hours.
Isoetharine, 0.5 ml of 1 percent solution
(5 mg) in 2 to 3 ml total volume, every 4 hours.
Isoproterenol, 0.5 ml of an 0.5 percent solution
(2.5 mg) in 2-3 ml total volume, every 2 to 4 hours.

In ARF these agents are delivered more reliably by a hand-held compressor-driven or compressed-air-driven nebulizer than by a commercial metered-dose device. Patients often use the latter incorrectly when they are stable, and seldom can do so effectively when acutely dyspneic or confused. IPPB is difficult to administer in ARF and increases dyspnea in many patients; it is not a preferred method of bronchodilator administration. The inhaled route is preferable to oral administration in acutely ill patients because of a higher therapeutic-effect-to-toxicity ratio and uncertain gastric absorption. Terbutaline, which is not approved for inhalation in the United States, has characteristics similar to those of metaproterenol and is given by subcutaneous injection, 0.25 mg every 4 to 6 hours, in some centers. Whichever beta-agonist is used, it is best to increase the dose of this single agent in inhaled form if the effect is clinically submaximal, rather than to add a second agent by another route. Because of their lack of beta-2-receptor specificity in relation to the drugs listed above, ephedrine and epinephrine should not be used in COPD patients with ARF.

Some patients with severe chronic airflow limitation that cannot be reversed acutely with beta-agonists improve with inhaled atropine sulfate, at least when they are stable.[102] Although no data are currently available to show a similar effect in ARF, atropine is occasionally given on an empirical trial basis in severe refractory airflow limitation. A dose of 0.02 mg/kg, aerosolized in a fluid volume of 2 to 3 ml given every 4 to 6 hours, is used. Tachycardia and the drying of secretions, frequent side effects of parenteral atropine, are less apparent clinically with aerosol delivery of the drug. Atropine's maximum bronchodilator effect may not occur for 60 minutes after a dose, making bedside spirometry at 10 and also at 60 minutes appropriate if objective measurements are used in gauging therapy.

Corticosteroids

High-dose corticosteroid therapy is a standard part of the management of status asthmaticus,[103] but has been controversial in COPD. However, a recent study of ARF in COPD, from which patients with asthmatic features were carefully excluded, showed faster improvement in pulmonary function under a comprehensive respiratory care regimen plus methylprednisolone (0.5 mg/kg i.v. every 6 hours, for 72 hours) as compared with placebo.[104] Patients with a history of variable airflow obstruction or known bronchodilator reversibility, and those chronically taking corticosteroids, would be appropriate candidates for short-term, high-dose parenteral methylprednisolone; on the basis of the study just referred to, patients without such a history might also be helped by such therapy. The ideal or minimum effective dose is unknown, but methylprednisolone at 2 mg/kg/24 hours, or its equivalent in other steroid preparations for 72 hours, would be a reasonable choice.[97,104]

Antibiotics

Benefit from antibiotic therapy in acute exacerbations of COPD has been difficult to show using well-designed, placebo-controlled studies.[105] Because COPD patients, whether acutely decompensated or not, are usually colonized with *Streptococcus pneumoniae* and *Hemophilus influenzae*, isolation of one or both of these organisms from the sputum does not necessarily have clinical importance.[106] Nonetheless, clinical experience suggests that antibiotics shorten and perhaps ameliorate acute episodes of the disease. Studies comparing tetracycline, ampicillin or amoxicillin, and trimethoprim-sulfamethoxazole have failed to demonstrate a clinical advantage of any one over the others.[105] Considering cost and availability, ampicillin or tetracycline, in a dose of 500 mg given every 6 hours, would be reasonable empirical therapy, assuming that an identified specific infection (pneumonia, urinary tract infection) is not present.[52,97]

Digitalis

Because of hypoxemia, acidosis, and frequent diuretic-induced hypokalemia, patients with ARF complicating COPD are at increased risk for ventricular arrhythmias and other manifestations of digitalis toxicity. Digitalis is clinically ineffective in cor pulmonale, and should be given only for specific indications, such as left ventricular failure or supraventricular arrhythmias.

Chest Physiotherapy

With few exceptions, chest percussion and postural drainage should be given a trial in an acute exacerbation of COPD. This should follow beta-agonist aerosol inhalation, and should be focused on the dependent areas of the lungs. Since airway obstruction by inspissated secretions can add greatly to breathing work, successful chest physiotherapy can make a substantial difference clinically. The effectiveness of treatments should be assessed in terms of the volume of sputum produced and subjective changes in dyspnea. If no benefit is apparent in 12 to 24 hours, the treatments can be stopped.

ARF IN PATIENTS WITH BURNS

Respiratory complications account for the majority of fatalities among burned patients who survive to be admitted to the hospital. Aside from carbon monoxide poisoning,[4] several types of pulmonary injury leading to ARF are seen.[107,108] Acute pulmonary edema and ARDS can occur within a few hours of a burn, as a result of direct respiratory tract injury by products of incomplete combustion. This acute fulminating form of ARF is often associated with bronchospasm, upper airway obstruction, or both, and is usually fatal. Pulmonary edema may also occur hours to days after the burn, and may be exacerbated by vigorous fluid administration.

Bacterial pneumonia is a later complication in burned patients, and most get it at some time during their course in the hospital. Usually hematogenous, this pneumonia may be caused by a wide variety of endogenous and hospital-acquired pathogens. Along with sepsis, it adds to the ventilatory demand of the burned patient, in whom CO_2 production is often already twice normal, leading to what may be called "high output" ARF.[109] Such patients often require prolonged mechanical ventilation despite having spontaneous ventilatory parameters that would ordinarily predict successful weaning. A period of several weeks may be required before the resting ventilatory demand decreases to 10-15 L/min for normal CO_2 elimination. Patients with severe surgical sepsis may present similar problems, particularly if peritoneal soilage, wound dehiscence, or multiple abdominal explorations are involved.

COMPLICATIONS OF ARF AND ITS MANAGEMENT

Virtually every aspect of ARF and its treatment in the ICU setting is associated with potentially life-threatening complications. Table 4–9 lists the most important of these, several of which have been discussed in earlier sections. That complications occur commonly in ARF was demonstrated by one prospective study of patients ventilated at a major respiratory care center.[27] Nearly one complication or situation considered a potential complication occurred per patient. Clearly, complications of ARF must be anticipated and active measures taken to prevent them whenever mechanical ventilation or other ICU care becomes necessary.

Pulmonary barotrauma (pneumothorax, pneumomediastinum, subcutaneous emphysema) complicating mechanical ventilation is related more directly to the maximum distending volume than to the peak inspiratory pressure. As shown in Table 4–3, PEEP/CPAP therapy is more likely to result in barotrauma if it is used when the lung compliance is high or if the lung volume (FRC) is already normal or high when the therapy is begun. The static compliance curve popularized by Bone[29] can be a useful aid in detecting potentially dangerous lung inflation, with or without PEEP/CPAP. Although the static hold pressure is sufficient for monitoring many patients, the presence of a high risk of barotrauma during ventilator therapy makes it important to have equipment at the bedside for emergency tube thoracostomy, since tension pneumothorax during mechanical ventilation can be rapidly fatal.

Acute lobar or whole-lung atelectasis is a common complication in patients with ARF, particularly in quadriplegia and comatose states. It can result in severe hypoxemia, and if allowed to persist can lead to pneumonia. Although bronchoscopy has constituted the major part of management of such atelectasis in some

Table 4–9. Complications of Acute Respiratory Failure and Its Management

Oxygen toxicity
Complications related to tracheal intubation (see Chapter 2)
Barotrauma: pneumothorax, pneumomediastinum, subcutaneous emphysema, bronchopleural fistula
Nosocomial pneumonia and other infections
Lobar atelectasis
Cardiac arrhythmias
Aspiration of gastric contents
Pulmonary embolism
Mechanical failure of ventilators and alarms
Complications of ICU care:
Fluid overload
Electrolyte and metabolic disturbances
Malnutrition
Physical deconditioning
Depression; "ICU psychosis"

centers,[110] a prospective, randomized study has shown that bronchoscopy for the removal of plugs and secretions is unnecessary in ARF if the patient can be given vigorous chest physiotherapy.[111] Effective respiratory therapy in this study consisted of sustained maximal inspirations for 3 minutes by the manual bag or incentive spirometer technique, encouragement of coughing and expectoration, bronchodilator inhalation, and chest percussion and postural drainage of the affected lobe; this regimen was performed every 4 hours and was continued for 48 hours. Although the recurrence of lobar collapse is common when fiberoptic bronchoscopy constitutes the primary therapy for atelectasis, there were no recurrences in the patients whose atelectasis resolved during the study.[111] Bronchoscopy becomes necessary when lobar atelectasis does not improve after 24 to 48 hours of chest physiotherapy, as described, or if the patient is prevented by traction, multiple rib fractures, or other circumstances from being positioned and clapped upon.

Measures to facilitate the removal of secretions are most likely to succeed in re-expanding a collapsed lobe if the major bronchi are filled with secretions. A branching air bronchogram within the area of atelectasis implies that the major airways are patent and that collapse is not due to large mucous plugs. Figure 4–8 shows the chest radiograph of a young man with left lower-lobe atelectasis complicating a severe, traumatic brainstem injury. Within the area of collapse there is a branching air bronchogram. Chest physiotherapy and other measures failed to re-expand the lobe, and pneumonia developed in the affected area over the next several days. In the study described earlier, atelectasis without an air bronchogram responded favorably to treatment within 48 hours in 83 percent of the patients, while it resolved in only 45 percent of those with air bronchograms regardless of the therapy used.[111]

Other important complications of ARF include cardiac arrhythmias[112,113] and acute gastrointestinal bleeding,[114] the latter of which can be largely prevented by antacid titration of the gastric pH.[115] A number of pulmonary and cardiovascular complications can be detected and should be sought actively on chest radiographs taken in the ICU.[116] Finally, it must be remembered that the catheters and other

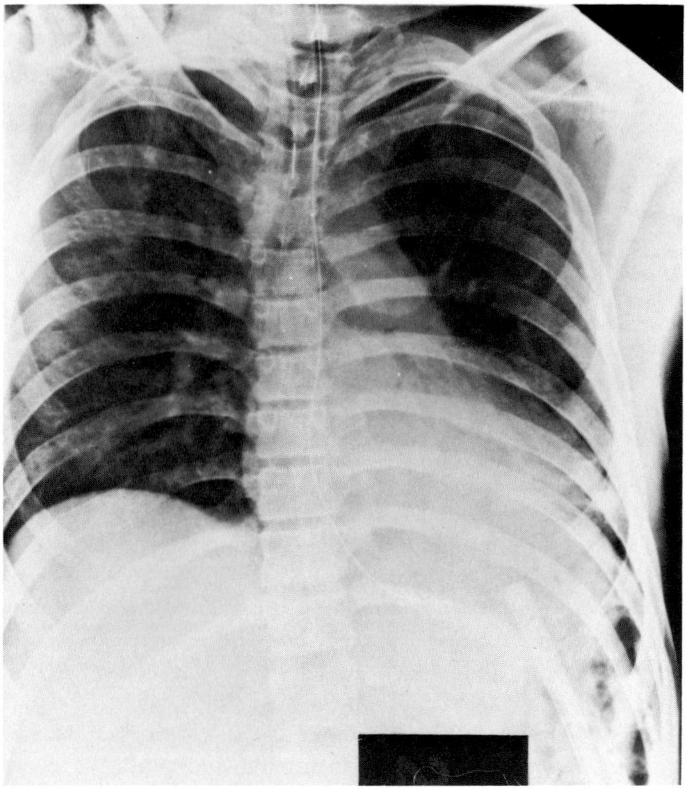

Figure 4–8. Acute atelectasis of left lower lobe. A branching air bronchogram can be seen through the heart shadow, indicating that the lobar bronchus is patent. When this finding is present, mucous plugging and copious secretions are seldom found at bronchoscopy, and the atelectasis responds poorly to therapy.

devices used in monitoring the course and management of ARF can be sources of complications. Thrombosis, ischemia, and cerebral embolization are known complications of radial artery cannulation,[117] and the first two of these increase with the duration of cannulation. Arterial catheters are usually necessary only for pressure monitoring; leaving them in place for several days for convenience in drawing ABG specimens can seldom be justified in view of the risks involved. Pulmonary artery catherization has proved invaluable in the management of severe ARF. However, the Swan-Ganz catheter frequently causes arrhythmias during insertion, and may also lead to subclavian vein thrombosis and catheter-related sepsis.[118] As with all monitoring procedures, the value of the information to be obtained from the pulmonary artery catheter, and the use to which it will be put in clinical management, must be weighed against the hazards of its use.

PROGNOSIS OF ARF

As defined in this chapter, ARF, if untreated, would be fatal in the great majority of patients. Reviews of mixed populations of ARF patients show that across-the-board acute survival with intensive respiratory care has been stable for the last decade at about 75 percent.[54] The prognosis obviously depends upon the underlying health of the patient as well as on the cause and severity of the acute insult. The reported survival rate in ARF complicating COPD ranges from 66 to 76 percent, based upon widely differing management regimens in different areas of the world.[119] Recently, however, it has been suggested that over 90 percent of decompensated COPD patients can be managed successfully, with a 2-year survival that is about the same as that previously reported at the time of hospital discharge.[20] This represents a potential overall improvement in the management of ARF in COPD.

The reported survival rates of patients with the adult respiratory distress syndrome (ARDS) varies with the criteria used in different centers for definition of the syndrome. One estimate made by the National Heart and Lung Institute indicated an average ARDS mortality rate of 40 percent among 150,000 cases in this country each year.[120] Application of more rigorous diagnostic criteria undoubtedly would raise the mortality rate; patients meeting the strict entry criteria for the multi-center ECMO study had an overall survival of 8 percent.[12] Patients who do survive, however, appear to have a good prognosis for the eventual return of their pulmonary function to pre-ARDS levels, although 1 to 2 years may be necessary for this to occur.[121]

REFERENCES

1. Comroe JH Jr, Botelho S: The unreliability of cyanosis in the recognition of arterial anoxemia. Am J Med Sci 214:1, 1947.
2. Mithoefer JD, Bossman OG, Thibeault DW, et al: The clinical estimation of alveolar ventilation. Am Rev Resp Dis 98:868, 1968.
3. Ralph D, Robertson HT: Respiratory gas exchange in adult respiratory distress syndrome. Sem Respir Med 3:114, 1981.
4. Winter PM, Miller JN: Carbon monoxide poisoning. JAMA 236:1502, 1976.
5. Deneke SM, Fanburg BL: Normobaric oxygen toxicity of the lung. N Engl J Med 303:76, 1980.
6. Clark JM, Lambertsen CJ: Pulmonary oxygen toxicity: A review. Pharmacol Rev 23:37, 1971.
7. Greenbaum DM, Miller JE, Eross B, et al: Continuous positive airway pressure without tracheal intubation in spontaneously breathing patients. Chest 69:615, 1976.
8. Smith RA, Kirby RR, Gooding JM, et al: Continuous positive airway pressure (CPAP) by face mask. Crit Care Med 8:483, 1980.
9. Covelli HD, Weled, BJ, Beekman JF: Efficacy of continuous positive airway pressure administered by face mask. Chest 78:513, 1980.
10. Hopewell PC: Adult respiratory distress syndrome. Basics Resp Dis 7(4): 1, 1979.

11. Hudson LD: Ventilatory management of patients with adult respiratory distress syndrome. Sem Respir Med 2:128, 1981.
12. Zapol WM, Snider MT, Hill JD, et al: Extracorporeal membrane oxygenation in severe acute respiratory failure. JAMA 242:2193, 1979.
13. Bendixen HH, Bullwinkel B, Hedley-White J, et al: Atelectasis and shunting during spontaneous ventilation in anesthetized patients. Anesthesiology 25: 297, 1964.
14. Carrico CJ: Pulmonary response to injury. Bull NY Acad Med 55:175, 1979.
15. Hudson LD: Ventilatory management. In ed. Shires GT, Care of the Trauma Patient, 2nd Ed New York, McGraw-Hill, 487, 1979.
16. Crockard HA, Coppel DL, Morrow WFK: Evaluation of hyperventilation in treatment of head injuries. Br Med J 4:634, 1973.
17. Becker DP, Miller JD, Ward JD, et al: The outcome from severe head injury with early diagnosis and intensive management. J Neurosurg 47:491, 1977.
18. Christensen MS, Paulson OB, Oleson J, et al: Cerebral apoplexy (stroke) treated with an without artificial hyperventilation. I. Cerebral circulation, clinical course, and cause of death. Stroke 4:568, 1973.
19. Martin RJ, Rogers RM: The treatment of acute respiratory failure without mechanical ventilation. Med Times 106:31, 1978.
20. Martin TR, Lewis SW, Albert RK: Prognosis of patients with chronic obstructive pulmonary disease after an episode of acute respiratory failure. Chest 78:529, 1980.
21. Bone RC, Pierce AK, Johnson RL Jr: Controlled oxygen administration in acute respiratory failure in chronic obstructive pulmonary disease: A reappraisal. Am J Med 65:896, 1978.
22. Ringel SP, Carroll JE: Respiratory complications of neuromuscular disease. In Respiratory Dysfunction in Neurological Disease, ed. Weiner WJ, Mount Kisco, NY, Futura, 133, 1980.
23. Bendixen HH, Hedley-White J, Laver MB: Impaired oxygenation in surgical patients during general anesthesia with controlled ventilation. A concept of atelectasis. N Engl J Med 269:991, 1963.
24. Egbert LD, Laver MB, Bendixen HH: Intermittent deep breaths and compliance during anesthesia in man. Anesthesiology 24:57, 1963.
25. Visick WD, Fairley HB, Hickey RF: The effects of tidal volume and end-expiratory pressure on pulmonary gas exchange during anesthesia. Anesthesiology 39:285, 1973.
26. Bergman NA: Effect of varying respiratory waveforms on distribution of inspired bas during artificial ventilation. Am Rev Resp Dis 100:518, 1969.
27. Zwillich CW, Pierson DJ, Creagh CE, et al: Complications of assisted ventilation. Am J Med 57:161, 1974.
28. Pontoppidan H, Geffin B, Lowenstein E: Acute respiratory failure in the adult. N Engl J Med 287:690, 743, 799, 1972.
29. Bone RC: Monitoring respiratory function in the patient with the adult respiratory distress syndrome. Sem Respir Med 2:140, 1981.
30. Downs JB, Klein EF Jr, Desautels D, et al: Intermittent mandatory ventilation: A new approach to weaning patients from mechanical ventilators. Chest 64:331, 1973.
31. Klein EF Jr: Weaning from mechanical breathing with intermittent mandatory ventilation. Arch Surg 110:345, 1975.
32. Luce JM, Pierson DJ, Hudson LD: Intermittent mandatory ventilation: A critical review. Chest 79:678, 1981.

33. Williams MH Jr: IMV and weaning. Chest 78:804, 1980.
34. Rochester DF, Braun NMT: The respiratory muscles. Basics Resp Dis 6(4):1, 1978.
35. Ashutosh K, Gilbert R, Auchincloss JH, et al: Asynchronous breathing movements in patients with chronic obstructive pulmonary disease. Chest 67:553, 1975.
36. Sharp JT, Goldberg NB, Druz WS, et al: Thoracoabdominal motion in chronic obstructive pulmonary disease. Am Rev Resp Dis 115:47, 1977.
37. Gilbert R, Ashutosh K, Auchincloss JH, et al: Prospective study of controlled oxygen therapy. Poor prognosis of patients with asynchronous breathing. Chest 71:456, 1977.
38. Downs JB, Perkins HM, Modell JH: Intermittent mandatory ventilation: An evaluation. Arch Surg 109:519, 1974.
39. Rochester DF, Braun NMT, Laine S: Diaphragmatic energy expenditure in chronic respiratory failure: The effect of assisted ventilation with body respirators. Am J Med 63:223, 1977.
40. Hudson LD: Diagnosis and management of acute respiratory distress in patients on mechanical ventilators. In Respiratory Emergencies, eds. Shibel EM, Moser KM, St. Louis, CV Mosby, 207, 1977.
41. Roizen MF, Feeley TW: Pancuronium bromide. Ann Intern Med 88:64, 1978.
42. Lakshminarayan S, Sahn SA, Hudson LD: Treatment of status asthmaticus (Letter). Br Med J 1:611, 1973.
43. Birnbaum ML, Cree EM, Rasmussen H, et al: Effects of intermittent positive-pressure breathing on emphysematous patients. Am J Med 41:552, 1966.
44. Sukumalchantra Y, Park SS, Williams MH Jr: The effect of intermittent positive-pressure breathing in acute ventilatory failure. Am Rev Resp Dis 92:885, 1965.
45. Hudson LD: Is IPPB effective: A controversy in respiratory therapy. Primary Care 5:529, 1978.
46. Pierson DJ: Respiratory stimulants: Review of the literature and assessment of current status. Respir Care 18:549, 1973.
47. Canter HG, Luchsinger PC: The treatment of respiratory failure without mechanical assistance. Am J Med Sci 106:206, 1964.
48. Edwards G, Leszczynski SO: A double-blind trial of five respiratory stimulants in patients with acute ventilatory failure. Lancet 2:226, 1967.
49. Moser KM, Luchsinger PC, Adamson JS, et al: Respiratory stimulation with intravenous doxapram in respiratory failure: A double-blind study. N Engl J Med 288:427, 1973.
50. Wolfson BE, Siker ES, Ciccarelli OO: A double-blind comparison of doxapram, ethamivan, and methylphenidate. Am J Med Sci 249:391, 1965.
51. Winnie AP, Collins VJ: The search for a pharmacologic ventilator. Anesthesiology 26:265, 1965.
52. Bone RC: Treatment of respiratory failure due to advanced chronic obstructive lung disease. Arch Intern Med 140:1018, 1980.
53. Ohi M, Nakashima M, Heki S, et al: Doxapram hydrochloride in the treatment of acute exacerbation of chronic respiratory failure. Chest 74:453, 1978.
54. Petty TL, Lakshminarayan S, Sahn SA, et al: Intensive respiratory care unit: Review of ten years' experience JAMA 233:34, 1975.
55. Zwillich CW, Kryger M, Weil JV: Hypoventilation: Consequences and management. Adv Intern Med 23:287, 1978.
56. Shibel EM: Acute respiratory failure with hypercapnia. In Respiratory Emergencies, eds. Shibel EM, Moser KM, St. Louis, CV Mosby, 85, 1977.

57. Sjöstrand U: High-frequency positive-pressure ventilation (HFPPV): a review. Crit Care Med 8:345, 1980.
58. Sjöstrand U ed.: Experimental and clinical evaluation of high-frequency positive-pressure ventilation. Acta Anaesthesiol Scand (Suppl) 64:1, 1977.
59. Carlon GC, Ray C Jr, Klain M, McCormack PM: High-frequency positive-pressure ventilation in management of a patient with bronchopleural fistula. Anethesiology 52:160, 1980.
60. Kirby RR: High-frequency positive-pressure ventilation (HFPPV): What role in ventilatory insufficiency? Anesthesiology 52:109, 1980.
61. Sahn SA, Lakshminarayan S, Petty TL: Weaning from mechanical ventilation JAMA 235:2208, 1976.
62. Bowser MA, Hodgkin JE, Burton GG: Techniques of ventilator weaning. In Respiratory Care, eds. Burton GG, Gee GN, Hodgkin JE, Philadelphia, JB Lippincott, 664, 1977.
63. Gilbert R, Auchincloss JH Jr, Peppi D, et al: The first few hours off a respirator. Chest 65:152, 1974.
64. Milbern SM, Downs JB, Jumper LC, et al: Evaluation of criteria for discontinuing mechanical ventilatory support. Arch Surg 113:1441, 1978.
65. Schachter EN, Tucker D: The impact of intermittent mandatory ventilation on the weaning of patients in respiratory failure. (Abstract). Chest 76:366, 1979.
66. Newman JH, Neff TA, Ziporin P: Acute respiratory failure associated with hypophosphatemia. N Engl J Med 296:1101, 1977.
67. Blackburn GL, Maini BS, Pierce EC Jr: Nutrition in the critically ill patient. Anesthesiology 47:181, 1977.
68. Doekel RC, Zwillich CW, Scoggin CH, et al: Clinical semi-starvation: Depression of hypoxic ventilatory response. N Engl J Med 295:358, 1976.
69. Pflug AE, Murphy TM, Butler SH, et al: The effects of postoperative peridural analgesia on pulmonary therapy and pulmonary complications. Anesthesiology 41:8, 1974.
70. Sahn SA, Lakshminarayan S: Bedside criteria for discontinuation of mechanical ventilation. Chest 63:1002, 1973.
71. Zwillich CW, Pierson DJ: Nasal necrosis: A complication of nasotracheal intubation. Chest 64:376, 1973.
72. Wanner A: Clinical aspects of mucociliary transport. Am Rev Resp Dis 116:73, 1977.
73. Conference on the scientific basis of in-hospital respiratory therapy. Am Rev Resp Dis (Suppl)122:1, 1980.
74. Chopra SK, Taplin GV, Simmons DH, et al: Effects of hydration and physical therapy on tracheal transport velocity. Am Rev Resp Dis 115:1009, 1977.
75. Forbes AR: Humidification and mucous flow in the intubated trachea. Br J Anaesth 45:118, 1973.
76. Conference on the scientific basis of respiratory therapy. Am Rev Resp Dis (Suppl)110:1, 1974.
77. Tisi GM: Preoperative evaluation of pulmonary function. Am Rev Resp Dis 119:293, 1979.
78. Thorén L: Post-operative pulmonary complications: Observations on their prevention by means of physiotherapy. Acta Chir Scand 107:193, 1954.

79. Stein M, Cassara EL: Preoperative pulmonary evaluation and therapy for surgery patients. JAMA 211:787, 1970.
80. Murray JF: The ketchup-bottle method. N Engl J Med 300:1155, 1979.
81. Graham WGB, Bradley DA: Efficacy of chest physiotherapy and intermittent positive-pressure breathing in the resolution of pneumonia. N Engl J Med 299:264, 1978.
82. Anthonisen P, Riis P, Sogaard-Andersen T: The value of lung physiotherapy in the treatment of acute exacerbations in chronic bronchitis. Acta Med Scand 175:715, 1964.
83. Campbell AH, O'Connell JM, Wilson F: The effect of chest physiotherapy upon the FEV_1 in chronic bronchitis. Med J Aust 1:33, 1975.
84. Leading article: Mechanical chest physiotherapy. Lancet 2:129, 1979.
85. Maxwell M, Redmond A: Comparative trial of manual and mechanical percussion technique with gravity-assisted bronchial drainage techniques in patients with cystic fibrosis. Arch Dis Child 54:542, 1979.
86. Remolina C, Khan AU, Santiago TV, et al: Positional hypoxemia in unilateral lung disease. N Engl J Med 304:523, 1981.
87. Zack MB, Pontoppidan H, Kazami H: The effect of lateral positions on gas exchange in pulmonary disease: A prospective evaluation. Am Rev Resp Dis 110:49, 1974.
88. Fishman AP: Down with the good lung. N Engl J Med 304:537, 1981.
89. Douglas WW, Rehder K, Beynen FM, et al: Improved oxygenation in patients with acute respiratory failure: The prone position. Am Rev Resp Dis 115:559, 1977.
90. Urban BJ, Weitzner SW: Avoidance of hypoxemia during endotracheal suction. Anesthesiology 31:473, 1969.
91. Petersen GM, Pierson DJ, Hunter PM: Arterial oxygen saturation during nasotracheal suctioning. Chest 76:283, 1979.
92. Shim C, Fine N, Fernandez R, et al: Cardiac arrhythmias resulting from tracheal suctioning. Ann Intern Med 71:1149, 1969.
93. Fineberg C, Cohn HE, Gibbon JH Jr: Cardiac arrest during nasotracheal aspiration. JAMA 174:410, 1960.
94. LeFrock JL, Klainer AS, Wu W-H, et al: Transient bacteremia associated with nasotracheal suctioning. JAMA 236:1610, 1976.
95. Hodgkin JE, ed: Chronic obstructive pulmonary disease. Park Ridge, IL, American College of Chest Physicians, 1979.
96. Burrows B: Course and prognosis of advanced disease. In Chronic Obstructive Pulmonary Disease, ed. Petty TL, New York, Marcel Dekker, 23, 1978.
97. Hudson LD, Pierson DJ: Comprehensive respiratory care for patients with chronic obstructive pulmonary disease. Med Clin North Am 65:629, 1981.
98. Paterson JW, Woolcock AJ, Shenfield GM: Bronchodilator drugs. Am Rev Resp Dis 120:1149, 1979.
99. Webb-Johnson DC, Andrews JL: Bronchodilator therapy. N Engl J Med 297:476, 758, 1977.
100. Powell JR, Vozah S, Hopewell P, et al: Theophylline disposition in acutely ill hospitalized patients. Am Rev Resp Dis 118:229, 1978.
101. I.V. dosage guidelines for theophylline products. FDA Drug Bull 10:4, 1980.
102. Marini JJ, Lakshminarayan S: The effect of atropine inhalation in "irreversible" chronic bronchitis. Chest 77:591, 1980.

103. Scoggin CH, Sahn SA, Petty TL: Status asthmaticus. A nine-year experience. JAMA 238:1158, 1977.
104. Albert RK, Martin TR, Lewis SW: Controlled clinical trial of methylprednisolone in patients with chronic bronchitis and acute respiratory insufficiency. Ann Intern Med 92:753, 1980.
105. Tager I, Speizer FE: Role of infection in chronic bronchitis. N Engl J Med 292:563, 1975.
106. Gump DW, Phillips CA, Forsyth BR, et al: The role of infection in chronic bronchitis. Am Rev Resp Dis 113:465, 1976.
107. Fein A, Leff, A, Hopewell PC: Pathophysiology and management of the complications resulting from fire and the inhaled products of combustion: Review of the literature. Crit Care Med 8:94, 1980.
108. Pierson DJ: Respiratory complications in the burned patient: Pathophysiology and management. Respir Care 21:123, 1976.
109. Burke JF, Pontoppidan H, Welch CE: High output respiratory failure: An important cause of death ascribed to peritonitis or ileus. Ann Surg 158:581, 1963.
110. Mahajan VK, Catron PW, Huber GL: The value of fiberoptic bronchoscopy in the management of pulmonary collapse. Chest 73:817, 1978.
111. Marini JJ, Pierson DJ, Hudson LD: Acute lobar atelectasis: A prospective comparison of fiberoptic bronchoscopy and respiratory therapy. Am Rev Resp Dis 119:971, 1979.
112. Hudson LD, Kurt TL, Petty TL, et al: Arrhythmias associated with acute respiratory failure in patients with chronic airway obstruction. Chest 63:661, 1973.
113. Holford FD, Mithoefer JC: Cardiac arrhythmias in hospitalized patients with chronic obstructive pulmonary disease. Am Rev Resp Dis 108:879, 1973.
114. Harris SK, Bone RC, Ruth WE: Gastrointestinal hemorrhage in patients in a respiratory intensive care unit. Chest 72:301, 1977.
115. Hastings PR, Skillman JJ, Bushnell LS, et al: Antacid titration in the prevention of acute gastrointestinal bleeding. N Engl J Med 298:1041, 1978.
116. Eaton RJ, Senior RM, Pierce JA: Aspects of respiratory care pertinent to the radiologist. Radiol Clin North Am 11:93, 1973.
117. Brodsky J: Radial artery cannulation. West J Med 131:234, 1979.
118. Elliott CG, Zimmerman GA, Clemmer TP: Complications of pulmonary artery catheterization in the care of critically ill patients. Chest 76:647, 1979.
119. Pierson DJ: When to hospitalize the COPD patient. Chest 73:126, 1978.
120. Respiratory Diseases: Task force report on problems: Research approaches and needs. NIH Publication No. 73–432. Department of Health, Education, and Welfare, Washington DC, 171, 1972.
121. Lakshminarayan S, Hudson LD: Pulmonary function following the adult respiratory distress syndrome (ARDS). Semin Respir Med 2:160, 1981.

5

Acute Asthma and Status Asthmaticus

Charles H. Scoggin, M.D.

INTRODUCTION

Asthma is a ubiquitous respiratory disorder, occurring in the elderly as well as the young and middle aged. Both sexes are affected, although for reasons that are not clear, women tend to have more severe asthma than men.

In this chapter we will consider the most severe form of asthma, acute asthma, and its possible sequela, status asthmaticus. Fortunately, most asthmatics never experience a life-threatening attack of acute asthma; however, for those patients in whom such asthma occurs, skillful medical attention may mean the difference between life and death. The clinical strategies for the management of these patients should be based upon an understanding of the factors that may precipitate acute asthma, the pathophysiologic basis of the attacks in this condition, the clinical manifestations of the disorder, the rational use of the laboratory in the assessment of the patient, the therapeutic modalities used to treat asthma, and errors to be avoided in treating acute asthma and status asthmaticus.

UNDERSTANDING ASTHMA

Asthma results in airflow obstruction characterized by episodic shortness of breath, usually accompanied by wheezing and coughing.[1] Patients with asthma have hyperirritable airways. Stimuli to such airways accentuate the normal reactivity of the tracheobronchial tree. Irritant receptors within the airways, when stimulated, lead to the reactions of cough and bronchoconstriction. The abnormalities of asthma may be precipitated by a number of causes. Acute attacks may be brought on by infection (usually viral), exercise, allergies, emotional stress, environmental factors such as cold and wind, occupational exposures, pharmacologic agents (such as aspirin) and maneuvers which lead to distortion of the airways, such as coughing and laughing.

HOW MAY ACUTE ATTACKS OF ASTHMA BE PRECIPITATED?

As mentioned to above, respiratory tract infection, particularly viral, is probably the most important precipitating factor in acute asthma.[2] Although such bacterial infections as pneumonia may be seen in association with asthma, these are usually the consequence rather than the cause of acute asthma. A common occurrence is that a patient predisposed to asthma will develop a viral upper respiratory infection and have a 2- to 3-day "grace period" during which the asthma remains stable. Subsequently, the asthmatic develops a cough with associated wheezing and shortness of breath. It is our practice to recommend to patients with known asthma that they commence bronchodilator therapy upon the emergence of lower respiratory tract symptoms such as a cough. Other factors that may lead to an acute asthmatic attack include emotional upset, inhalation of substances which are irritating to the airways, such as cold air or gases like chlorine, exposure to pollens or dust to which the patient is sensitive, physical factors such as exercise or the breathing of cold air, and certain drugs, usually nonsteroidal and anti-inflammatory medications such as aspirin.

HOW DOES THE EXPOSURE TO A PRECIPITATING EVENT LEAD TO AN ACUTE ATTACK OF ASTHMA?

It is the hyperirritability of the tracheobronchial tree that predisposes asthmatics to acute attacks. Exogenous or endogenous stimuli lead to a cascade of either neurogenically or chemically mediated events which result in airways obstruction. Airways obstruction not only is due to bronchial smooth-muscle constriction, but also to mucosal edema of the airways.[3] A particularly important and sometimes unappreciated factor promoting airways obstruction is the excessive production of mucus.[4] Because mucus may be a prominent factor in airflow limitation, physical measures such as chest percussion, the inhalation of moisture, and supervised coughing are important in improving airflow when excessive mucus is produced. It is also likely that there is a physical distortion of the airways of asthmatic patients as a consequence of air trapping. Trapped air in the lung does not actively participate in gas exchange, and may infringe upon the contiguous airways, further impairing pulmonary function.

As a consequence of airflow obstruction, four physiologic abnormalities occur which are reflected in the arterial blood gases:[5] (1) a mismatching of blood flow and ventilation (V/Q abnormalities), leading to arterial hypoxemia; (2) if the asthmatic attack progresses, airways resistance increases which contributes to alveolar hypoventilation; (3) when alveolar hypoventilation occurs, the arterial PCO_2 rises and respiratory acidemia results ($pH < 7.35$ with $PCO_2 > 45$ mmHg); and (4) as the work of breathing increases due to the marked airways resistance and trapped air, particularly in the face of arterial hypoxemia, lactic acid is generated by the respiratory muscles and a combined metabolic and respiratory acidosis occurs. This is the hallmark of life-threatening asthma. Thus, uncontrolled asthma can lead to a cascade of potentially fatal events, with systemic acidosis superimposed upon arterial hypoxemia. The result is a potential disaster, characterized by central nervous system depression, cardiovascular instability, cardiac arrhythmias, and death.

MANAGEMENT OF ACUTE ASTHMA

As with any life-threatening illness, the management of acute asthma necessitates an organized approach. Since time is of the essence, certain measures directed toward stabilizing the patient require immediate initiation upon establishing the diagnosis of acute asthma.

Initial Management

The first-step in the management of acute asthma is to ensure that the patient is oxygenated adequately, since all patients with acute asthma will have some degree of hypoxemia from V/Q mismatching. Oxygen (2 to 6 L/min by nasal prongs) should be administered. Since patients with asthma do not as a rule develop carbon dioxide retention as a consequence of high-flow oxygen, oxygen usually can be administered safely in this setting. The carbon dioxide retention that can occur in asthma usually is due primarily to mechanical hypoventilation rather than to the depression respiratory drives.

Establishing the Diagnosis

Fortunately, most patients with asthma will never experience an acute, life-threatening attack. In those patients who do, the disorder tends to be recurrent; thus, the majority of patients who suffer an acute attack will be able to equate their symptomatology with uncontrolled asthma. A small minority of patients will not have experienced such symptoms previously and will, therefore, not be able to identify their problem as related to asthma. The history and physical examination will help substantiate the diagnosis. Important symptoms to be sought are cough, wheezing, a previous history of such episodes, and a family history of asthma. Some other points of the history are also important.

Importance of the History

The following four historical points should be obtained initially.

1. Can a precipitating factor for the acute asthmatic attack be identified? A recent history of respiratory tract infection is strong circumstantial evidence as to the etiology. Other factors, such as emotional stress or a change in the drugs used to manage chronic asthma should not be overlooked.
2. What are the medications that the patient has been taking? In drug-associated asthma, the history of recent ingestion of a medication such as aspirin may give a clue as to what precipitated the acute asthmatic attack. It is vital

that patients be questioned about medications they may have been taking for their asthma. For instance, if the patient has been taking a theophylline compound prior to coming to the emergency room or clinic, intravenous aminophylline should not be administered in a loading dose; instead, maintenance therapy should be begun and continued until the serum theophylline level can be documented. When an excessive amount of beta-adrenergic stimulants has been used, often in inhaled form, then the suspicion of drug tachyphylaxis should be considered.[6] If tachyphylaxis is suspected, early corticosteroid therapy should be given.

3. Does the patient have any known allergies? This is particularly important if antibiotics are going to be used. Although it is rare, some patients also have allergic reactions to corticosteroids[7]: thus, a corticosteroid preparation to which these patients are not sensitive should be employed.
4. Are there any coexisting medical conditions that might be influenced by management of the asthma? This is particularly important in older patients. The use of medications such as isoproterenol, which have appreciable cardiac side-effects, may aggravate other conditions such as coronary artery disease. It is also important to consider other medical conditions that may masquerade as asthma. For instance, a patient who appears to have asthma may in fact be experiencing congestive heart failure as a result of primary cardiac disease.[8] Rarely, other disorders, such as pulmonary embolism[9] and tracheal carcinoma, may masquerade as asthma.

Physical Examination

As with the history, a complete physical examination should not be performed initially; thorough evaluation should be reserved until the patient is stable. Particular aspects of the examination should be done because the findings from these will have an impact on patient management.

The respiratory rate, heart rate, and temperature should be recorded as part of the initial evaluation of asthma. A respiratory rate of greater than 32/min and a heart rate of greater than 120/min are signs of severe asthma. The presence of fever suggests that infection may be the cause of the exacerbation. The blood pressure is also important in the evaluation of asthma. It has been observed that a pulsus paradoxus of greater than 20 mmHg is an indication of severe asthma, usually requiring hospitalization.[10] Hypertension is often associated with an acute attack of asthma. This usually resolves with therapy and does not necessarily mean that the patient has chronic hypertension.

Attention should also be paid to the upper airway of patients with acute attacks of asthma. Rarely, upper airway obstruction due to tumor, goiter, or even a foreign body may present with symptoms identical to those in asthma.[11] Compromise of the upper airway may lead to expansion of the thorax due to trapping of air within the lungs. Auscultation over the larynx and trachea of such patients will usually disclose localized wheezing. In contrast, the lung sounds may be so diminished so as to be inaudible. It is important to inspect the nose for nasal polyps. Should the necessity arise to intubate the patient, the presence of large nasal polyps is a contraindication to the nasal tracheal route of intubation. An association apparently exists between sinusitis and worsening asthma.[12] If there are physical findings of sinusitis, part of the management of the patient should include nasal decongestants and antibiotics.

Examination of the chest in acute asthma may be misleading. Because of severe airways obstruction, patients may not be moving a large enough volume of air to generate the sounds of wheezing. In fact, in these patients, the emergence of wheezing is actually a good prognostic sign. It denotes that enough air is entering and leaving the thoracic cavity to generate breath sounds. In most asthmatics, wheezing should be heard diffusely; localized wheezing suggests a bronchial lesion; and the absence of wheezing on one side of the chest may indicate a pneumothorax. Finally, if rales are heard in the chest, either congestive heart failure or pneumonia should be considered.

Laboratory Examination

An important philosophy to be maintained in utilizing the laboratory in the assessment of acute asthma is whether the data obtained will influence management of the patient. Careful selection of tests will increase the cost-effective utilization of the laboratory, decrease expensive and often painful procedures, and also minimize laboratory-associated complications. Diagnostic tests such as chest radiographs and arterial blood measurements gas are probably overutilized. In fact, both the cost and discomfort associated with such studies may cause some patients to defer seeking medical attention until their asthma is out of control.

Because asthma is a disorder characterized by airflow obstruction, tests designed to measure the amount of such airflow obstruction are the most important means for managing and assessing acute asthma. Two types of tests may be practically employed. These are the peak flow rate, and the forced vital capacity (FVC) and forced expiratory volume in the first second (FEV_1). Both tests have their limitations, in that they are effort-dependent; however, when properly instructed, the majority of patients are cooperative, and the results obtained are therefore medically valid. These tests are noninvasive, easily performed at the bedside, and give immediate, useful information. They not only provide information which is important in assessing the severity of asthma, but also provide a measure by which the response to therapy may be followed. Each type of test will be briefly discussed below.

Peak Expiratory Flow Rate

This may be measured using a simple, hand-held, inexpensive device. In Table 5–1 we have presented a method of classifying the severity of asthma according to either the peak expiratory flow rate or the FEV_1. This classification is of clinical use, since the three stages shown in the table have been demonstrated to correlate with blood gas abnormalities.[5] Patients with stage 1 asthma may show arterial hypoxemia, but rarely have carbon dioxide retention with respiratory acidemia.

Table 5–1. Noninvasive Assessment of Acute Asthma in Adults

Stage	Respiratory Parameters
1	FEV_1 > 2 L, PEFR > 200 L/min
2	FEV_1 1–2 L, PEFR 80–200 L/min
3	FEV_1 < 1 L, PEFR < 80 L/min

Stage 2 asthma is associated with either a normal or elevated carbon dioxide tension in the arterial blood. When stage 3 asthma has been reached, respiratory failure and acidemia are present, and the asthma may be rightfully regarded as life-threatening. The peak expiratory flow rate has certain advantages over the FEV_1; it does not require the patient to expel the entire vital capacity. In contrast, in order to derive a value for the FEV_1, the patient must inspire maximally and expel the inspired volume as rapidly as possible. This may result in irritation of the airways and the further provocation of bronchial spasm.[13]

Bedside Spirometry

The term "bedside spirometry" does not downgrade the important role of simple spirometry; rather, spirometry at the bedside provides useful information. The FVC and FEV_1 are important indices of pulmonary function. An improvement in the FEV_1 is a good prognostic sign, indicating that the patient is responding to treatment; however, it should be remembered that in some patients, the improvement in the FEV_1 may lag behind the improvement in the FVC.[14] This means that the patient has less trapped air in the lungs but still has airway obstruction. As the FVC continues to improve, it is reasonable to expect that the FEV_1 will follow suit. It should be emphasized that regardless of which bedside test of airflow is performed, its importance revolves about its noninvasive nature, convenience of performance, and capacity to demonstrate trends of improvement which correlate with the clinical response to therapy. While no improvement in pulmonary function may be seen initially in patients with severe asthma, even though they are apparently responding to therapy, a consistent lack of improvement in pulmonary function tests should lead the clinician to suspect that all is not well. For this reason, the evaluation of oxygenation and carbon dioxide elimination remain important in many patients.

Arterial Blood Gases

Arterial blood gas measurements are used to determine the efficiency of oxygen transport across the lung, CO_2 homeostasis, and acid-base balance. Since stage 1 asthma is rarely associated with respiratory acidemia, and supplementary oxygen usually serves to correct stage 1 hypoxemia, patients in this stage of asthma do not need routine arterial blood gas determinations. The situation is different in stages 2 and 3 asthma. If the patient with stage 2 asthma does not respond to therapy within the first 30 minutes to 1 hour, an arterial blood gas determination should be done; at this point the patient may be developing carbon dioxide retention and require hospitalization. In stage 3 asthma, carbon dioxide retention and acidemia are almost universally present; even the use of high-flow oxygen does not necessarily assure that the patient will be normoxemic. If the patient with stage 2 or stage 3 asthma shows blood gas abnormalities, the blood gas determination should be repeated only if the patient does not appear to be responding to therapy or is deteriorating. Thus, the clinical strategy in stage 3 asthma would be to measure an arterial blood gas, initiate therapy, and only perform a second arterial blood gas or serial arterial blood gas determinations if the patient does not improve or deteriorates.

The patient with chronic obstructive lung disease may represent a different situation. These patients may have an asthmatic component to their disorder, and present with acute respiratory failure that is analogous to acute asthma. In this setting, low-flow oxygen should be given and the response documented with an arterial blood gas determination. Correction of hypoxemia in these patients may lead to changes in their respiratory drive as well as pulmonary circulation which result in carbon dioxide retention and acidemia.[15] Because these changes may not be clinically apparent, the documentation of responses by arterial blood gas determination is important.

Chest Radiograph

Like the arterial blood gas determination, the chest radiograph is overutilized in the assessment of acute asthma. Routine chest radiographs should not be obtained in all asthmatics presenting with acute asthma; however, if fever or pleurisy is present, or there is reason to suspect some other diagnosis, such as congestive heart failure, a chest radiograph should be done. Because of the extremely lability of asthma, it is important that such patients be accompanied to the radiology department by a nurse or some other health-care professional. In the majority cases of acute asthma, the chest radiograph shows only hyperinflation.[16] As with the arterial blood gas determination, the chest radiograph should be done only if there is a suspicion that the findings will appreciably change the management of the patient.

Blood Tests

If infection is suspected or hospitalization is anticipated, a complete blood count should be done on the acutely asthmatic patient. An elevation of the leukocyte count may represent the response to stress, acute hypoxemia, or the effect of medication, such as subcutaneous epinephrine or intravenous corticosteroids. The degree of eosinophilia may be important. It has been reported that some individuals with asthma may show a relative resistance to systemic corticosteroid therapy which correlates with the persistence of peripheral blood eosinophilia.[17] Correlation of the remission of asthma with the disappearance of eosinophilia may be a measure by which a beneficial response to corticosteroid therapy is inferred. While not specific, an elevation of the hematocrit may signal dehydration and indicate a need for vigorous fluid replacement.

Sputum Examination

While cough is often a prominent feature in an uncomplicated acute asthmatic attack, sputum production is usually scanty. The mucus produced in acute asthma may be so tenacious as to prevent easy expectoration. When bronchodilator therapy is used in combination with chest physiotherapy, many patients begin to produce sputum. The production of sputum in this setting is a good prognostic sign. It indicates that substantial bronchodilatation has occurred, allowing an amount of air to be inhaled that is adquate to generate an effective cough. Patients who have a cough productive of purulent sputum should be suspected of having an infection. Examination of the sputum using the Gram-stain technique is helpful. The finding of a predominant bacterial organism such as *Streptococcus pneumoniae* in association with polymorphonuclear leukocytes should suggest either acute bronchitis or pneumonitis. It is important to remember that some patients with allergic asthma may have a marked sputum eosinophilia, and that a "purulent" sputum may result as a consequence of eosinophilia. Examination of the sputum by the Wright or Hansel stain should establish such a condition. A finding which may occur in the sputum of asthmatics is that of bronchial casts. These have been named "Curschmann's spirals," and represent the consequence of inspissated bronchial mucus.

TREATMENT

Once oxygen therapy has been initiated to correct hypoxemia, the necessary history and physical information have been obtained as outlined above, appropriate laboratory evaluations have been initiated, and the diagnosis of asthma has been established, specific treatment to control the acute attack of asthma should begin.

An approach to the management of the patient with acute asthma is outlined in Table 5-2. This revolves around the so-called "ABC's of asthma." That is, intravenous aminophylline, beta-adrenergic medications, and corticosteroids. The use of these medications in the treatment of asthma is analogous to the use of antihypertensive medications in controlling blood pressure; they should be added in stepwise fashion. If an agent fails to control an acute attack of asthma, it should not be abandoned, but rather another class of medications should be added.

Beta-Adrenergic Medications

Recent information suggests that the beta-adrenergic medications are superior to theophyllines as first-line drugs for controlling acute asthma.[18] These medications have the advantage over intravenous aminophylline because they are administered easily, may be given by a variety of routes, and have absorption and clearance characteristics that do not require the monitoring of blood levels. Because of the irritable nature of the asthmatic airway, some patients cannot tolerate inhaled forms of these medications. In this case, the subcutaneous (or in

Table 5–2. Emergency Treatment of Acute Asthma

Start nasal oxygen at 2 to 6 L/min
(oxygen may alternatively be delivered by mask)

Administer beta-adrenergic medication
Epinephrine 1:1000 subcutaneously
$<$ 60 kg body weight = 0.3 ml
60–80 kg body weight = 0.4 ml
$>$ 80 kg body weight = 0.5 ml
or
Terbutaline sulfate subcutaneously 0.25 mg
or
Inhaled isoetharine mesylate 0.5 ml via nebulizer diluted 1:3 with saline or water
or
Inhaled metaproterenol sulfate 0.3 ml via nebulizer diluted 1:3 with saline or water

If no improvement in 15 to 30 minutes, repeat beta adrenergic medication

If no better in 15 to 30 minutes, insert intravenous line and start aminophylline
If patient taking theophylline preparation, start i.v. infusion at 0.6 mg/kg/hr
If patient not taking theophylline preparation load with iv aminophylline 3–5 mg/kg in dextrose and water over 20 minutes and start maintenance infusion as above
Decrease maintenance dosage and infusion rate by one-half for patients with heart disease or liver disease
If patient fails to improve or if theophylline toxicity suspected, use serum theophylline level to guide therapy

If no improvement in 1 to 2 hours after first starting intravenous aminophylline add either:
Inhaled atropine 1 to 3 mg via nebulizer (usually used in patients with cough as prominent complaint)
or
Intravenous corticosteroids (100 mg hydrocortisone or equivalent or more q 6 hrs)

Continue beta adrenergics (usually as q. 4 h. treatments by inhalation) and intravenous aminophylline

other countries, intravenous) route is the mode of choice. In at least one study, no discernable difference could be established in the tolerance to intravenous versus inhaled beta-adrenergic drugs.[18] There are no absolute contraindications to the use of the beta-adrenergic medications. However, because even the relatively selective beta-2 adrenergic medications may have some effect on the cardiovascular system, beta-adrenergic medications should be given with caution to patients with underlying cardiac disease or to those with heart rates greater than 130 beats per minute.[19]

The approach to the average-sized adult, who has been taking no medications and presents in the emergency room with acute asthma, would be to administer either 0.4 ml of 1:1000 epinephrine subcutaneously, or terbutaline sulfate 0.25 mg subcutaneously. An alternative approach would be to give either isoetharine 0.5 ml by nebulizer, diluted with saline or water for inhalation, or inhaled metaproterenol solution 0.3 cc by nebulizer. If no improvement occurs within 15 to 30 minutes, the medication should be repeated. As will be discussed below, tachyphylaxis may occur in patients who have been using excessive amounts of beta-adrenergic agents in an attempt to control their asthma.[6] In such patients it may not be necessary to abandon the use of beta-adrenergic drugs, but only to restore

Table 5–3. Factors Which Influence the Metabolism of Theophylline (Aminophylline)

Increase Metabolism	Decrease Metabolism
Cigarette smoking	Liver disease
Childhood	Congestive heart failure
	Chronic obstructive lung disease
	Pneumonia

responsiveness to them by the use of corticosteroids. In the patient who fails to respond to beta adrenergic medications, intravenous aminophylline should be begun.

Aminophylline

Aminophylline is the intravenous form of theophylline. Its mechanism of action is thought to be through inhibition of the enzyme phosphodiesterase, which breaks down 3′, 5′-cyclic adenosine monophosphate (cAMP)—a compound thought to promote bronchodilation.[20] The use of aminophylline in the treatment of acute asthma is well established: Both the toxicity and the efficacy of theophylline are related to its serum blood levels[21]; the metabolism of theophylline varies from one individual to another, and is influenced by coexisting clinical conditions. Table 5-3 outlines some of the factors known to influence theophylline metabolism. Some points relative to the use of this medication deserve emphasis.

Patients taking a theophylline compound at the time of an acute asthmatic attack should not receive a loading dosage of this medication. Although such patients may not have therapeutic levels of theophylline, the blind administration of a loading dose—without a direct measurement of the serum theophylline level—may lead to theophylline toxicity in patients who have therapeutic theophylline levels. Ideally, it would be desirable to be able to rapidly measure the theophylline level and to formulate a clinical judgement on this basis; however, even under ideal circumstances, it takes approximately 30 minutes to 1 hour to obtain a serum theophylline level, and in most patients it may therefore be necessary to begin theophylline therapy prior to the return of serum level results from the laboratory. In such a case, maintenance theophylline therapy should be started and the rate of administration adjusted when the baseline theophylline level is obtained. In certain clinical conditions the loading dose of theophylline must be reduced. This is particularly important in patients with liver disease or hepatic congestion secondary to heart failure. In addition, such patients also should have their maintenance rate of theophylline infusion decreased, as outlined in Table 5-4. It should be emphasized that general recommendations for the loading and maintenance doses of theophylline may vary from one individual to another. Thus, the only way to be absolutely certain that a patient is receiving either a therapeutic and nontoxic dose of theophylline is to measure the serum theophylline level.

Table 5–4. Maintenance Aminophylline Infusion to Obtain Theophylline Concentration of 10 μg/ml

Normal	0.6 mg/kg/hour
Smoker	0.8 mg/kg/hour
Congestive heart failure	0.2 mg/kg/hour
Pneumonia	0.2 mg/kg/hour
Severe chronic obstructive lung disease	0.4 mg/kg/hour

Adapted from Powell JR, Vozeh S, Hopewell P, et al: Theophylline disposition in acutely ill hospitalized patients. The effect of smoking, heart failure, severe airway obstruction, and pneumonia. Am Rev Resp Dis 118:229–238, 1978.

Once this level is determined, the rate of theophylline administration can be manipulated as shown in Table 5-5 to approach the desired level.

In general, the side effects of intravenous theophylline correlate with serum theophylline levels. However, some patients display a surprising degree of tolerance to high levels, while others have symptoms with subtherapeutic levels. Some patients may have no side effects with serum theophylline levels of 30 μg/ml, while others will develop severe symptoms with levels below 15 μg/ml. The side effects of theophylline include nausea, vomiting, diarrhea, tachycardia, tachyarrhythmias, insomnia, central nervous excitation, and seizures. These side effects are unusual with serum theophylline levels below 20 μg/ml.[22] If one suspects theophylline toxicity, the infusion of theophylline should be discontinued and a serum theophylline level obtained. This protocol will be sufficient to prevent continuing toxicity in almost all cases. The only way to promote theophylline clearance is by hemodialysis, using an activated charcoal column.[23] Hemodialysis should be considered only if the serum theophylline level exceeds 50 μg/ml, or if the patient has had a theophylline-induced seizure or cardiac tachyarrhythmia.

Table 5–5. Formula for Adjustment of Aminophylline Infusion Rate Based upon Measured Serum Theophylline Concentration

$$\text{Adjusted aminophylline infusion rate} = \text{Initial aminophylline infusion rate} \times \frac{(\text{Target serum theophylline level})}{(\text{Measured serum theophylline level})}$$

Example:

Initial aminophylline infusion rate = 0.6 mg/kg/hr

Measured serum theophylline level = 5 μg/ml

Target serum theophylline level = 15 μg/ml

$$\text{Adjusted aminophylline infusion rate} = 0.6\ \text{mg/kg/hr}\ \frac{15\ \mu\text{g/ml}}{5\ \mu\text{g/ml}}$$

Adjusted aminophylline infusion rate = 1.8 mg/kg/hr

Table 5–6. Procedures and Medications to Avoid in Acute Asthma

Sedation
Ultrasonic nebulizers
Inhaled steroids
Cromolyn
Acetylcysteine
IPPB
Cool mist
Transtracheal aspiration

Fluids

Many patients with acute asthma have some degree of dehydration. This may be evidenced clinically by poor skin turgor, the absence of axillary sweat, by postural hypotension, or by hemoconcentration as reflected in an elevated blood hematocrit. Patients with acute asthma may be dehydrated as a consequence of poor fluid intake or excessive fluid loss through the lungs as a result of continued hyperventilation. Most patients with asthma will tolerate fluid replacement of 3 to 5 liters over 24 hours. This should be in the form of glucose and water. In patients with underlying cardiac disease, fluid replacement should be done cautiously.

Procedures and Medications to Be Avoided

Table 5-6 outlines some therapeutic modalities which are contraindicated in the setting of acute asthma. At our institution, we observed an association between the inappropriate use of sedatives and the need for mechanical ventilation.[24] Patients with an acute exacerbation of asthma are often agitated, with the agitation being the result primarily of physiologic and not neuropsychiatric conditions. What should be treated aggressively is the patient's asthma, and not the agitation. The inappropriate use of drugs such as diazepam may depress respiratory drives and literally turn a patient who "can't breathe" into a patient who in addition "won't breathe." Some medications such as morphine promote histamine release and, at least on theoretical grounds, may worsen asthma.[25] Because of the irritable airways of the acute asthmatic, particulant medication such as cromolyn or inhaled steroids usually worsen the situation. Acetylcysteine (Mucomyst) is also irritating to the airways and is contraindicated in acute asthma.

It is well established that the mechanism by which exercise induces asthma is related to the flux of heat and water across the respiratory epithelium.[26] The inhalation of cool mist in some patients may result in symptoms of chest tightness and coughing. Because of this, it is recommended that only warm mist be administered to patients with asthma. The use of ultrasonic nebulizers, which generate particles of water of 5 μ in diameter or less, are very effective for delivering moisture to the airways; however, the nature of these particles makes them irritating, and for this reason the use of nebulizers in the setting of acute asthma is not condoned. Intermittent positive pressure breathing (IPPB) has been associated with mortality in asthma.[27] Acute asthma is associated with hyperinflation of the lungs; IPPB may create more hyperinflation in some patients. IPPB also may decrease cardiac output and induce barotrauma. Furthermore, IPPB produces turbulent airflow which may further promote bronchospasm. Finally, although it has been argued that IPPB is an effective way to deliver aerosolized bronchodilators in asthma, most of the airflow with this technique unfortunately goes to the areas in the lung with the lowest resistance, whereas one would ideally like to deliver medication to points of obstruction rather than to less involved areas. On occasion, we have used IPPB in acute asthma, but this has been solely as a means of respiratory support in patients with marked hypoventilation. In this situation, IPPB delivered by mask has been used as an alternative to mechanical ventilation requiring an endotracheal tube. Such a strategy can only be used for a short time while waiting for the pharmacologic form of therapy to become effective, so as to avoid the need for intubation and mechanical ventilation.

STATUS ASTHMATICUS

There is no universally accepted definition of status asthmaticus. However, an operational-pharmacologic definition based upon the clinical setting in which status asthmaticus occurs is useful. By this definition, status asthmaticus is an acute attack of asthma which is refractory to therapy with beta-adrenergic agents, intravenous aminophylline, and rehydration. When this occurs, it is absolutely critical that another pharmacologic agent be added. It can be said about status asthmaticus that it is a battle about to be lost. There is no oversimplification in saying of status asthmaticus that "the longer it lasts, the worse it gets, and the worse it gets, the longer it lasts."

When the clinician makes the diagnosis of status asthmaticus, two therapeutic options exist. In a small number of patients, inhaled atropine will be effective; but in a much larger number of patients, the use of intravenous corticosteroids will be necessary.

Inhaled Atropine

It is now appreciated that the cholinergic nervous system plays an important role in mediating bronchial tone, and may play a role in acute asthma.[28] Atropine is an anticholinergic medication which when given by inhalation has few systemic side effects but serves to block the cholinergic aspect of bronchospasm. An important indicator of the patient who is likely to benefit from inhaled atropine is the presence of cough as a prominent symptom. Atropine and its congener, ipratropium bromide (SCH 1000), have been used in other countries for a number of years for the treatment of asthma.[29] In the coming decade, these drugs may find the same sort of acceptance in this country. At present, however, the use of

Table 5–7. Use of Inhaled Atropine

Indications:	Acute attacks of asthma with cough as a predominant symptom	
Administration:	Solution:	1 mg delivered by hand bulb or powered nebulizer
	Tablets:	Dissolve two 0.6 mg tablets in sterile water (0.5 to 1 cc) and nebulize
Frequency:	TID or q. 3–4 h.	
Cautions:	Avoid spraying in eye Keep out of reach of children	

inhaled atropine is usually reserved for patients who have proven to be refractory to conventional forms of therapy with beta-adrenergic medication and theophylline compounds. Surprisingly, atropine does not appear to produce a drying of bronchial secretions. While localized dryness of the mouth may occur, at least one study has documented that inhaled atropine promotes rather than inhibits mucociliary clearance.[30] When given by inhalation, systemic side effects of atropine, such as tachycardia and bladder outlet obstruction, are unusual.

Table 5-7 details a method for the administration of atropine. A disadvantage of atropine is its relatively short duration of action (approximately 3 hours). Congeners of the drug, such as ipratropium bromide, have the advantage of a longer duration of action and a possibly decreased incidence of side effects. When atropine is administered by inhalation, the patient must be cautioned to avoid spraying it into his or her eyes, since this will result in prolonged pupillary dilation. Inhaled atropine may be combined with inhaled beta-adrenergic therapy. The combined use of these medications[31] has been shown both in asthma and in chronic bronchitis to benefit some patients as judged by increased bronchodilatation.

Corticosteroids

The role of corticosteroids in both the chronic and acute treatment of asthma is well established.[32] The mechanism of action of these drugs probably relates to their antiinflammatory effect as well as to their effect of increasing the sensitivity to beta-adrenergic medications. In fact, in experimental situations in which refractoriness to beta-adrenergic therapy has been induced, as little as a single dose of corticosteroids has been shown to restore this responsiveness.[33]

Once a patient has been judged to be in status asthmaticus, 100 mg of hydrocortisone or its equivalent should be given intravenously. This dosage should be repeated every 6 hours until the asthma has been brought under control. Should the patient not respond to the initial dosage of intravenous corticosteroids, the dose should be doubled until control has been established. While clinical studies have not been done to document the superiority of this particular approach over the use of more conventional pharmacologic dosages of corticosteroids, there is anecdotal evidence to support it. For one thing, regardless of intellectual arguments, those who care for the asthmatic patient would agree that the major side effects of corticosteroids are not related to the absolute amount of any given single

Table 5–8. Use of Intravenous Isoproterenol in Status Asthmaticus

Generally should be reserved for young and those without heart disease
Cardiac arrhythmias and myocardial necrosis are major complications
Usual initial dosage is 0.1 μg/kg/min, but may be titrated upwards as long as heart rate less than 130 beats/min
Maintain arterial PO_2 above 60 mmHg
Monitor pulse and blood pressure
Monitor cardiac enzymes daily, particularly more cardiac-specific CPK-MB isoenzyme

dosage, but rather to the duration of corticosteroid therapy. Put another way, status asthmaticus is more dangerous than "industrial strength" corticosteroid therapy. Likewise, prolonged corticosteroid administration because of uncontrolled asthma is worse than acute high-dose therapy which results in controlled asthma.[34] Furthermore, although a response has been demonstrated within an hour of the initiation of treatment[35] in some studies of corticosteroid administration in chronic asthma, it probably takes as long as 6 hours to see a clinical effect in patients with status asthmaticus. For this reason, it is important to start corticosteroid therapy sooner rather than later. Translated into clinical terms, this would mean initiating corticosteroid therapy within 1 to 2 hours if there is no response to the standard initial therapy. This implies that theophylline and beta-adrenergic drugs can be gauged as successful if they produce at least a clinical trend toward improvement without necessarily completely controlling an asthmatic attack.

The side effects of corticosteroids are well known to most clinicians. As mentioned above, they relate mainly to the duration of therapy. It is controversial whether acute, moderate dose corticosteroid therapy can produce gastrointestinal hemorrhage. When high-dose corticosteroid therapy is employed, it is prudent to use either antacid therapy or cimetadine to decrease the likelihood of gastrointestinal hemorrhage.

OTHER FORMS OF THERAPY FOR ACUTE ASTHMA AND STATUS ASTHMATICUS

Intravenous Isoproterenol

Anecdotal evidence exists to support the use of intravenous beta-adrenergic medication such as isoproterenol in acute asthma.[36] This route of drug administration should be used for the most severe asthmatic attacks not responsive to conventional beta-adrenergic therapy, intravenous aminophylline, atropine, and corticosteroids. The guidelines for intravenous administration of beta-adrenergic agents are presented in Table 5-8. Major complications of the technique are tachyarrhythmias and myocardial necrosis.[37] The possibility of intravenous isoproterenol-associated complications may be increased in the setting of hypoxemia. Myocardial toxicity may be reflected in an elevation of the MB isoenzyme band of creatinine phosphokinase (CPK) in the serum. The success of the more selective

Table 5–9. Use of Rectal Ether in Acute Asthma

Life-threatening asthma not responding to beta-agonists, intravenous aminophylline, or large doses of corticosteroids.
Need to gain time (15 to 60 minutes) to allow other more definitive agents (corticosteroids) to become effective.
Dose = 45 cc for < 60 kg 60 cc for 60–80 kg 90 cc for > 90 kg dissolved in mineral oil; infused by rectal tube over 3–5 minutes as a retention enema.
May require immediate intubation and mechanical ventilation.

beta-2 adrenergic agents, such as salbutamol, given via the intravenous route has been documented in other countries; it is likely that this approach is superior to the intravenous use of isoproterenol.[38]

Rectal Ether

In Table 5-9 the guidelines for use of rectal ether have been outlined. Like intravenous isoproterenol, rectal ether administration should be reserved for the most severe cases of acute asthma and status asthmaticus. We do not employ this form of therapy but present this information for the use of those practitioners who may wish to employ it as a "last resort." It should be emphasized that because of the respiratory depressant effect of rectally administered ether, one should be prepared to intubate and place the patient on mechanical ventilation.

Bronchopulmonary Lavage

Anecdotal experience with bronchopulmonary lavage has been reported in both chronic and acute asthma.[49] We have not had to resort to this type of therapy, but would accept that it may have benefit in selected patients. It would appear that its usefulness would be in those patients in whom the excessive production and retention of bronchopulmonary secretions exists and other forms of conventional physiotherapy have been unsuccessful in relieving this mechanical form of airways obstruction.

General Anesthesia

Certain inhaled general anesthetics such as halothane are bronchodilators. As a last resort, patients with severe status asthmaticus may have general anesthesia induced either at the bedside or in the operating room. This may result in control of the bronchospasm even after the effects of the general anesthesia have waned. However, some patients may simply relapse into severe bronchospasm once the effect of this medication has dissipated.

Table 5–10. Indications for Mechanical Ventilation in Status Asthmaticus

Cardiopulmonary arrest
Progressive increase in arterial carbon dioxide tension as defined by serial arterial blood gases
Mental obtundation and coma
Clinical deterioration despite vigorous medical therapy
Advancing fatigue and impending exhaustion

Table 5–11. Principles of Mechanical Ventilation of Patients with Status Asthmaticus

Use large endotracheal tube (8-mm internal diameter or greater in adults)
Intubate by oral route
Employ volume ventilator
Ensure adequate humidification
Attempt to obtain lowest cycling pressure
Keep respiratory rate slow
Avoid hypocapnia
Suppress ventilation with sedation or paralyze if necessary

SPECIAL CONSIDERATIONS IN ACUTE ASTHMA AND STATUS ASTHMATICUS

Mechanical Ventilation

In patients with status asthmaticus refractory to medical therapy, respiratory failure may progress to the point at which life support through mechanical ventilation will be necessary. In this setting it is important to remember that mechanical ventilation is used to support the patient while other forms of treatment directed primarily at the asthma are continued. The use of mechanical ventilation in status asthmaticus should not be undertaken lightly; it has both a high mortality (up to 40 percent) and a high morbidity (major complications occur in approximately 80 percent of all patients).[24]

Indications for the use of mechanical ventilation in status asthmaticus are outlined in Table 5-10, while important principles in the ventilation of patients with status asthmaticus are detailed in Table 5-11. Volume ventilators must be used. This is because the increased airways resistance in status asthmaticus demands very high pressures in order to deliver an adequate tidal volume. Ventilators which can deliver the large pressures necessary for ventilating such patients include the Ohio Critical Care, Bennett MA2, and Bourn's Bear ventilators. It should be emphasized that patients in status asthmaticus represent extremely difficult management problems. The introduction of the artificial airway in such patients may result in trauma to the oral or nasal mucosa, with hemorrhage. In addition, such artificial devices may irritate receptors within the airways and lead to further bronchospasm.[40] Patients undergoing intubation for status asthmaticus may be combative. For this reason neuromuscular blocking agents such as pancuronium bromide have been used.[41] This makes intubation easier and allows the patient to be ventilated more efficiently with a self-inflating bag.

Because both the hyperventilation and hypoventilation of patients with asthma

Table 5–12. Considerations for Weaning from Mechanical Ventilation Following Recovery from Status Asthmaticus

Is the patient getting better?
Is the fraction of inspired oxygen 50 percent or less?
Is the patient's resting minute ventilation less than 10 liters?
Is the patient able to double the resting minute ventilation?
Can the patient generate 25 cmH_2O or more of negative inspiratory pressure?
Is the patient awake, alert, and coordinated?

may result in serious ventilator-associated complications, blood gases must be monitored frequently, particularly within the first few hours of mechanical ventilation. The high pressures necessary to deliver adequate tidal volumes may result in barotrauma. A chest tube taped to the respirator or to the head of the patient's bed will not only make this available, should the need for it arise, but will also serve to remind those caring for the patient that barotrauma may occur. Because asthma represents a condition characterized by obstruction of airflow both into and out of the chest, adequate time for expiration must be allowed. The appropriate settings for the ventilator cannot be dictated "cookbook" style but must be individualized for each patient.

Weaning the Patient from Mechanical Ventilation

Once asthma has been controlled, it is appropriate to consider the discontinuation of mechanical ventilation. Control of the asthmatic attack usually will be reflected by a decrease in peak cycling pressure, a decrease in minute ventilation, and improvement in the arterial blood gas concentrations. Table 5-12 outlines factors to be considered when weaning patients from the mechanical ventilator. One factor which may discriminate the patient with asthma from the usual patient being weaned from the ventilator is the effect of tracheobronchial reflexes initiated by the endotracheal tube.[40] It has been shown in normals that the presence of an artificial airway leads to increased airway resistance; this may be more impressive in the asthmatic. The added burden of having to breathe through an endotracheal tube may make weaning even more difficult for the patient with increased airways resistance. Many of the agents used to control asthma are effective in blocking reflex-associated bronchospasm.

Because of the combined effects of airways resistance and endotracheal-tube-associated airways resistance, the measures designed to determine whether or not a patient may be successfully weaned from the ventilator and extubated should be brief.[42] The fraction of inspired oxygen should be 50 percent or less, and hypercapnia should not exist. The patient should be able to generate an adequate tidal volume of at least 5 cc/kg, to demonstrate good ventilatory reserve, as indicated by the ability to at least double the resting minute ventilation, to show good respiratory muscle function, as reflected by the peak inspiratory pressure, and to be alert and cooperative enough to generate an effective cough after being extubated. If these criteria are met, the patient should be placed on a T-piece for approximately 15 to 30 minutes and allowed to breathe oxygenated, humidified air. If this trial is tolerated well and the arterial blood gas measurement at the end of this period

Table 5–13. Treatment of the Patient in the Recovery Phase of Acute Asthma

Clinical Situation	Clinical Strategy	Example
Acute asthma controlled by beta-adrenergic agent alone	Treat with oral (inhaled) beta-adrenergic agent	Metaproterenol 10–20 mg q.6h. Terbutaline 2.5–5mg q.8h.
Acute asthma controlled with aminophylline in addition to beta-adrenergic agent	Treat with combined oral (inhaled) beta-adrenergic agent plus oral theophylline	Oral metaproterenol or terbutaline plus 200–400 mg aminophylline q.6h. (or sustained release compound q.8–12h.)
Acute asthma controlled with beta-adrenergics, aminophylline, and corticosteroids	Continue oral steroids beyond acute phase to control asthma and decrease side effects of acute steroid withdrawal	See Table 5-14

shows no deterioration of respiratory function, as evidenced by either hypercapnia, respiratory acidemia or hypoxemia, the patient should be extubated. It should be emphasized that the use of mechanical measures such as intermittent mandatory ventilation (IMV) in the patient recovering from status asthmaticus would not only prolong the period of weaning and extubation, but may be very psychologically distressing to the patient.

THE RECOVERY PERIOD

Once asthma has been controlled it is important that a rational program be initiated to prevent its recurrence. It has been well documented that abnormalities of pulmonary function may persist for weeks following an acute attack of asthma, yet the patient may be unaware of any such pulmonary dysfunction.[43]

If the patient has used a beta-adrenergic agent alone, an oral preparation of such an agent or a theophylline compound should be added (Table 5-13). If treatment with a beta-adrenergic agent plus intravenous aminophylline has been necessary, a combination of these medications should be prescribed on an outpatient basis.

If corticosteroids have been necessary, the patient should be put on a tapering schedule of corticosteroids as outlined in Table 5-14. The tapering of corticosteroids is employed not only to prevent a re-exacerbation of asthma, but also to prevent the corticosteroid withdrawal syndrome.[44] This is a unique symptom complex not necessarily related to hypofunction of the adrenal glands. Its symptoms may vary from muscle pain to weakness, nausea, fatigue, and even fever. Patients should be advised of the possibility of this syndrome occurring and should be reassured that it does not necessarily mean that they are developing another illness.

ERRORS TO BE AVOIDED IN THE RECOVERY PHASE

There are two errors which occur during the management of the recovery phase of acute asthma. These are "too soon" and "too much." If treatment is stopped too soon, asthma may recur. This is best avoided by instituting a reasonable and

Table 5–14. Suggested Approach for Weaning Patients from Corticosteroids After Acute Attack of Asthma

Total number of 5 mg tablets of prednisone to prescribe = 78. Start with 12 tablets as single morning dosage and decrease by 1 tablet daily to effect following schedule:

Day	Tablets	mg Prednisone
1	12	60
2	11	55
3	10	50
4	9	45
5	8	40
6	7	35
7	6	30
8	5	25
9	4	20
10	3	15
11	2	10
12	1	5
13	0	0

If breakthrough occurs, return to day 1 dosage, add inhaled corticosteroids and recommence oral corticosteroid taper.

tolerable outpatient program of therapy. In treating patients with asthma, as with any illness, it is possible to be entirely rational while being completely unreasonable. The treatment regimen should be both tolerable from the standpoint of convenience as well as from cost and side effects. The use of a single oral preparation, either a beta-adrenergic drug or theophylline, will be accepted by most patients. It is important that the patient be educated as to the purpose of the continued therapy beyond the acute illness, so as to be motivated to continue with medications. The patient should also be counseled about the minor side effects that he may have temporarily from some of the medications. Hoerr's law that "it is hard to make an asymptomatic patient feel better" is true.[45] Likewise, an ounce of prevention saves an $150 emergency room visit. If the patient has required theophylline therapy in addition to beta-adrenergic therapy, the use of an oral theophylline agent plus an inhaled or oral beta-adrenergic agent on a regular basis for the first 2 to 3 weeks after recovery is often successful. If the patient requires corticosteriods, they may be used in combination with either an oral or an inhaled beta-adrenergic agent plus a theophylline.

SUMMARY

The treatment of acute asthma is in many ways like the treatment of diabetic ketoacidosis. When the condition is properly and intelligently managed, a satisfactory outcome may be rapidly achieved, with a minimum both of discomfort to the patient and of therapeutic misadventure. Understanding how to accomplish this depends not only upon experience but upon an appreciation of the role of the various forms of pharmacologic therapy which are available for asthma. In addition, it is important to avoid making a bad situation worse by the use of inappropriate treatment modalities. The successful management of both acute and chronic asthma should result in a patient who can return to a gainful and enjoyable existence. Given this, the treatment of asthma is both a worthwhile and satisfactory endeavor.

REFERENCES

1. Gross NJ: What is this thing called love?—Or, defining asthma. Am Rev Resp Dis 121:203, 1980.
2. Hudgel DW, Langston L, Selner JC, et al: Viral and bacterial infections in adults with chronic asthma. Am Rev Resp Dis 210:393, 1979.
3. Messer JW, Petero GA, Bennett WA: Causes of death and pathological findings in 304 cases of bronchial asthma. Dis Chest 38:616, 1960.
4. Keal EE, Reid L: Pathological alterations in mucous in asthma with and without the cell. In New Directions in Asthma, ed. Stein M, Park Ridge, IL, American College of Chest Physicians, 1975.
5. McFadden ER, Lyons HA: Arterial blood gas tensions in asthma. Engl J Med 278:773, 1974.
6. Reisman RE: Asthma induced by adrenergic aerosols. J Allergy Clin Immunol 46:162, 1970.
7. Leading article: Allergy to corticosteroids. Br Med J 4:551, 1974.
8. Collins JV, Clar TJH, Brown DJL: Airway function in healthy subjects and patients with left heart disease. Clin Sci Mol Med 49:217, 1975.
9. Windebank WJ, Boyd G, Moran FL: Pulmonary thromboembolism presenting as asthma. Br Med J 1:90, 1973.
10. Kelsen SG, Kelsen DP, Fleegen BF: Emergency room assessment and treatment of patients with acute asthma. Am J Med 64:220, 1978.
11. Shim C, Corro P, Park S, et al: Pulmonary function studies in pathins with upper airway obstruction. Am Rev Resp Dis 106:233, 1972.
12. Slavin RG, Cannon RE, Fiedman WH, et al: Sinusitis and bronchial asthma. J Allergy Clin Immunol 66:250, 1980.
13. Orehek J, Charpin D, Velarocchi JM, et al: Bronchomotor effect of bronchoconstriction-induced deep inspirations in asthmatics. Am Rev Resp Dis 121:297, 1980.
14. Woolcock AJ, Read J: Improvement in bronchial asthma not reflected in forced expiratory volume. Lancet ll:1323, 1965.
15. Aubier M, Murciano D, Melic-Emili J, et al: Effects of the administration of O_2 on ventilation and blood gases in patients with chronic obstructive pulmonary diseases during acute respiratory failure. Am Rev Resp Dis 122:747, 1980.
16. Zelefsky M, Swain BK: The nature of the increased lung volume in asthma. Br J Dis Chest 65:39, 1971.
17. Schwartz H, Lowell FC, Melby SC: Steroid resistance in bronchial asthma. Ann Intern Med 69:493, 1968.
18. Rossing TH, Fanta CH, Goldstein DH, et al: Emergency therapy of asthma: comparison of the acute effects of parenteral and inhaled sympathomimetics and infused aminophylline. Am Rev Resp Dis 122:365, 1980.
19. Josephson GW, Kennedy HL, MacKenzie, EJ, et al: Cardiac dysrhymias during the treatment of acute asthma. Chest 78:429, 1980.
20. Paterson JW, Woolcock AJ, Shenfield GM: Bronchodilator drugs. Am Rev Resp Dis 120:1149, 1979.

21. Mitenko PA, Ogilvie RI: Rational intravenous doses of theophylline. N Engl J Med 289:600, 1973.
22. Zwillich CW, Sutton FD Jr, Neff TA, et al: Theophylline-induced seizure in adults: Correlation with serum concentrations. Ann Intern Med 82:784, 1975.
23. Russo ME: Management of theophylline intoxication with charcoal-column hemoperfusion. N Engl J Med 300:24, 1979.
24. Scoggin CH, Sahn SA, Petty TL: Status asthmaticus: A nine year experience. JAMA 238:1158, 1977.
25. Blumberg MZ: Morphine for severe asthma. N Engl J Med 288:50, 1973.
26. Deal EC Jr, McFadden ER Jr, Ingram RH Jr, et al: Role of respiratory heat exchange in production of exercise-induced asthma. J Appl Physiol 46:467, 1979.
27. Karetsky MS: Asthma mortality associated with pneumothorax and intermittent positive-pressure breathing. Lancet 1:828, 1975.
28. Ingram RH Jr, Wellman JJ, McFadden ER Jr, et al: Relative contributions of large and small airways to flow limitations in normal subjects before and after atropine and isoproterenol. J Clin Invest 59:696, 1977.
29. Storms WW, DoPico BA, Reed CL: Aerosol SCH 1000: An anticholinergic bronchodilator. Am Rev Resp Dis 111:419, 1975.
30. Chopra SK: Effect of atropine on mucocilliary transport velocity in anesthetized dogs. Am Rev Resp Dis 118:367, 1978.
31. Brady RE, Easton JG: The value of atropine in the documentation of reversible airways obstruction. Ann Allergy 42:211, 1979.
32. Chakrin LW, Krell RD: Pathophysiology and pharmacotherapy of asthma: an overview. J Pharm Sci 69:236, 1980.
33. Ellub-Mically R, French FF: Effect of intravenous prednisolone in asthmatics with diminished adrenergic responsiveness. Lancet 2:1269, 1975.
34. Tuft L: Steroid-phobia in asthma management. Ann Allergy 42:152, 1979.
35. Ellub-Mically R, French FF: Intravenous prednisolone in chronic bronchial asthma. Thorax 30:312, 1975.
36. Klaustermeyer WB, Rosario L, Di Bernaardo L, et al: Intravenous isoproterenol: Rationale for bronchial asthma. J Allergy Clin Immunol 55:325, 1975.
37. Kurland G, Williams J, Lewiston N: Fatal myocardial toxicity during continuous infusion of intravenous isoproterenol therapy of asthma. J Allergy Clin Immunol 63:407, 1979.
38. Johnson AJ, Spiro SG, Pidgeon Bateman S, et al: Intravenous infusion of salbutamol in severe acute asthma. Br Med J 1:1013, 1978.
39. Millman M, Goodman AH, Goldstein IM, et al: Bronchoscopy and lavage for chronic bronchial asthma. Immunol Allergy Pract 3:10, 1981.
40. Gal TJ: Pulmonary mechanics in normal subjects following endotracheal intubation. Anesthesiology 52:27, 1980.
41. Levin N, Dillion J: Status asthmaticus and pancuronium bromide. JAMA 22:1158, 1977.
42. Sahn SA, Lakshminarayan S, Petty TL: Bedside criteria for discontinuation of mechanical ventilation. Chest 63:1002, 1973.
43. Rubinfeld AR, Pain MCF: Preception of asthma. Lancet 1:882, 1976.
44. Dixon RB, Christy NP: On the various forms of corticosteroid withdrawal syndrome. Am J Med 68:224, 1980.
45. Hoerr SD: Hoerr's law. Am J Surg 103:411, 1962.

6

Pulmonary Edema

Richard K. Albert, M.D.

INTRODUCTION

Pulmonary edema is an abnormal accumulation of extravascular water or solute in the lung. It occurs whenever more fluid is filtered from the pulmonary vessels than can be removed by vascular resorption and lymphatic clearance. The movement of fluid across a vessel wall in either direction is related to the hydrostatic and osmotic pressure gradients of the fluid, as well as to the permeability characteristics of the vessel wall. Using the notation suggested by Staub, as applied to the lung:

$$Qf = Kf\,[(Pmv - Ppmv) - \sigma(\pi mv - \pi pmv)] \quad (1)$$

where Qf is the net volume of fluid flow; Kf is the filtration coefficient or transvascular conductance; Pmv and Ppmv are the microvascular and perimicrovascular hydrostatic pressures, and πmv and πpmv are the microvascular and the perimicrovascular osmotic pressures; and σ is the reflection coefficient or sieving tendency of the vessel wall for protein.[1,2] The term *microvascular* was chosen to avoid implying that all fluid and protein exchange occurs across alevolar capillaries. The term perimicrovascular allows for the presence of different interstitial spaces and interstitial pressures.[3] Pulmonary edema can occur if any of the variables in Equation 1 are altered in the direction favoring increased fluid filtration.

This chapter will summarize the causes, clinical manifestations, and pathophysiology of both normal- and increased-permeability pulmonary edema and will discuss the current recommendations for the treatment and the short- and long-term prognosis for this condition.

ETIOLOGY

Pulmonary edema can be classified by the permeability characteristics of the vascular endothelium (Fig. 6–1). When permeability is normal, edema will develop if the hydrostatic gradient favoring fluid filtration increases or if the oncotic

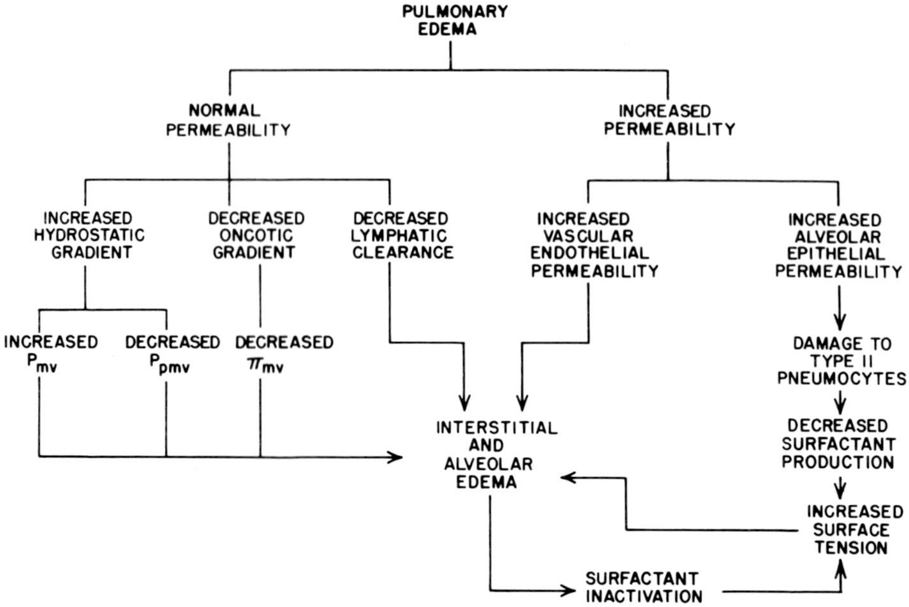

Figure 6–1. Mechanisms of pulmonary edema formation. Pmv and Ppmv are the microvascular and perimicrovascular hydrostatic pressures, respectively. πmv is the microvascular oncotic pressure.

gradient favoring fluid resorption decreases. Hydrostatic edema is the result of either an increased Pmv or a decreased Ppmv. Additionally, edema may rarely occur (or at least may increase more rapidly) when lymphatic clearance is impaired. Vascular endothelial and alveolar epithelial permeability may be altered in association with many types of disease. Because the clinical presentations and patterns of diffuse lung injury are similar regardless of the specific cause, all of the conditions that increase endothelial or epithelial permeability (or both) are commonly grouped under the heading of the adult respiratory distress syndrome (ARDS).[4,5,6]

Normal Permeability

Increased Hydrostatic Gradient

Increased Pmv

Cardiogenic edema is said to occur whenever the Pmv is increased; it is the most common cause of excess extravascular lung water. While elevation of the left ventricular end-diastolic pressure (LVEDP) is the major cause of an increased Pmv, it is important to realize that several noncardiac problems may also increase the Pmv (Table 6–1).

When the left ventricle is failing from any cause, an elevated LVEDP is required either to increase the left ventricular end-diastolic volume, or to keep

Table 6–1. Conditions That Increase Intravascular Hydrostatic Pressure

Increased left ventricular end-diastolic pressure
Aortic valve disease
Hypertension
Coronary artery disease
Cardiomyopathy (congestive, restrictive, or hypertrophic)
High output states (thyrotoxicosis, systemic AV fistula, beriberi, severe anemia)
Arrhythmias
Intravenous fluid overload
Constrictive pericarditis
Increased left atrial pressure
Mitral valve disease
Left atrial myxoma
Increased pulmonary venous pressure
Pulmonary veno-occlusive disease
Fibrosing mediastinitis
Congenital cardiovascular abnormalities
Neurogenic edema
Head trauma
Seizures
Cerebrovascular accidents
High-altitude pulmonary edema

this volume constant when left ventricular compliance is decreased. Left atrial, pulmonary venous, pulmonary capillary, and pulmonary arterial diastolic pressures all increase as a result of an increased LVEDP. A similar sequence of events occurs if the left atrial pressure is elevated secondary to outflow obstruction or regurgitation from the left ventricle. Several unusual conditions can raise the pulmonary vascular pressures farther upstream by obstructing pulmonary venous drainage into the left atrium (Table 6–1).

The pathogenesis of neurogenic edema is debated. While early studies suggested that alveolar and vascular permeability were increased in this condition, others have suggested that the causative problem is a massive sympathetic discharge occurring in response to midbrain hypoxia. This causes: (1) systemic arterial vasoconstriction, which raises the blood pressure and shifts blood to the thorax; (2) a decrease in left ventricular compliance with an increase in the LVEDP; and (3) pulmonary venous constriction.[7,8] These changes could increase pulmonary arterial, venous, and capillary pressure. High protein concentrations in the edema fluid might result from the loss of vascular integrity secondary to the hydrostatic stress created by these pressures.[9,10,11] Marked vascular pressure swings in such a patient have recently been observed; the systemic blood pressure went from 210/110 to 410/200 mmHg, the pulmonary artery pressure from 40/2 to 110/60 mmHg, and the pulmonary arterial wedge pressure from 4 to 48 mmHg.[12]

The mechanism of high-altitude pulmonary edema (HAPE) is also debated. The pulmonary arterial wedge pressure in this condition is known to be normal, while the pulmonary arterial pressure is markedly elevated.[13,14,15] Characteristically, patients who develop HAPE are young and otherwise healthy. Many have previously lived for some time at high altitude. After moving closer to sea-level and

Table 6–2. Conditions That Decrease Interstitial Hydrostatic Pressure

Mechanical ventilation
Positive end-expiratory pressure breathing
Surfactant depletion
Re-expansion edema
Acute upper airway obstruction
Neoplasm
Intubation

living under such conditions for 6 to 9 months, they become ill within the first 36 hours after reascending to an altitude greater than 10,000 feet (2750 meters). Heavy physical exertion frequently precipitates the edema. Previous living at a high altitude may augment these individual's normal pulmonary vasoconstrictive response to hypoxia. Patients who develop HAPE have a greater increase in pulmonary artery pressure (Ppa) when exposed to hypoxia than do normal subjects.[16] The hydrostatic stress that results from this increased Ppa might cause fluid leakage from precapillary vessels,[17] despite a normal permeability of these vessels. The low alveolar fluid protein concentration observed in one patient with HAPE supports this mechanism.[18] Alternatively, the high Ppa might increase vascular permeability.[9,10,11] Others suggest that capillary permeability is altered in HAPE as a result of the increased blood flow and nonuniform hypoxic vasoconstriction.[19,20,21]

Decreased Ppmv

The hydrostatic gradient favoring fluid filtration is a *transmural* pressure. It can be increased by increasing the Pmv or by decreasing the Ppmv (Table 6–2). The Ppmv is markedly influenced by the mechanical effects of lung inflation (see "Pathophysiology").

Perivascular edema has been shown to develop with mechanical ventilation at high inspiratory pressures and a zero end-expiratory pressure.[22,23] Both perivascular and alveolar edema can result when a positive end-expiratory pressure (PEEP) is used.[23,24,25] The large lung volume produced by either high inspiratory pressures or PEEP increases the transmural pressure across certain vessels in the lung by decreasing the surrounding Ppmv (see "Pathophysiology, Extra-alveolar interstitium"). When a zero end-expiratory pressure is used, the Ppmv might also be decreased as a result of surfactant depletion (see "Pathophysiology, Surface Tension").

Pulmonary edema may develop during the re-expansion of a lung that has been collapsed for at least several days by a pleural effusion or a large pneumothorax (>50 percent). The edema is seen only in the re-expanded lung.[26] The pathophysiology of the edema is thought to involve a large, negative pleural pressure and Ppmv, which occur when the lung is inflated after surfactant has been inactivated by atelectasis or by interrupted perfusion.[27,28] An alternative explanation for the development of edema is that lack of perfusion to the collapsed lung increases vascular permeability, so that when blood flow is restored, excessive transvascular fluid filtration occurs at a normal transmural pressure.

Table 6–3. Conditions Associated with ARDS

Trauma
Shock
Infection
Drug overdose
Aspiration
Inhalation
Pancreatitis

Pulmonary edema may also be seen with upper airway obstruction secondary to neoplasms[29] or intubation.[30] In both of these, a large, negative pleural pressure could decrease the Ppmv. The large pleural-pressure swings noted in asthma have similarly been related to increased lung water.[31]

Decreased Oncotic Gradient

Decreased πmv

Anasarca and ascites are frequently seen with severe, chronic hypoproteinemia, but pulmonary edema in this condition is unusual. Presumably, this is because both the πmv and πpmv are decreased, so that the osmotic gradient remains unchanged. Nonetheless, edema can result from a rapid decrease in πmv (intravenous fluid replacement) and, when the πmv is low, edema will develop at a lower hydrostatic gradient.[32]

Decreased Lymphatic Clearance

Water and protein are both cleared by pulmonary lymphatics. Smooth muscle fibers are present in the lymphatic walls, and pressures up to 25 mmHg can be generated to assist in the clearance of these substances. Ventilatory movements are also thought to increase lymphatic transport.[2,33]

Lymphatic obstruction from a variety of conditions may cause or contribute to pulmonary edema. Among these conditions are pneumoconioses, lymphangitic carcinomatosis, elevated systemic venous pressures, and an unusual disease of young women called lymphangiomyomatosis.[34,35] However, since collateral lymphatic channels can develop rapidly, it is unusual for decreased lymphatic drainage to be the primary cause of pulmonary edema.

Increased Permeability

Vascular and alveolar permeability may be increased by a variety of insults to the endothelial or epithelial surfaces. While these insults may be grouped into general categories (Table 6–3), the mechanism of injury may vary both between and within categories.

ARDS was first associated with wartime trauma.[36,37] It may result from direct thoracic trauma with lung contusion or from nonthoracic trauma complicated by fat emboli, shock, or sepsis. All forms of shock (cardiogenic, hemorrhagic, anaphylactic, and septic) have been associated with ARDS. In addition, sepsis without

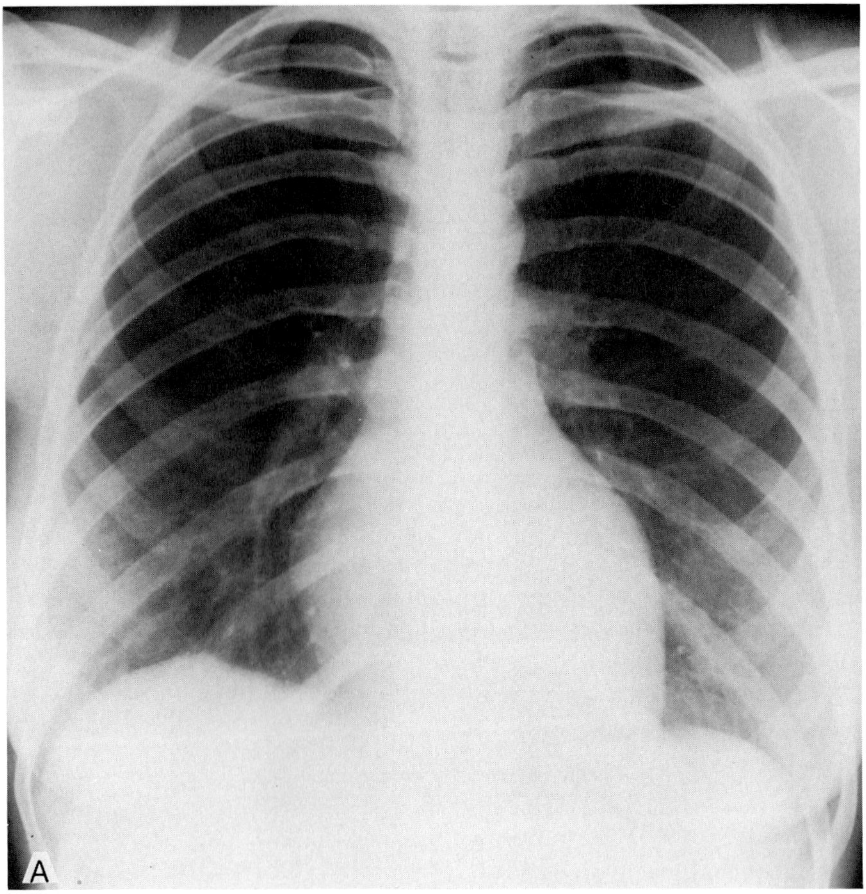

Figure 6–2. (A) Chest roentgenogram 1 month prior to heart failure.

shock can cause ARDS[38]; the syndrome has been caused by various types of pneumonitis, including viral (influenza and varicella), bacterial, mycobacterial, fungal, and parasitic.

Up to 50 percent of patients hospitalized for drug overdoses will develop ARDS.[39,40,41] Most commonly, heroin is the associated agent, but other narcotics (methadone, propoxyphene), barbiturates, colchicine, salicylates, and ethchlorvynol have also been implicated. The aspiration of various substances may also cause ARDS. Gastric aspiration is discussed in Chapter 12. Near-drowning victims can aspirate gastric juice, fresh or salt water, and other foreign material. In animal models of near drowning, the aspiration of large volumes of fresh water (>22 ml/kg) results in a hypotonic load; water is absorbed into the vasculature, causing hemolysis and profound electrolyte shifts.[42] The hypertonicity that results from salt-water aspiration causes transudation of fluids into the lung.[43] Problems result-

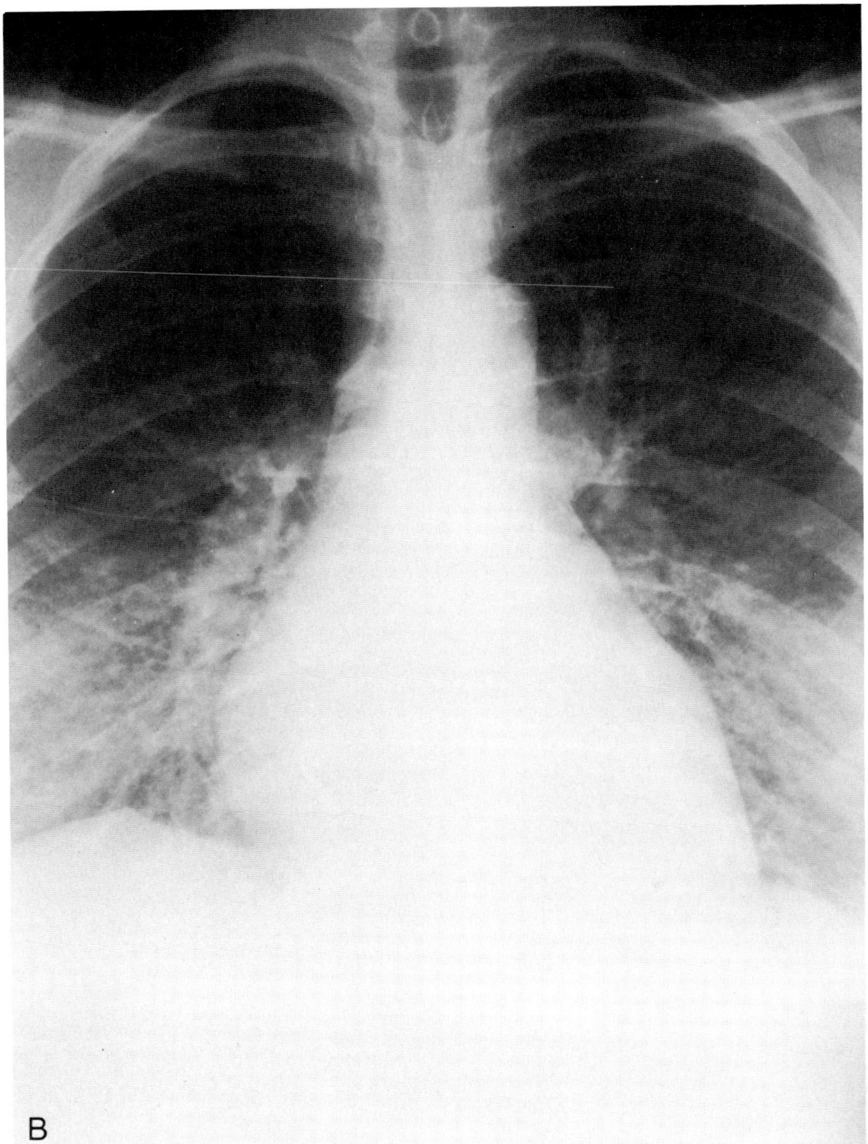

Figure 6–2 (continued). (B) Repeat film showing enlargement of the upper lobe pulmonary vessels. (Courtesy Dr. M. Figley, University of Washington.)

ing from hypo- and hypertonicity have not been observed in patients with near-drowning, but these may be less severe in survivors who reach medical attention. Hydrocarbon aspiration is seen with gas siphoning, suicide attempts, inadvertent ingestions, and rarely in professional entertainers using lighter fluid to produce the illusion of breathing fire.

(Text continues on p. 158.)

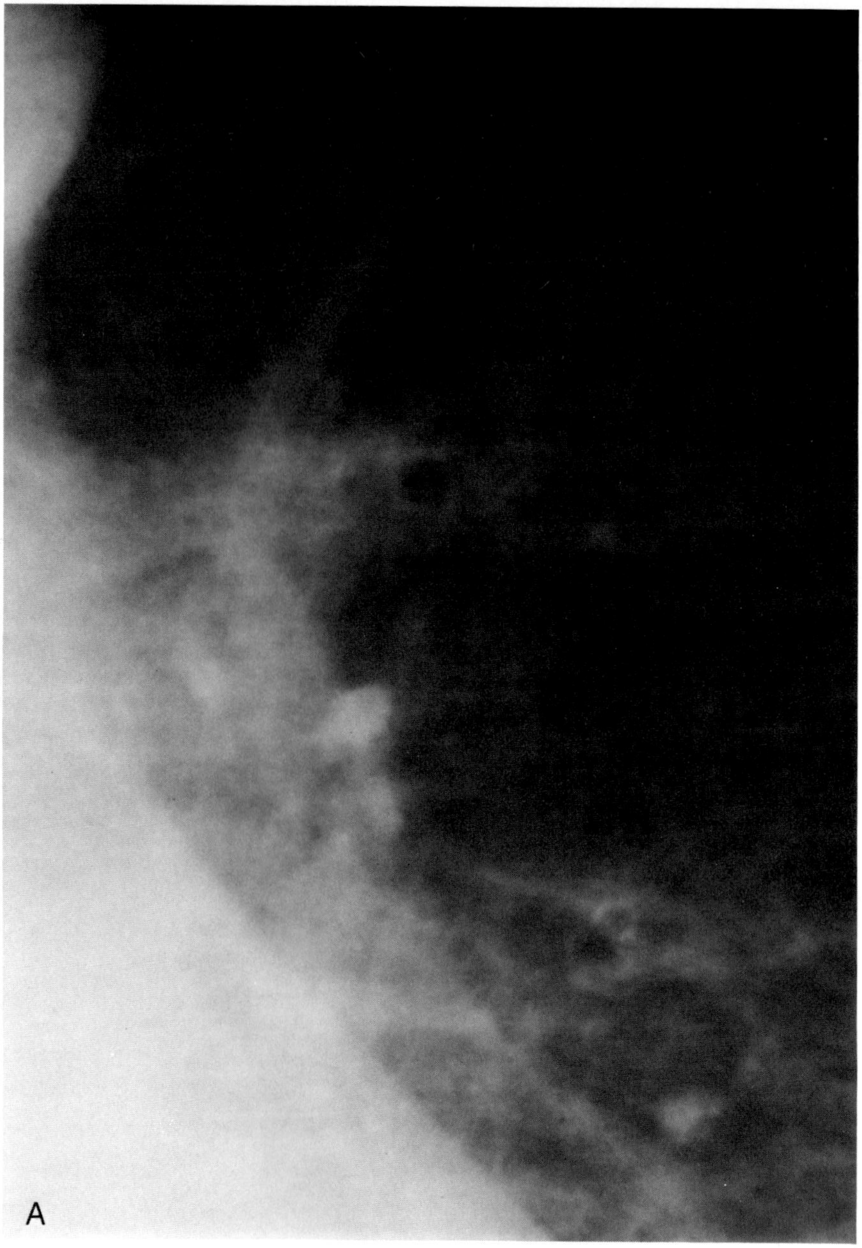

Figure 6–3. Bronchus seen end-on prior to (A) and following development of pulmonary edema (B). Note thickening of the bronchial wall. (Courtesy of Dr. M. Figley, University of Washington.)

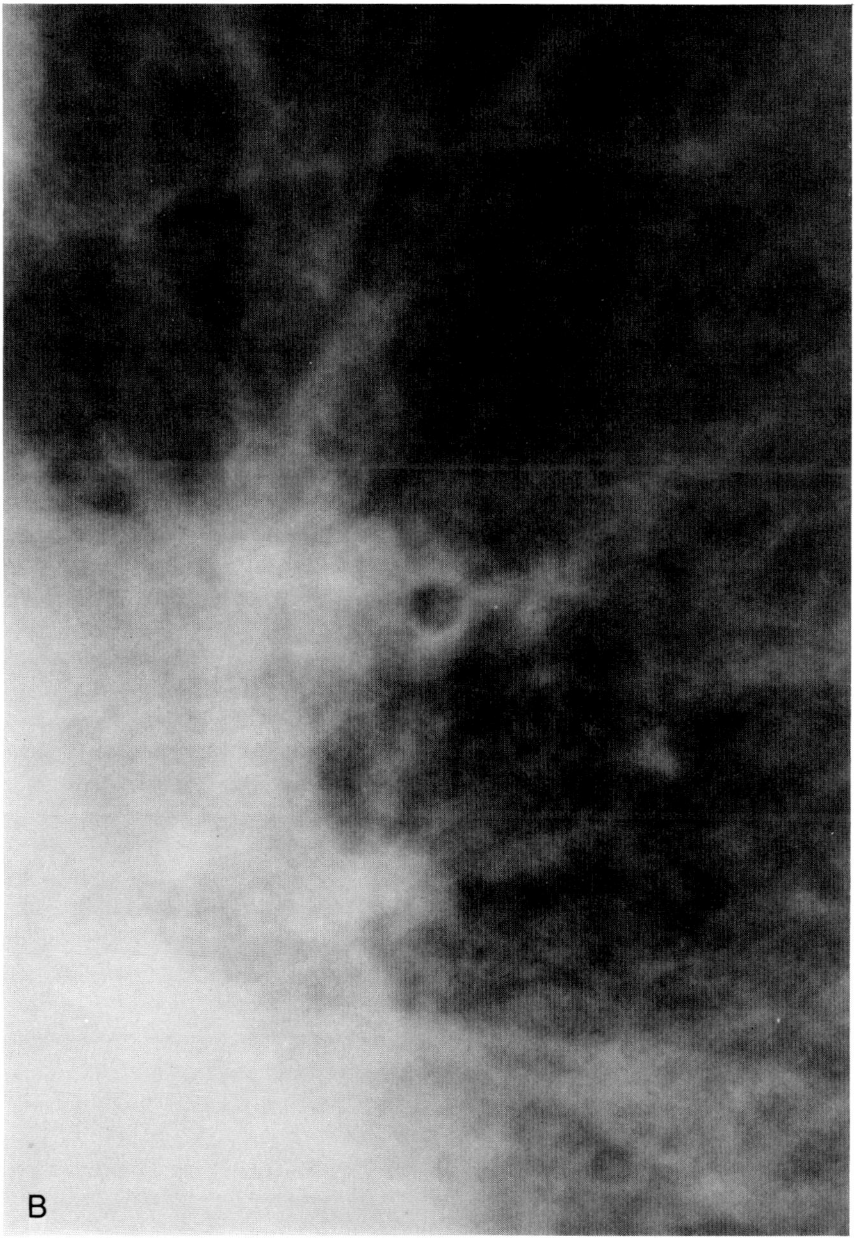

Figure 6–3 (continued).

Inhalation of toxic chemicals is a common cause of ARDS (see Chapter 13). The list of injurious agents includes chlorine gas, ammonia, cadmium, sulfur dioxide, ozone, phosgene, and high concentrations of oxygen. Silo filler's disease is caused by inhaling the nitrogen oxides produced by stored grain.

Approximately 20 percent of patients with acute pancreatitis will develop ARDS. Other associated conditions include uremia, paraquat ingestion, eclampsia, post-cardioversion, radiation pneumonitis, disseminated intravascular coagulation, massive transfusion, and post-cardiopulmonary bypass.

DIAGNOSIS

It is critical to recognize pulmonary edema because the inadequate tissue oxygenation that results may be fatal but can also often be markedly improved by augmenting the inspired oxygen concentration. Separating hydrostatic edema from increased-permeability edema is important because the therapy for each condition differs in many respects. The presentation of either form of edema may be sufficiently distinctive to permit a diagnosis from clinical data alone. However, in many instances, the signs and symptoms overlap to such a degree that right-heart catheterization is required for the measurement of several hemodynamic variables that can accurately distinguish normal- from increased-permeability edema. Occasionally, both types of edema may be present simultaneously.

Normal-Permeability (Hydrostatic) Edema

Patients with normal-permeability edema present with dyspnea and a cough that is frequently productive of clear, watery, or blood-tinged sputum. The presence of blood in the sputum is characteristic of normal-permeability edema. Symptoms of an acute myocardial infarction may be present. The past history may suggest chronic left ventricular failure (paroxysmal nocturnal dyspnea and orthopnea), previous cardiac decompensation, or angina pectoris. The patient may have a history of hypertension, rheumatic fever, or a previously known heart murmur. Tachypnea and tachycardia are usually observed, and signs of cardiac decompensation (pedal edema, jugular venous pressure elevation, rales, and an S_3 gallop) may be found.

Routine laboratory studies generally are of little value. An arterial blood gas determination may show respiratory alkalosis or acidosis, but frequently, metabolic acidosis is present secondary to tissue oxygen deficiency and consequent lactate production.[44] Hypoxemia is uniformly present and the $PaCO_2$ may be low, normal or, in up to 20 percent of patients, elevated.[45] The ECG may document an acute myocardial infarction, cardiac ischemia, left ventricular hypertrophy, various tachy- or bradyarrhythmias or, rarely, may be normal. The P wave morphology may suggest left atrial enlargement.

Cardiomegaly may be present on the chest roentgenogram, but left ventricular

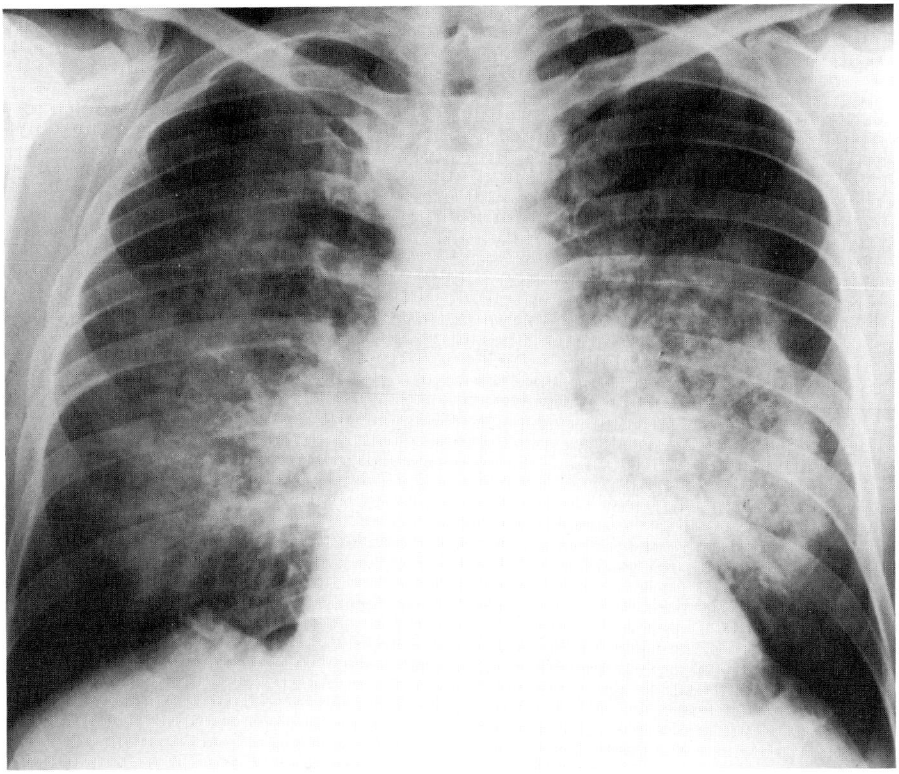

Figure 6–4. Butterfly distribution of pulmonary edema. (Courtesy of Dr. M. Figley, University of Washington.)

failure can occur with a normal heart size, particularly in the setting of an acute myocardial infarction, left atrial myxoma, or restrictive cardiomyopathy. If a lateral chest radiograph can be obtained, aortic and mitral valve calcification should be sought. Occasionally, calcified coronary vessels may be seen. Pleural effusions may occur and are usually indicative of both pulmonary and systemic venous hypertension. With pulmonary venous hypertension, blood flow is redistributed to the upper lung zones, increasing the caliber of upper-lobe vessels (Fig. 6–2 A and B). When pulmonary edema develops, fluid first accumulates in the interstitial space around larger vessels and airways (see "Pathophysiology, Sequence of edema formation"). This blurs the vascular markings and will increase the bronchial wall thickness of those bronchi that can be seen end-on (Fig. 6–3 A and B). With progressive edema, alveolar flooding occurs. This causes air bronchograms and silhouette signs and may distribute in a perihilar "butterfly" fashion (Fig. 6–4).

Increased-Permeability (ARDS) Edema

ARDS usually occurs in the setting of an obvious event known to be associated with the syndrome (Table 6–3). Commonly, respiratory symptoms will be delayed, sometimes for as long as 24 hours.[46,47,48] Presenting symptoms and signs include not only those of pulmonary dysfunction, but also those of the underlying problem.

Pinpoint pupils, needle tracks, and hypoventilation may be found on the physical examination if the cause of ARDS was an overdose of heroin. Evidence of trauma, burns or sepsis may be obvious. Conjunctival and axillary petechiae may be seen with fat emboli. A laboratory evaluation may establish the diagnosis of pancreatitis, smoke inhalation (elevated carboxyhemoglobin values), or disseminated intravascular coagulation. Gram stains and cultures may confirm sepsis or pneumonitis. Symptoms of the underlying problem do not define the presence of ARDS, but merely suggest a predisposition to development of the syndrome. Indeed, many patients with the diseases mentioned here never have substantial pulmonary dysfunction.

The presenting characteristic of ARDS is arterial hypoxemia due to a shunt that may be severe and progressive. Tachypnea may be accompanied by a respiratory alkalosis early in the syndrome, but a variably compensated metabolic acidosis is frequently found on arterial blood gas analysis. The ECG may show a variety of arrhythmias. The chest roentgenogram shows diffuse alveolar filling, but the heart size is usually normal. Pleural effusions are rare in the absence of bacterial pneumonia, pancreatitis, or chest trauma.

When the clinical information does not allow differentiation of hydrostatic from increased-permeability edema, hemodynamic data are needed. During its insertion, a triple-lumen, flow-directed catheter will allow measurement of the right atrial pressure and of the pulmonary arterial and wedge pressures (Ppaw) when it is properly positioned. The cardiac output and mixed venous oxygen tension (or saturation) can also be determined. In pulmonary edema secondary to an increased Pmv, the Ppaw generally exceeds 20 to 25 mmHg.[49] The cardiac output is usually low in the presence of left ventricular failure. In ARDS, the cardiac output is generally increased except in the setting of shock. Pulmonary hypertension and a decrease in the pulmonary vascular bed have been documented in ARDS.[50] These are thought to result from vascular obstruction (see "Pathophysiology, Platelet or Platelet-Fibrin Microemboli"), rather than hypoxic vasospasm, since vasodilating agents have no effect.

The ratio of alveolar-to-serum protein has been used to distinguish normal- from increased-permeability edema.[2,51,52,53] Obtaining an accurate alveolar fluid protein concentration is difficult; protein may selectively concentrate in the foam–air interfaces, the protein concentration may artifactually increase with fluid evaporation or drying, or the specimen may be contaminated by airway, oral, or gastric secretions.[2] The presence of hemoglobin will make standard protein determinations inconclusive, and makes immunoelectrophoretic comparison of the alveolar and serum proteins necessary.[54] Additionally, both the alveolar and serum protein concentrations will change over time regardless of the lung permeability. Because isolated samples of alveolar fluid and serum will not take this time factor into account, multiple paired samples are needed.[55] When copious amounts of edema fluid are pouring out of the trachea, measurements of edema fluid-to-serum protein ratios are more likely to be reliable. With smaller volumes of fluid, the data may be inaccurate. With high vascular pressures, the endothelial permeability may increase, and the distinction between normal and increased permeability may be lost.[9,10,11]

A variety of nonspecific abnormalities in tests of pulmonary function result from pulmonary edema. While these tests are impractical to perform on an acutely ill patient, their results do tend to correlate with the amount and distribution of edema. When the Pmv is elevated, the pulmonary blood volume increases. This will increase the carbon monoxide diffusion capacity, since the latter depends in part upon the blood volume. When interestitial edema is present, the PaO_2 drops, as a result of ventilation/perfusion mismatching (low $\dot{V}_A/\dot{Q}$). The airways are narrowed, as demonstrated by a change in the maximum expiratory flow-volume curve and an increased closing volume. With alveolar flooding, a shunt develops, the PaO_2 drops further, and wasted ventilation increases. The total lung capacity and vital capacity are reduced.[56]

PATHOPHYSIOLOGY

Sequence of Edema Accumulation

Whether the vascular permeability is normal or increased, the first evidence of excessive pulmonary fluid is the appearance of cuffs of edema around large vessels and bronchi[49] (Figs. 6–5 A and B; 6–6). A volume of fluid up to 35 percent of the lung weight can be accommodated in these cuffs before alveolar edema is observed. With further edema accumulation, alveoli either remain air-filled, have a small amount of edema in the corners, or become completely flooded (Fig. 6–7).

This sequence of edema accumulation can be explained by mechanical influences of the lung on the Ppmv in each of two compartments.

A Two-Compartment Lung

The pulmonary vessels and the interstitium immediately surrounding them can be divided into alveolar and extra-alveolar compartments on the basis of the way in which lung inflation affects the vessels within each compartment. Macklin,[57] and later Permutt et al.,[58] noted that when the vascular pressure was low and kept constant relative to the pleural pressure (Ppl), lung inflation compressed the alveolar vessels (AVs) and expanded the extra-alveolar vessels (EAVs) (Fig. 6–8).

Alveolar Interstitium

There are two types of AVs: those located in the corners of alveoli where adjacent septae join, and those located in the septum between two alveolar spaces. The alveolar septal vessels are compressed throughout their length in zone I when the

(Text continues on p. 164.)

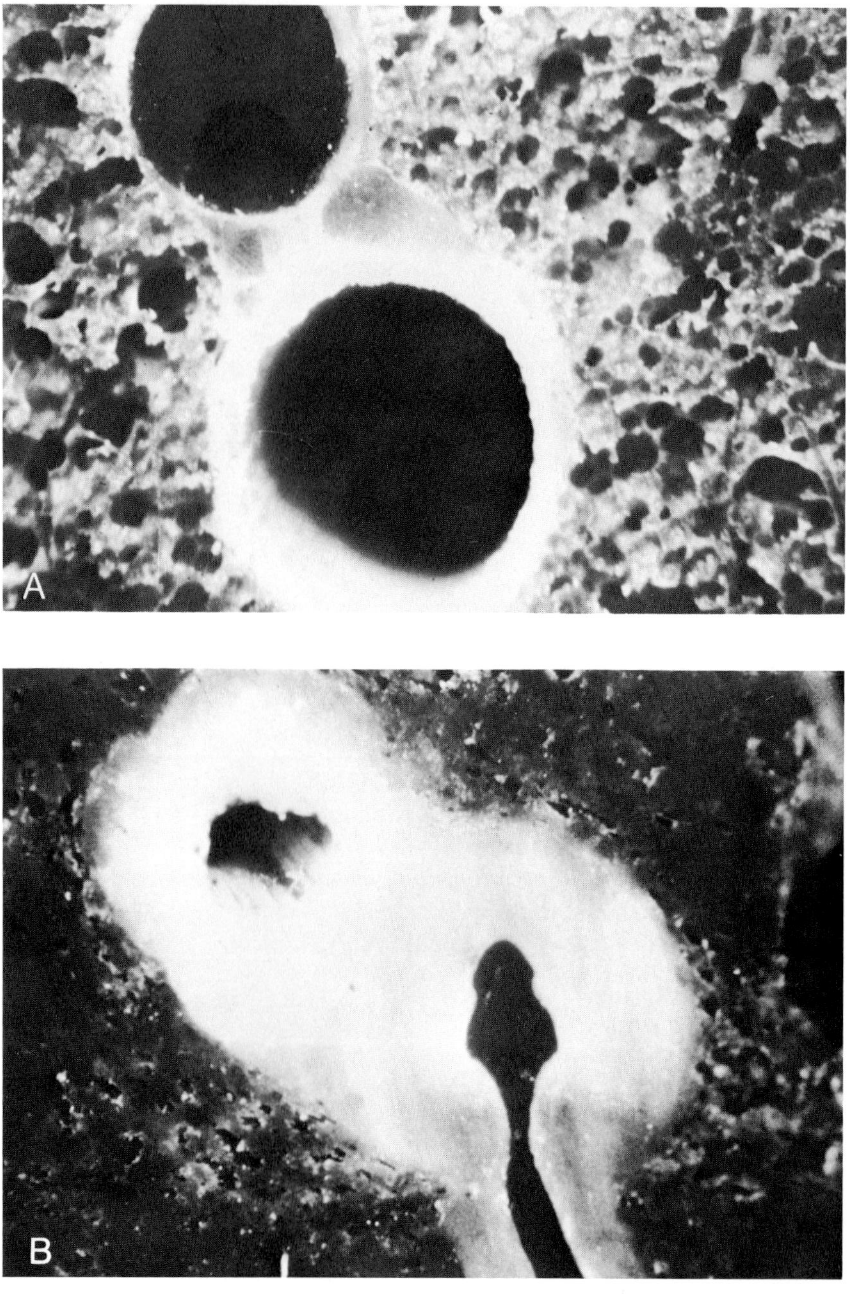

Figure 6–5. (A) Fresh-frozen section of lung showing the normal relationship of the interstitial cuff to the bronchovascular bundle. (B) Similar section under the same magnification after induction of pulmonary edema. (Figs. 6–5, 6–6, and 6–7 from Staub NC, Nagano, Pearce: Pulmonary edema in dogs. J Appl Physiol 22:227, 1967.)

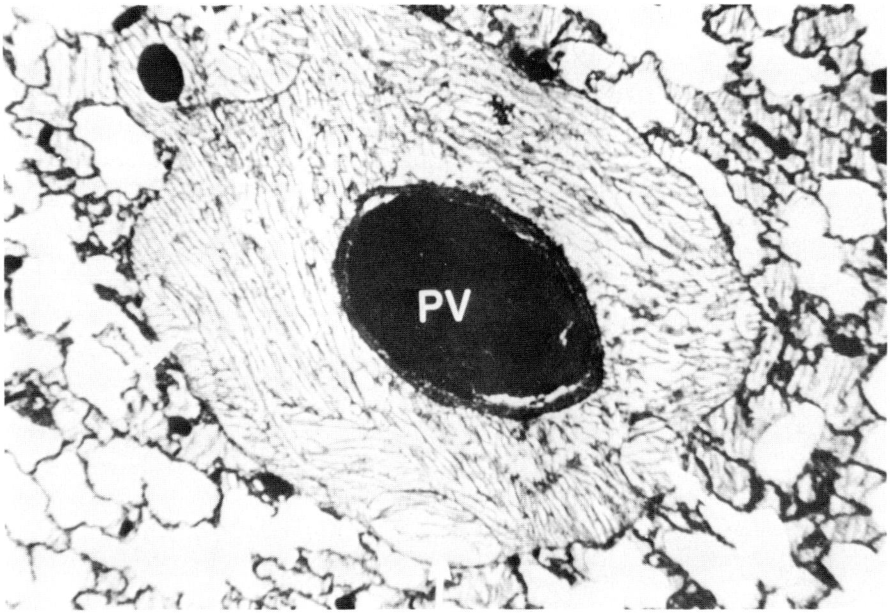

Figure 6–6. Microscopic appearance of perivascular cuffing. PV = pulmonary vein.

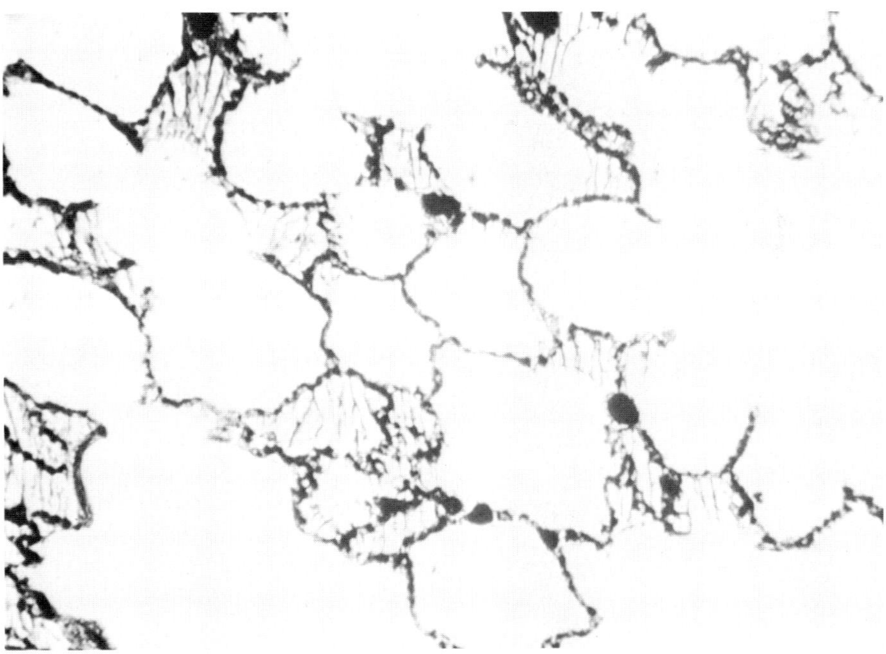

Figure 6–7. With progressive edema, alveoli are either completely flooded, remain air-filled, or have only a small amount of edema in the corners.

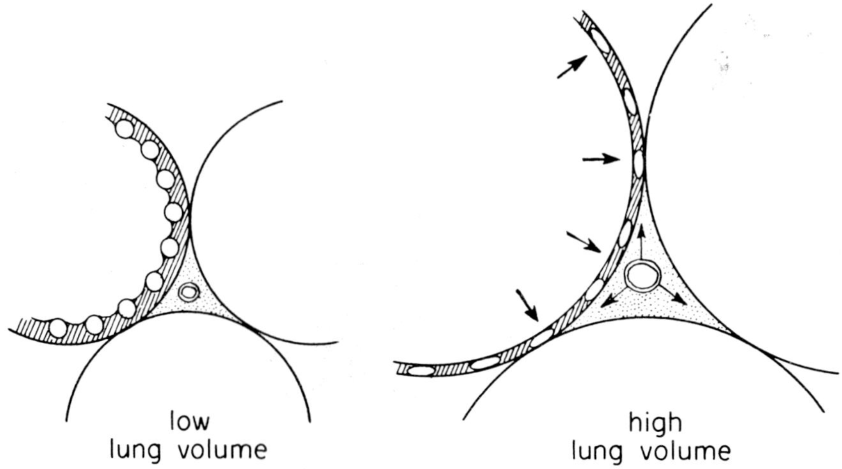

Figure 6–8. Alveolar and extra-alveolar vessels are distinguished by their response to lung inflation. When the transpulmonary pressure and lung volume are increased, and the vascular pressure is kept constant relative to the pleural pressure, alveolar vessels are compressed while extra-alveolar vessels are expanded.

alveolar pressure (P_A) is greater than either the pulmonary arterial or pulmonary venous pressure.[59] The corner vessels are partially exposed to the P_A, but may remain open in zone I[60,61,62] secondary to the effects of surface tension and interdependence properties of the lung[63,64] (Fig. 6–9).

When the lung is between 60 and 100 percent of its total capacity, the alveoli have a polyhedral shape, and the septae have smooth surfaces with only small degrees of curvature.[63] Consequently, surface forces acting on the septae will be low. In the corners of the alveoli, sharp angles are formed between the septae. The greater curvature found in these angles increases the pull, toward the center of the alveolus, due to surface tension. At the same vascular pressure and P_A, corner vessels can be dilated while septal vessels are compressed. This implies that the Ppmv in the corners is more negative than in the septum.[65]

The alveolar septum exposed to the P_A is thin and contains only a fused epithelial and endothelial basement membrane. Because a true interstitial space is lacking, it is reasonable to assume that the Ppmv in the septum approaches, but may be slightly more positive or negative than the P_A, depending upon the lung volume and vascular geometry.[63] The thick side of the septum is not directly exposed to the P_A; it is composed of an interstitial space containing cellular elements and connective tissue fibers which separate the basement membranes. The Ppmv on the thick side may be more negative than the P_A, primarily because the more negative Ppmv in the corner areas could be transmitted to the thick side of the septum via the connective tissue elements.[65]

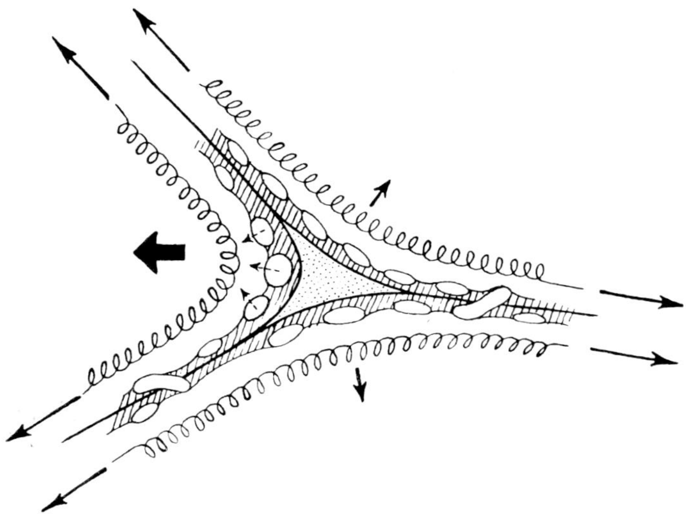

Figure 6–9. There are two types of alveolar vessels. Alveolar septal vessels lie in the flat portion of the septum. Surface tension in this portion of the alveolar wall has little, if any, net inward force. Alveolar septal vessels are subjected to most or all of the alveolar pressure, which is unopposed. Alveolar corner vessels are partially protected from the alveolar pressure, since surface tension in the curved portion of the alveolus provides a recoil pressure countering the alveolar pressure. Lung interdependence (due to the joining of alveolar septae) provides an additional force which lowers the perimicrovascular hydrostatic pressure.

Extra-alveolar Interstitium

Extra-alveolar vessel diameter and the transvascular fluid flux across these vessels should be influenced by the EAV transmural pressure (Ptm). The observation that EAVs expand with lung inflation when the vascular pressure is low and constant implies that the interstitial pressure around the EAVs decreases under such circumstances, causing the Ptm to increase.[57,66] Several estimates and direct measurements of the extra-alveolar interstitial pressure (both the fluid and the total pressure) have been made. Two qualitiatve trends are observed consistently: first, that the extra-alveolar interstitial pressure becomes more negative relative to the pleural pressure as the lung expands[67,68,69,70,71]; second, that the reduction in the extra-alveolar interstitial pressure with lung inflation is greater at lower vascular pressures.[69,70,71,72] From these findings, one would predict that an EAV Ptm sufficiently high to cause fluid transudation across these vessels might be produced by high lung volumes, even if the vascular pressures were low. With this as a hypothesis, we have recently demosntrated that: (1) EAV leakage can occur with a vascular pressure of 1 or 5 cmH_2O when the alveolar pressure is greater than 10 cmH_2O; and (2) that the rate of fluid flux from the EAVs increases directly with the P_A.[73]

Sites of Leakage

While the actual site of transudation has not been established, the fluid that causes pulmonary edema is thought to leak from AVs into the alveolar septum and to then move along connective tissue fibrils into juxta-alveolar areas, with subsequent displacement to the extra-alveolar interstitium.[65] However, several observations suggest that fluid transudation can occur directly from arterial and venous EAVs.[17,74,75,76,77] The extra-alveolar arteries and veins, studied separately,[78] have recently been shown to be a major site of fluid leakage in the early phase of normal-permeability edema, accounting for 41 and 32 percent, respectively, of the total transvascular fluid flux resulting from a hydrostatic stress. Preliminary data suggest a smaller but significant contribution from EAVs when the permeability of these vessels is increased by oleic acid.[79]

Perivascular cuffing might be the result of direct EAV leakage. This mechanism may also explain the edema that develops when the Ppmv is decreased from any cause (Table 6–2), as well as explaining other forms of edema (such as HAPE) occurring with normal left atrial or pulmonary capillary pressures.

Transmural Pressures

The vascular Ptm is the difference between the Pmv and Ppmv. Since the Ppmv surrounding AVs is not the same as that around EAVs, and because fluid seems to leak from both types of vessels, the Ptm for each type of vessel must be considered separately. The Pmv includes the pulmonary arterial, capillary, and venous pressures. The pulmonary capillary pressure is thought to be closer to the pulmonary venous pressure, and most of the pulmonary vascular resistance may be located within the capillaries.[80,81] The Ppmv varies with location. In the extra-alveolar interstitium, it is lower than the P_A and decreases (becomes more negative) with lung inflation or a reduction in the Pmv. The Ppmv approaches the P_A in the thin, flat portion of the alveolar septum. In the corners of alveoli, the Ppmv is more negative relative to the P_A because of surface tension and interdependence phenomena. Thus, when vascular pressures are normal, the Ptm is greatest for the extra-alveolar arteries and least for the alveolar septal vessels (capillaries). The Ptm for alveolar corner vessels and extra-alveolar veins should have a value between that of the extra-alveolar arteries and the septal vessels. Which is greater would depend on the specific vascular pressure and lung volume.

Safety Factors

The relationships explained above could provide a number of clinically important safety factors protecting against alveolar flooding when the forces in Equation 1 favor increased fluid filtration. First, a gradient of interstitial hydrostatic pressure seems to exist[65]; any fluid leaking from alveolar septal vessels should be pulled into the thick side of the septum and from there to the corner areas, rather than depositing in the alveoli themselves. If the alveolar and extra-alveolar interstitial spaces are continuous, the fluid should preferentially move into the peribronchial

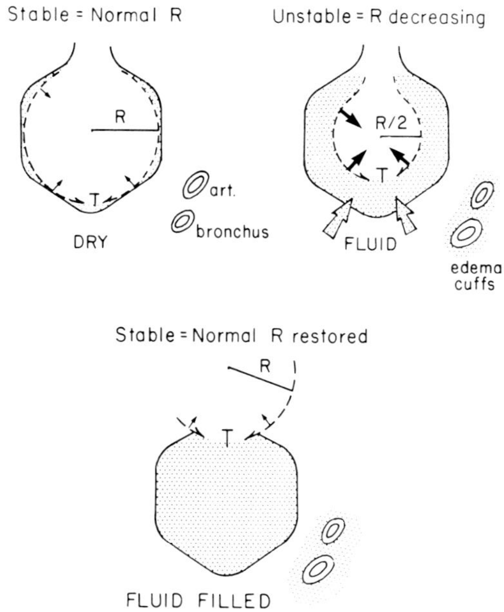

Figure 6–10. The "all-or-none" pattern of alveolar flooding (Fig. 6–7) may be explained by the Laplace relationship (P = 2T/R). Alveolar edema reduces R and progressively increases the recoil pressure. More fluid is pulled into the alveolus until complete flooding has occurred and R is restored to normal.

and perivascular cuffs in the extra-alveolar interstititum. Second, because of the small radius of curvatures in the angles at the corners of the alveoli, the Ptm will be greater in these corner areas, allowing fluid to accumulate there rather than in the alveolar septae. Alveolar areas where most of the gas exchange occurs will be kept dry. As fluid accumulates in the corner areas of the alveoli, their angles widen, increasing the radius of curvature. By the Laplace relationship (P = 2T/R where P = recoil pressure, T= surface tension and R = radius of curvature), recoil pressure is thereby decreased, reducing the Ptm and fluid leakage (Fig. 6–10). With further fluid accumulation, R decreases, causing the recoil pressure to increase. The Ptm rapidly increases, fluid is pulled into the alveolus, and R is decreased progressively until complete alveolar filling has occurred. This mechanism may account for the morphologic observation that in pulmonary edema, alveoli are either free of edema fluid, have a small amount of fluid in the corners, or are completely flooded.[49] It may serve as an additional safety factor by providing a greater number of functional alveoli during pulmonary edema and ARDS.

The observation that edema fluid accumulates in the extra-alveolar interstitium prior to alveolar flooding or alveolar septal edema not only supports the idea that the Ppmv is more negative in the extra-alveolar interstitium than in the alveolus or alveolar septum, but also suggests that the compliance of this space is high. A highly compliant extra-alveolar interstitium means that large volumes of edema can be accommodated without a rise in the extra-alveolar Ppmv or change in the gradient of the Ppmv that draws fluid away from the alveolar septae to the extra-alveolar interstitium. However, the extra-alveolar interstitial compliance will depend on lung inflation, the presence of edema, and the extra-alveolar vascular volume, since all of these affect the EAV Ppmv markedly.[67,68,70,71,82,83] At some volume of interstitial edema accumulation, the Ppmv will increase. This will reduce the Ptm, favoring transvascular fluid filtration across EAVs, and may help to limit edema formation.

Additional safety factors are related to the endothelial and epithelial membrane characteristics. Kf represents the permeability of the pulmonary vasculature to fluid. Highly permeable membranes will filter substantial volumes of fluid at low hydrostatic and osmotic driving pressures. Less permeable membranes will require higher gradients for filtration. Fluid filtration occurs across the vascular endothelium, as well as across the alveolar epithelium, and each cellular layer has its own Kf. For two membranes in series, fluid filtration will be limited more by the membrane with the smaller Kf. The alveolar epithelium is much less permeable than the vascular endothelium. This difference suggests that the driving pressure that produces alveolar edema will have to be much greater than that causing interstitial edema. This pressure difference may serve to keep the alveoli free of edema until a substantial volume of interstitial edema has developed, raising the Ppmv to the higher pressure needed to produce alveolar edema.

The reflection coefficient represents the ability of the pulmonary vasculature to sieve protein and maintain an osmotic gradient. If the membrane is freely permeable to protein, πmv equals πpmv, $\sigma = 0$, and the osmotic gradient drops out of Equation 1. If the membrane is totally impermeable to protein, $\sigma = 1$, and the osmotic gradient will contribute its full potential to transvascular fluid flux. Each osmotically active protein may have a different σ. Both πmv and πpmv depend upon the number rather than the kind of protein molecules present.

When Kf and σ are normal, the fluid leaking into the interstitium has a low protein content and dilutes the perivascular fluid, reducing the perivascular osmotic pressure.[84] πmv may become somehwat more concentrated. The effects on πmv and πpmv are a function of σ, and are greatest when the vessel is least permeable to protein. These changes will lower the forces favoring fluid filtration by increasing the osmotic gradient. Additionally, the hydrostatic gradient may be decreased as the Ppmv increases with interstitial edema accumulation. Once the edema has accumulated, these changes may contribute to the rapid rate of edema resorption that can be seen in conditions causing normal-permeability edema. In ARDS, Kf increases such that with normal hydrostatic and osmotic gradients, the rate of fluid filtration increases.[85] To minimize the forces favoring fluid filtration and maximize resorption of the interstitial fluid when permeability is either normal or increased, the Pmv should be reduced to the lowest value that allows maintenance of hemodynamic stability.

In the early phase of ARDS, large amounts of protein also leak across the vasculature.[52,55] Since σ approaches zero, πmv will equal πpmv, and the compensatory osmotic changes that are seen with normal-permeability edema will not occur. The use of osmotically active solutions during the phase of increased membrane permeability to protein therefore has no rationale (see "Treatment, Reduction of Pmv").

Surface Tension

Pattle[86] first suggested that a low surface tension might be needed to prevent surface forces of the fluid film constituting the alveolar lining layer from sucking fluid into the alveoli and causing pulmonary edema. Clements[87] and Guyton[88] postulated that the increased surface tension caused by surfactant depletion would cause the Ppmv to become more negative. This would increase the microvascular hydrostatic gradient and enhance fluid filtration. We recently have verified this hypothesis.[89] The effect of surfactant depletion favoring edema formation applies to both the infant and adult respiratory distress syndromes. In these settings, both qualitative and quantitative abnormalities in the alveolar surfactant have been documented.[4,90,91,92]

Surface tension may explain the observation that when the PEEP is reduced in a patient with ARDS and shunt increases, a return to the original PEEP level may not decrease the shunt to its former value.[93] Since the surface tension is higher upon inflation than upon deflation, the same transpulmonary pressure (returning to the former PEEP level) would produce a lower FRC.

Lung Ultrastructure

Electron microscopic examination of lungs with normal-permeability edema has shown interstitial edema widely separating the connective-tissue fibrils in the thick side of the alveolar septum. Red blood cells (but no fibrin) are present in the alveolar spaces and septal interstitium. The vascular endothelium and alveolar epithelium are intact, and no separtion of intercellular junctions is apparent unless very high vascular pressures are present.[9,11,94] The explanation for the appearance of red blood cells in the alveoli and interstitium is unknown, and the pathways for increased fluid movement have not been observed.[94] Potential pathways for such fluid migration include direct transcellular movement, vesicular transport, and diffusion through intercellular junctions or chains of intracellular vesicles.

Early studies of increased-permeability edema described primarily endothelial and sometimes alveolar epithelial injury.[4] When various agents are used to produce the syndrome in animal models, both endothelial and epithelial damage results. A recent report on the pathologic changes of ARDS in humans suggested that early in the disease process, the alveolar epithelium had extensive defects, but that the vascular endothelium and intercellular junctions were normal.[54] Platelet-fibrin thrombi were seen to cover the occasional endothelial defect. Nonetheless, because of the large amount of interstitial fibrin, temporary endothelial leaks were presumed to have existed.

Pathogenesis of ARDS

There are many potential mechanisms by which the vascular endothelium and alveolar epithelium could be damaged. These are listed in Table 6–4.

Table 6–4. Potential Mediators of Injury in ARDS

Platelets
Fibrin
Histamine
Complement system
Leukocyte proteases
Superoxide anions
Thromboxane A_2
Leukotrienes
Fibronectin

Platelet or Platelet-Fibrin Microemboli

Platelet aggregates or platelet-fibrin microemboli could cause nonuniform vascular obstruction and: (1) directly damage the vasculature; (2) release bioactive substances which cause lung injury indirectly; or (3) in combination with impaired fibrinolysis, produce fibrinogen fragments which could liberate histamine from mast cells, basophils, or platelets (Fig. 6–11).

Several investigators have noted widespread vascular thrombosis in histologic specimens from patients with ARDS.[95,96,97,98] In vivo ^{125}I-fibrinogen studies support these observations. Some have demonstrated a correlation between the amount of radiation emitted and the degree of hypoxemia.[97] However, others have found no such correlation and no evidence of platelet-fibrin thrombi in the lungs.[99,100,101] The infusion of platelet aggregates does not produce ARDS,[102] and the syndrome can be produced by thrombin infusion (with inhibition of fibrinolysis) in the absence of platelets or leukocytes.[103]

An inhibitor of plasminogen activator has been found in severely ill patients.[104] If fibrinolysis is blunted, the clearance of platelet-fibrin microemboli might be impaired, resulting in an increased exposure to fibrinogen degradation products (FDP). In an animal model,[105] the infusion of one of these FDP fragments (fragment D) can cause an ARDS which is blocked by the pre-administration of antihistamines.[106] However, neither fibrin nor fibrinogen degradation is needed to produce increased permeability in other models,[107] products of fibrinolysis are higher in patients with ARDS than in those with only the predisposing condition, and FDP (particularly fragment D) can be present in high concentrations in patients receiving thrombolytic therapy without ARDS developing. The deposition of platelet-fibrin microemboli in ARDS may be a response to injury rather than its cause.[108]

Fibronectin

Fibronectin, a nonimmune, cold insoluble, opsonizing globulin has been linked to the pathogenesis of ARDS. This substance is consumed in septic shock, and its levels can be returned toward normal by infusing cryoprecipitate. Since fibronectin functions as a "nonspecific vacuum cleaner" (Dr. T.M. Hyers, personal communication), reduced levels may impair the reticulo-endothelial clearance of cellular and particulate debris. The use of cryoprecipitate in one uncontrolled

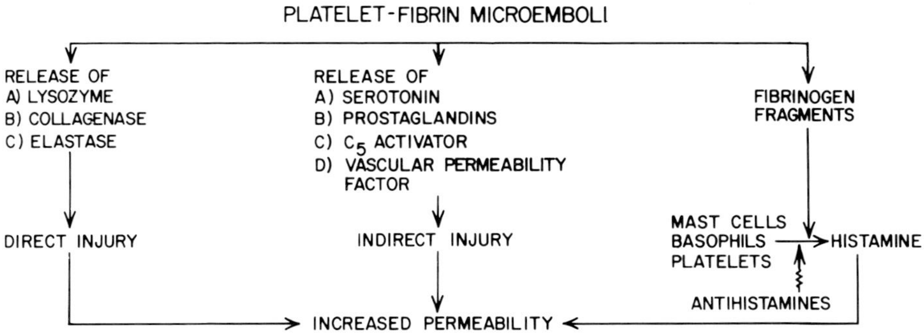

Figure 6–11. Potential mechanisms by which platelet-fibrin microemboli might increase vascular permeability and cause ARDS.

series seemed to improve the cardiopulmonary status of patients in septic shock.[109,110,111,112] However, fibronectin depletion is seen in many instances in which ARDS does not develop.[113]

Complement System-Leukocyte Aggregation

To test the hypothesis that complement-mediated aggregation of leukocytes accounted for the neutropenia and "hypoxemia" seen in renal dialysis patients, Craddock[114] infused cellophone- or zymosan-incubated plasma into normal animals. Leukopenia and hypoxia developed, along with pulmonary hypertension. Intravascular leukostasis and interstitial edema were observed. The syndrome could be prevented if the animals were made leukopenic or had their complement systems inactivated.

The activated third, fourth, and fifth fragments of complement are known to increase vascular permeability and to release histamine from mast cells, and may cause smooth-muscle contraction. C5a, which is increased in some conditions associated with ARDS,[15] attracts leukocytes. Pneumococci injected intravenously into guinea pigs will localize in the lung unless complement is previously depleted or congenitally deficient, or if the animals are made neutropenic.[116] C5a can also cause leukocytes to agglutinate. These leukocytes might then release both neutral (elastase and plasmin) and acid proteases (lysosyme and acid hydrolase) (Fig. 6–12), which in turn can cleave C5a (as do other substances). These leukocyte proteases can cause direct vascular injury, and have recently been found in the bronchoalveolar lavage fluid of ARDS patients.[118,119] Aggulatinated leukocytes also might cause endothelial damage through the generation of superoxide ions (H_2O_2, OH^- and O_2^-).[120,121] The leukocyte agglutination may be inhibited by certain corticosteroid preparations.[117]

While leukocytes are required to increase vascular permeability in several models of ARDS, [122,123,124] they are not needed in others (induced by ethchlorvynol or endotoxin).[125,126,127,128] Additionally, other diseases or substances can cause leukoag-

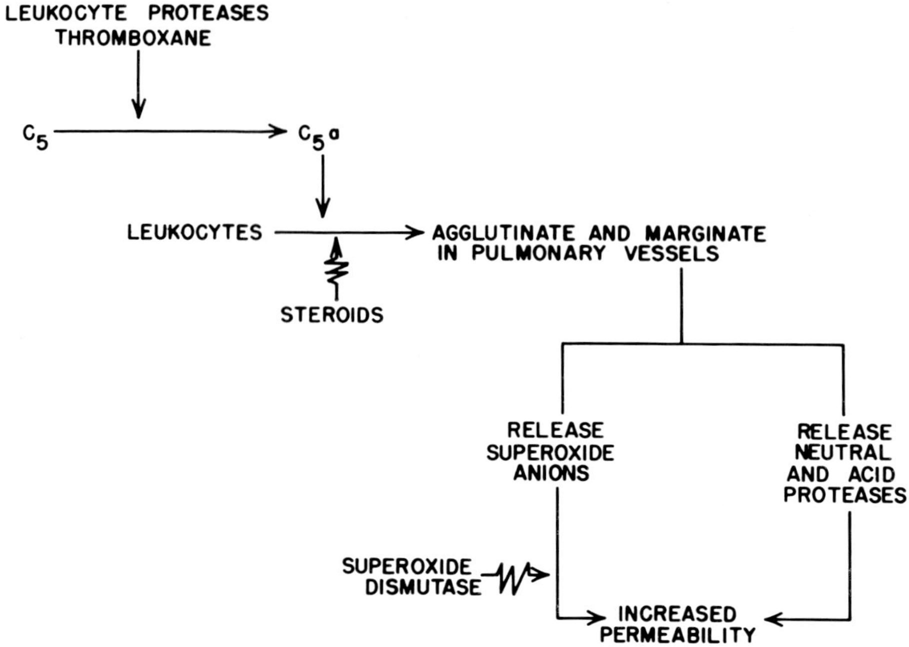

Figure 6–12. Potential mechanisms by which complement activation might increase vascular or alveolar permeability, or both, and cause ARDS.

glutination and sequestration in the lung without causing the type of injury seen in ARDS.[129,130] Finally, while the infusion of C5a does cause leukocyte sequestration in the pulmonary vasculature, increased vascular permeability is not observed.[131]

Prostaglandin System

Recent studies have implicated arachidonic acid derivatives in the pathogenesis of ARDS. One of these, thromboxane A_2 (TXA-2), can cause platelet aggregation, increase leukocyte adhesiveness, and produce vasoconstriction.[132] TXA-2 synthesis is increased in endotoxin-induced shock; the synthesis can be blocked, and mortality reduced, by pretreatment with imidazole or indomethacin, or by the restriction of free fatty acids, which limits endoperoxide synthesis (Fig. 6–13). Additionally, TXA-2 activates C5 (Fig. 6–12). Leukotrienes are also derived from arachidonic acid. These compounds are thought to be even more potent mediators of inflammation than TXA-2, and capable of regulating leukocyte function, causing smooth muscle contractions, and increasing vascular permeability.[133]

The prostaglandin and complement-activated leukocyte systems may work together to cause the marked increase in fluid and protein filtration that is characteristic of ARDS. C5a can cause leukoagglutination and sequestration in the pulmonary vasculature, with the release of proteases that increase vascular permeability. The volume of fluid filtration may then be increased markedly in the presence of a vasodilator prostaglandin.[134]

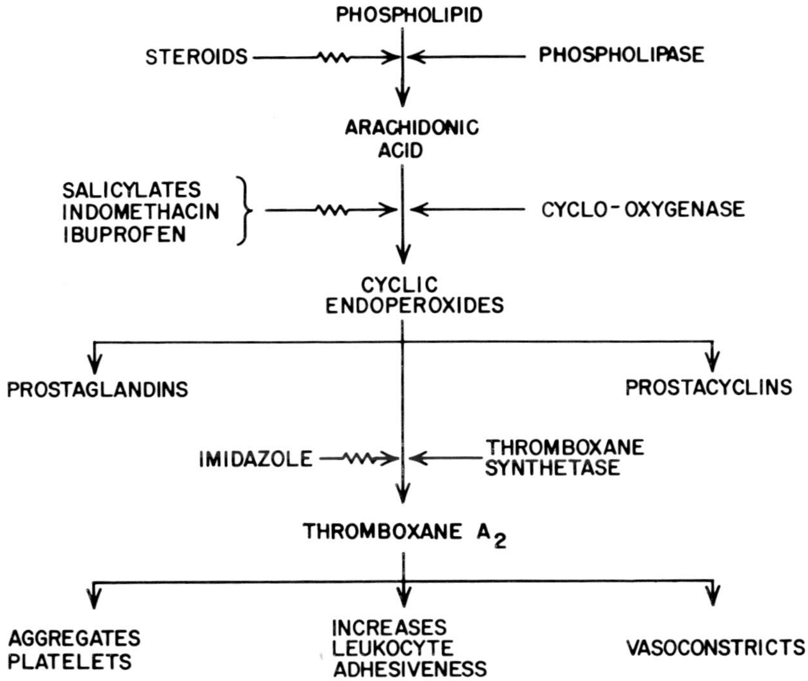

Figure 6–13. Arachidonic acid metabolites might cause ARDS. Thromboxane A_2 has many effects that could contribute to the pathophysiology. Leukotrienes (produced from arachidonic acid by lipoxygenase) are even more potent compounds that also increase vascular permeability and cause leukoagglutination.

THERAPY

Normal Permeability

Increased Pmv

Supportive Therapy

The first medication to administer is oxygen, either by mask or nasal cannula, at a high flow rate. There is no concern for suppressing the hypoxic drive of patients in pulmonary edema, while systemic hypoxemia may be lethal if untreated. Although the predominant physiologic causes of hypoxemia are shunt and a low cardiac output, areas of low $\dot{V}_A/\dot{Q}$ do exist. Augmenting the inhaled oxygen concentration will raise the oxygen content of blood coming from these low $\dot{V}_A/\dot{Q}$ units.

Some have suggested administering oxygen by positive pressure ventilation. If the intrathoracic pressure is sufficiently increased by this endeavor, venous return will decrease and the cardiac preload will be reduced. Applying tourniquets to three of four extremities and rotating these tourniquets every 15 minutes, as well as phlebotomy, have also been suggested as methods of reducing the preload. All of these interventions are being used less frequently as experience with vasodilating agents is gained.

Regardless of the cause, people immobilized for a period of days are at increased risk for deep venous thrombosis and subsequent pulmonary embolism. This risk may be increased by contraction of the intravascular volume secondary to the administration of diuretics. In the setting of acute myocardial infarction, the use of subcutaneous, low-dose heparin (5000 units twice daily) reduces the incidence of ^{125}I-fibrinogen-diagnosed deep venous thrombosis.[135,136] Complications of this treatment are infrequent and of minor consequence. Low-dose heparin should be equally effective as a prophylactic agent in patients with pulmonary edema.

Specific Therapy

The management of cardiogenic pulmonary edema should focus on reducing the cardiac workload and decreasing the excess fluid accumulation. Reduction of the ventricular afterload may be needed if the blood pressure is increased, and myocardial contractility may need improvement if the cardiac output is reduced.

Reducing Cardiac Work. The patient should be put at bed-rest to limit physical stress. The sitting position is generally preferred, since the supine posture minimizes gravitational changes in the Pmv and increases the venous return to an already overloaded central circulation. Having the patient sit upright lowers the Pmv in the upper portions of the lung.

Mental stress also should be minimized. Sedatives (such as chloral hydrate 0.5 to 1.0 g, phenobarbital 15 to 30 mg, or diazepam 2 to 10 mg orally, t.i.d. and at bedtime) and laxatives may be helpful in this regard. For extreme agitation, meperidine 50 mg, or morphine sulfate 10 to 15 mg i.v., may be used.

Reduction of Excess Fluid. Salt and water retention account for many of the symptoms of pulmonary edema. The commonly used diuretics increase sodium—and consequently water—excretion by the renal tubule. For acute pulmonary edema, diuretics that work primarily on the loop of Henle are preferred. These include furosemide and ethacrynic acid. These drugs will reduce the Pmv with little change in the cardiac output or heart rate. Furosemide should be administered orally or intravenously, in a dose of 20 to 50 mg, doubling the dose every 2 to 3 hours until a diuresis occurs. A single dose should not exceed 240 mg. With renal insufficiency, the drug should not be given at a more rapid rate than 4 mg/min so as to avoid causing a reversible hearing loss. Once the patient has stabilized, furosemide may be administered orally at a dose of 40 to 120 mg/day. Ethacrynic acid (50 mg) also may be used. It has no particular advantage over furosemide, but may have a higher incidence of ototoxicity. Patients given furosemide begin to improve before a diuresis occurs. This has been attributed to an immediate furosemide-induced decrease in venous tone.[137]

Commonly seen side effects from loop diuretics include volume depletion, hyponatremia, hypokalemia, and metabolic alkalosis. Additionally, the uric acid and glucose concentrations may rise.

Table 6–5. Common Arrhythmias Seen with Digitalis Toxicity

Ventricular premature contractions
Paroxysmal atrial tachycardia with block
Wenckebach second degree AV block
Complete heart block
Junctional tachycardias
Sinus bradycardia

It is important to recall that salt and water retention occur as a compensation for the reduced cardiac output in cardiogenic pulmonary edema. Expansion of the intravascular (and consequently the intraventricular) volume improves cardiac output. Thus, overly aggressive diuresis may actually reduce the cardiac output. In some instances, determining the cardiac output at different filling pressures may be necessary.

Increasing Myocardial Contractility. Digitalis increases the heart's contractile force such that a given stroke volume may be maintained at a lower left ventricular end-diastolic pressure. Shifting the ventricular function curve to the left improves cardiac performance.

Patients with pulmonary edema respond differently to digitalis depending upon the specific cause of the increased Pmv. There will be little or no effect of digitalis when left ventricular function is normal (such as in mitral stenosis or restrictive cardiomyopathy). In some conditions, the drug may actually increase the LVEDP (as in hypertrophic obstructive cardiomyopathy). However, when the increased Pmv is secondary to left ventricular dysfunction or to some superventricular tachycardias (atrial fibrillation, atrial flutter), digitalis is particularly effective. If left ventricular failure is secondary to acute ischemia, the use of digitalis may be limited by an additional problem: Digitalis-induced augmentation of myocardial contractility increases cardiac work; when myocardial blood flow is reduced, increased work may increase ischemia and extend the area of infarction.

The increased myocardial contractility seen with digitalis is linearly related to the dose. Thus, even subtherapeutic levels will have some effect. Doses needed to block the AV node are much higher than those required to treat congestive heart failure.[138] The therapeutic index of digitalis is low and the side effects are clinically important. Elderly patients or those with hypothyroidism, COPD, renal impairment, or hypokalemia are predisposed to toxicity. Digitalis blood levels are somewhat difficult to interpret since there is a wide overlap between toxic and nontoxic values. When blood levels of the drug are greater than 2 mg/ml and there are symptoms of nausea, vomiting, anorexia, or a variety of neuropsychiatric complaints, toxicity should be suspected. The major, and frequently the earliest sign of excess digitalis is the development of cardiac arrhythmias. Over 20 percent of hospitalized patients receiving digitalis may manifest cardiac toxicity during their hospitalization.[139,140] The combination of decreased AV conduction and ventricular premature contractions is highly suggestive of digitalis toxicity (Table 6–5).

Digitalis should be used intravenously only when pulmonary edema is life-threatening. This route of administration allows the maximum effect to be achieved in the shortest period of time, with an onset of action in 10 minutes and a peak effect within 1 hour. Additionally, when the cardiac output is reduced, absorption of digitalis may be decreased. The intravenous loading dose for patients not previously on digitalis is 0.75 to 1.0 mg. This dose should not be given at one time, since acute toxicity may result. The daily maintenance dose (0.125 to 0.375 mg) generally can be given orally. Loading may be done orally (0.5 to 0.75 mg), followed by 0.25 to 0.5 mg every 8 hours until the desired dose has been given. Oral digoxin is only 60 to 85 percent absorbed, which accounts for the need to use higher doses than when giving the drug intravenously. The need for rapid digitalization has diminished with the availability of loop diuretics. Some would reserve digitalis for the treatment of tachyarrhythmias which complicate or precipitate pulmonary edema, or for the patient with marked left ventricular dilatation.

Digoxin is eliminated primarily by renal excretion, and its rate of excretion is related to the creatinine clearance. When renal function is impaired, the maintenance dose should be 14 + (0.2 × the creatinine clearance in ml/min) expressed as a percentage and multiplied by the desired total body content of the drug (usually 0.01 to 0.02 mg/kg body weight). As an example, if the creatinine clearance is 25 ml/min, the daily maintenance dose for a 70 kg person would be

$$\frac{14 + (0.2 \times 25)}{100} \times (0.01 \times 70) = 0.125 \text{ mg}$$

Digitoxin is less acceptable as an intravenous digitalis preparation because it requires a longer period of time to achieve a maximal effect.

Isoproterenol, norepinephrine, and dopamine are also other intropic agents that can decrease the Pmv and increase the cardiac output. These medications have variable effects on the alpha- and beta-adrenergic receptors. Isoproterenol primarily stimulates beta receptors, causing sympathetic vasodilation. Dopamine and norepinephrine are beta stimulators when administered in low doses (less than 2 mg/min) but alpha stimulators (causing vasoconstriction) at higher doses. Dopamine is particularly useful when pulmonary edema is present along with a reduced cardiac output and hypotension. Norepinephrine should be used for the immediate treatment of life-threatening hypotension.[141]

Afterload Reduction. Vasodilator therapy is generally reserved for those patients with left ventricular failure in the setting of an acute myocardial infarction or for those patients with pulmonary edema who do not respond to diuretics and digitalis. When cardiac output falls, the renin–angiotensin and adrenergic nervous systems are activated in an attempt to increase blood pressure and stroke volume. This increases the systemic vascular resistance which, in turn, increases the left ventricular end-diastolic volume and pressure, and can result in a further reduction of cardiac output. Depending upon which vasodilating agent is used, the venous capacitance may be increased, the arterial resistance can be reduced, or both effects can occur (Table 6–6). These agents are particularly helpful for left

Table 6–6. Vasodilator Administration

	Dosage	Route	Interval	Site of Action
Nitrates				
Nitroglycerin ointment	½″–4″	Cutaneously	q.6h.	Veins
Isosorbide dinitrate	20–40 mg	Oral	q.4h.	
	2.5–10 mg	Sublingual	q.1–2h.	
Hydralazine	50–75 mg	Oral	q.6h.	Arteries
Nitroprusside	15 μg/min increasing to 400 μg/min maximum	Intravenous	Continuous infusion	Arteries and veins

ventricular failure secondary to coronary artery disease, hypertension, cardiomyopathy, mitral regurgitation, and aortic regurgitation.

Nitrates (nitroglycerin ointment or isosorbide dinitrate) primarily act on the venous capacitance vessels. As a result, the intravascular volume is redistributed. Cardiac output is minimally improved, but the pulmonary arterial wedge pressure may be significantly reduced. If central congestion is not present, nitrates may decrease the cardiac output.

Hydralazine primarily works on the arterial side of the circulation. Systemic vascular resistance is reduced, left ventricular emptying is improved, and the cardiac output is increased. Since blood pressure is the product of the cardiac output multiplied by the systemic vascular resistance, the blood pressure drops only slightly and the heart rate is unchanged when hydralazine is given. However, hydralazine may, although rarely, cause a reflex tachycardia, and may increase angina. Therefore, the drug should be used cautiously in the setting of acute cardiac ischemia.

Nitroprusside affects both the capacitance and the resistance vessels. It will increase cardiac output while simultaneously reducing the pulmonary arterial wedge pressure. This agent should not be used when the wedge pressure is less than 12 to 15 mmHg. It should not be given in doses greater than that which reduces the blood pressure by more than 20 mmHg, or below 100 mmHg.

The major complication encountered when using vasodilators is hypotension. This may occur suddenly and be quite severe, and has led to the recommendation that arterial lines and Swan-Ganz catheters be used whenever a patient is so severely ill that nitroprusside is needed. Hydralazine may cause a lupus-like syndrome in doses greater than 200 mg daily. With discontinuation of the medication the syndrome will reverse. The prolonged use of nitroprusside (greater than 48 hours) may result in thiocyanate toxicity manifested by nausea, anorexia, singultus, changes in mental status, and occasionally hyperthyroidism.

The treatment of normal-permeability edema has classically included morphine sulfate, and this may be the most important agent available for the condition. Its exact mechanism of action is unknown, but several effects are thought to contribute to the excellent response observed. Morphine may reduce the venous tone and shift blood from the central to the peripheral circulation as a reflex response to (1) reduced anxiety; (2) an improved ventilatory pattern; or (3) direct central nervous system effects.[142,143,144] Additionally, morphine may affect the distribution of ventilation by relaxing airway smooth muscle.

The decision to use diuretics, inotropic agents, or vasodilators depends upon the hemodynamic status of each patient. In general, if pulmonary edema is present when the cardiac output and blood pressure are normal, diuretics are indicated. If the blood pressure is increased, vasodilators should be used. If the cardiac output is decreased, inotropic agents should be used when the blood pressure is reduced and vasodilators when it is elevated.[141]

The condition causing pulmonary edema must be identified before treatment is undertaken (Table 6–1). In addition to treatment for reducing the edema, additional meausres may be needed to treat the underlying problem. For example, surgical intervention may be required to successfully reverse the increased Pmv caused by aortic stenosis. If there is left ventricular failure secondary to anemia or hypertension, transfusions or antihypertensive medications should be given. In some patients with chronic left ventricular disease controlled with a variety of medications, acute episodes of pulmonary edema may be the result of noncompliance with a diet or drug regimen. The cause of left ventricular failure may be as obvious as complete heart block presenting with a heart rate of 20 to 40 beats per minute, or as subtle as apathetic hyperthyroidism manifested by heart failure and lethargy.

Decreased Ppmv

The tendency for patients who are being mechanically ventilated to retain fluid and increase their lung water content must be kept in mind. These patients' fluid balance must be meticulously followed. The increased lung water that occurs with high levels of PEEP is a theoretical argument favoring use of the lowest effective level of PEEP (see "Increased Permeability, Supportive Therapy"). However, there have been no clinical studies comparing survival using various levels of end-expiratory pressure.

In a patient who presents with chronic pneumothoraces or effusions, the possibility of re-expansion edema should be considered prior to therapeutic intervention. In general, pressures more negative than -10 cmH_2O should not be used when evacuating the pleural space. When a chronic effusion is present, no more than 750 ml of fluid should be removed at a time. If re-expansion edema develops, recollapsing the affected lung may be of benefit.[145]

The edema seen with acute upper airway obstruction resolves when the occlusion is removed and large, negative pleural pressures are no longer generated.

Increased Permeability

Because the pathophysiology of ARDS is poorly understood, treatment is largely supportive and focuses on providing adequate oxygenation and minimizing the

Pmv. Since clinical studies are lacking, specific therapy can be based only on theoretical considerations.

Supportive Therapy

Oxygenation

The immediate, life-threatening problem in ARDS is inadequate oxygen delivery to the tissues. Oxygen delivery is determined by the amount of oxygen in the blood (the O_2 content) and the cardiac output (CO).

$$O_2 \text{ delivery} = CO \times O_2 \text{ content} \tag{2}$$

Each variable must be considered separately.

Since CO = heart rate × stroke volume (SV), bradyarrhythmias could limit the CO and, therefore, reduce O_2 delivery. Tachyarrhythmias and other conduction abnormalities also could reduce O_2 delivery by lowering the SV. The SV is determined by the ventricular end-diastolic volume (LVEDV or preload), the systemic vascular resistance (SVR or afterload), and the intrinsic myocardial contractility. When the myocardial contractility is constant, a substantial reduction in the LVEDV will decrease the SV, CO, and consequently O_2 delivery. This usually is manifested by a low end-diastolic filling pressure (depending on the ventricular compliance), which in turn usually results in a low left atrial pressure and consequently a low pulmonary arterial wedge pressure (Ppaw). Central venous pressure has been used to estimate the Ppaw, but it may be inaccurate when there is acute dysfunction of the left or right ventricle or when there is significant pulmonary disease causing pulmonary arterial hypertension.

Since the Ppaw frequently determines subsequent therapeutic interventions, it is important to review those situations in which the Ppaw may not accurately reflect the left atrial pressure or LVEDP. First, when left atrial function is good, the mean left atrial pressure may underestimate the LVEDP.[146] Second, the relationship between the LVEDV and LVEDP (ventricular compliance) may not be constant, such that changes in the LVEDP may not reflect changes in ventricular filling. Third, when PEEP therapy is used, the Ppaw may not be the same as the left atrial pressure. A patent column of blood must extend from the left atrium to the tip of the catheter in the pulmonary arteriole. This condition will not exist if the P_A is greater than the pulmonary venous pressure. In this circumstance, the Ppaw will be the same as the alveolar pressure.[147] Fortunately, because the Swan-Ganz catheter is flow-directed, it almost always lodges in zone III of the lung, where the P_A is less than either the pulmonary arterial or venous pressures.[4,148] Nonetheless, whenever the pressure recorded by the wedged catheter is the same as or somewhat below the P_A, the absence of a patent blood column from the left atrium to the catheter tip should be considered.

The stroke volume (SV) is inversely related to ventricular afterload or the amount of tension that must be developed in the heart wall over a given radius to overcome the SVR.

$$\text{SVR} = \frac{(\text{Mean arterial pressure}^* - \text{CVP}) \times 80}{\text{CO}}$$

If the SVR is increased, vasodilators may be needed to increase O_2 delivery. If the SV is low despite an adequate preload—the afterload and heart rate being normal—then the ejection fraction must be reduced, implying intrinsic cardiac disease. Maximizing the cardiac output and O_2 delivery in this instance might include trials of digoxin or other inotropic agents or increasing the preload.

The O_2 content of the blood includes oxygen that is bound to hemoglobin, as well as that dissolved in plasma. The O_2 content is a function of the hemoglobin (Hgb) concentration, the degree to which the Hgb molecule is saturated with oxygen, and the partial pressure of oxygen (PaO_2), which determines the volume of oxygen dissolved in the plasma, as follows:

$$O_2 \text{ content} = 1.39 \times \text{Hgb concentration} \times \text{percent saturation} + 0.003 \times PaO_2 \quad (3)$$

Where the constant 1.39 is the volume of oxygen that can combine with 1 gm of Hgb, and the constant 0.003 is the volume of oxygen that is dissolved in the plasma (by Henry's law, a function of the partial pressure).

Under normal conditions (assuming an Hgb of 15 gm percent, an O_2 saturation of 95 percent, and a PaO_2 of 95 mmHg):

$$\begin{aligned} O_2 \text{ content} &= 1.39 \times 15 \times 0.95 + 0.003 \times 95 \\ &= 20.1 \text{ ml oxygen/100 ml blood} \end{aligned}$$

Inability of the lungs to oxygenate the blood is the primary cause for decreased O_2 delivery in ARDS. The physiologic cause of the hypoxemia is a shunt (with a small component due to a low $\dot{V}_A/\dot{Q}$). Since shunted blood is unaffected by the alveolar oxygen tension, low fractions of inspired oxygen (FIO_2) cannot restore adequate oxygenation, and higher fractions (0.5 to 1.0) of oxygen almost always are needed. Intubation is required to insure a constant high FIO_2.

Although tracheitis may develop with as little as 6 hours of exposure to 95 percent oxygen,[149] patients with otherwise normal lungs seem able to tolerate 100 percent oxygen for 24 to 72 hours without clinically important physiologic abnormalities.[150,151] The precise concentration of oxygen that is toxic to the lung probably depends on many factors, including age, nutritional and endocrinologic status, and previous exposure to oxygen.[152] Forty percent oxygen can be tolerated for several weeks.[153] Concentrations between 60 and 100 percent may cause lung damage when given over longer periods of time, and the risk seems proportional to the FIO_2. There is experimental evidence suggesting that lung injury changes the susceptibility to O_2 toxicity.[154,155,156] Therefore, it seems prudent to use the lowest FIO_2 that produces an adequate O_2 content.

$$^*\text{Mean arterial pressure} = \frac{\text{systolic pressure} + 2 \times \text{diastolic pressure}}{3}$$

PEEP or CPAP breathing has been employed effectively in ARDS to increase the PaO_2 and allow reduction of the FIO_2, thereby lowering the risk of O_2 toxicity.[157,158,159] With interstitial edema, pulmonary compliance is decreased, the functional residual capacity (FRC) is reduced, airway resistance is increased, and ventilation/perfusion mismatching occurs. PEEP restores the FRC, thus improving airway resistance and compliance either by shifting the lung to a different volume on the same compliance curve or by opening atelectatic areas and shifting to a new curve entirely. Alveolar edema is associated with atelectasis and shunt. PEEP reduces both of these, perhaps by expanding partially collapsed, edema-filled alveoli with the effect that the amount of edema present is spread over a larger area (a greater R), which will convert areas of shunt to ones of low or normal $\dot{V}_A/\dot{Q}$. The recoil pressure also will be decreased. The end result is that O_2 content is increased and the FIO_2 can be reduced.

An additional rationale for the use of PEEP may be the circular pattern of injury noted in Figure 6–1. Alveolar edema impairs the pulmonary surfactant, which causes an increase in surface tension and predisposes to more edema. Experimental data suggest that PEEP may conserve surfactant and interrupt this cycle.[23] Two poorly controlled clinical studies support the early use of low levels of PEEP to prevent ARDS.[160,161]

There is considerable debate about the appropriate amount of PEEP to use. Some investigators have suggested that the "best PEEP" level produces the greatest oxygen delivery. The "best" level has been correlated with the level of best pulmonary compliance, such that when the tidal volume/(expiratory hold airway pressure—PEEP) begins to fall, depression of cardiac output and reduction of oxygen delivery is likely.[162] Others suggest using the lowest level of PEEP that allows reduction of the FIO_2 to less than 0.6 ("least PEEP")* while still providing enough oxygen to meet tissue demands. Still others employ extremely high levels of PEEP (super-high end-expiratory pressure or "SHEEP") in an attempt to reduce the venous admixture (shunt plus low $\dot{V}_A/\dot{Q}$) to its lowest value. These investigators have used from 15 to 60 cmH_2O CPAP along with intermittent mandatory ventilation (IMV).[163,164,165,166,166a]

While there have been no comparative studies, the "least PEEP" approach seems to be the most reasonable approach for several reasons. First, in most instances, low levels of PEEP (less than 15 cmH_2O) will reverse most of the shunt.[100,167] Even SHEEP supporters find it necessary to use these high levels for only approximately 10 percent of ARDS patients. Second, if vascular pressures are kept constant relative to the pleural pressure as the PEEP is increased (which generally occurs until the cardiac output falls), the lung water will increase.[23,24,25] Third, cardiac output is progressively reduced with higher levels of PEEP, and while it can be restored by fluid administration, the latter will elevate the Pmv and also increase the lung water content. Fourth, at higher levels of PEEP, areas of high $V_A/\dot{Q}$ and dead space develop. When this occurs, the minute ventilation

---

*Courtesy Dr. L.D.H. Wood.

must increase to maintain a constant $PaCO_2$.[164,168] Fifth, relying on the venous admixture to adjust the PEEP may be misleading. Venous admixture may improve if pulmonary function improves or if the pulmonary venous oxygen tension or cardiac output fall.

Regardless of the level of PEEP used, it is important, when evaluating its effect on the PaO_2, cardiac output, mixed venous oxygen tension, or lung compliance, to measure these variables immediately before, and within 30 minutes after changing the PEEP. If the effect of a given PEEP is to be accurately determined, measurements of the physiologic variables must colsely bracket alterations in the PEEP level.

If the O_2 content is reduced because of anemia, the transfusion of red blood cells to a patient with ARDS will be markedly effective. For example, when the Hgb = 10 gm percent, O_2 saturation = 87 percent and the PaO_2 = 47 mmHg,

$$\begin{aligned} O_2 \text{ content} &= 1.39 \times 10 \times 0.87 + 0.003 \times 47 \\ &= 12.2 \text{ ml oxygen/100 ml blood} \end{aligned}$$

By raising the Hgb to 12 gm percent

$$\begin{aligned} O_2 \text{ content} &= 1.39 \times 12 \times 0.87 + 0.003 \times 47 \\ &= 14.7 \text{ ml oxygen/100 ml blood} \end{aligned}$$

or a 20 percent increase in the O_2 content. Additional hemoglobin may augment O_2 delivery more than manipulations of the FIO_2 or PEEP. For example, if the PaO_2 is increased to 95 mmHg and results in an oxygen saturation of 95 percent in the same anemic patient,

$$\begin{aligned} O_2 \text{ content} &= 1.39 \times 10 \times 0.95 + 0.003 \times 95 \\ &= 13.5 \text{ ml oxygen/100 ml blood} \end{aligned}$$

This represents only an 11 percent increase in the O_2 content (about one-half the increase seen with transfusion). Additionally, if higher levels of PEEP are needed to improve the O_2 content, O_2 delivery may even decrease as a result of PEEP-induced cardiac-output reductions.

Oxygen delivery must be interpreted relative to tissue needs. When the delivery is less than the demand, more oxygen should be extracted from hemoglobin, keeping the tissue oxygen uptake constant. If this occurs, the mixed venous oxygen tension (MVO_2) and saturation will fall. Some have suggested using the MVO_2 as a guide for FIO_2 reduction, reasoning that unless the MVO_2 falls, oxygen delivery is adequate for tissue needs.[169] However, the tissue oxygen uptake of patients with ARDS seems to decrease when oxygen delivery drops. This may result from abnormal regulation of peripheral blood flow or from diffuse cellular injury limiting the ability to utilize the oxygen delivered.[170] Regardless of the mechanism, this observation suggests that the MVO_2 may not accurately reflect tissue oxygenation.

The two major complications of PEEP therapy are barotrauma and depression of cardiac output. Barotrauma includes pneumothorax and subcutaneous or mediastinal emphysema or both.[171,172,173] It occurs in up to 18 percent of patients treated with PEEP, but the incidence does not clearly relate to the level of PEEP employed. Presumably, the risk of barotrauma depends on the end-inspiratory airway pressure and regional lung inflation. The end-inspiratory airway pressure is a function of the tidal volume, the functional residual capacity (FRC), the total pulmonary compliance, and the PEEP level used. Lung parenchymal factors will influence the alveolar pressure. Large alveoli have smaller recoil pressures than small ones (the Laplace relationship) and therefore, will be more likely to rupture at any given P_A. When the surfactant is reduced, the alveoli will have a higher recoil pressure acting against the alveolar pressure. The amount of alveolar pressure transmitted to the tissue will be reduced.

PEEP therapy reduces the cardiac output by at least two mechanisms: a decreased venous return and an increased pulmonary vascular resistance. The former depends upon the change in pleural pressure induced by PEEP therapy. The pleural pressure also depends on lung compliance and the lung volume present relative to the total lung capacity when a PEEP is applied. Pulmonary vascular resistance (PVR) is a function of the P_A as it relates to the Pmv. PVR also may increase if the vessels are lengthened by the increase in lung volume. The effects on the PVR of increasing the PEEP may depend upon the lung volume, as well as the alveolar pressure, and will affect extra-alveolar vessels (EAVs) differently than alveolar vessels (AVs). Some suggest that PEEP therapy primarily affects the myocardium.[174,175,176] This interpretation depends upon an accurate assessment of left and right ventricular transmural pressures.[177] A reduction in cardiac output by PEEP therapy can be reversed by infusing additional volume.[178] However, this will be at the expense of increasing the Pmv, which will increase the lung water content. Alternative methods for returning the cardiac output to normal following a PEEP-induced reduction in the output include the infusion of dopamine[179] or nitroprusside.[180]

In some circumstances, a PEEP may actually decrease the PaO_2. If lung damage is nonuniform and areas of varying compliance are present, PEEP therapy could overdistend normal alveoli before expanding diseased ones. This would increase pulmonary vascular resistance and decrease blood flow to the normal alveoli, potentially increasing blood flow through the diseased alveoli and resulting in an increased shunt.[181]

Reduction of Pmv

When vascular permeability is increased, a greater amount of transvascular fluid filtration occurs for any given hydrostatic gradient. To minimize edema formation, under such circumstances, the Pmv should be reduced as low as possible without impairing cardiac output. This may be accomplished with diuretics, vasodilators, the restriction of volume replacement or all three.

Some suggest that colloids will increase the πmv and pull fluid from the interstitium into the pulmonary vasculature. When increased permeability is present, the πmv will either equilibrate with, or at least closely approximate, the

πPmv (depending on σ). No beneficial effects of increasing the πmv would therefore be expected; and in studies in which the πmv was increased, the lung water content also increased.[182] As the repair process begins, in recovery from ARDS, vascular permeability decreases. This suggests that at some time during this process, it might be possible to produce an oncotic gradient. However, it is currently impossible to tell when the vascular permeability is improving. Newer techniques that measure this variable at the bedside have been described recently,[183] and may contribute substantially to our ability to diagnose and manage ARDS in the future.

Additional Measures

Antacids and low-dose subcutaneous heparin are reasonable additions to therapy for ARDS in an attempt to reduce stress-induced upper GI bleeding and deep venous thrombosis with possible pulmonary emboli.

Strict attention to the details of daily patient management is needed. Endotracheal and nasogastric tubes should be taped in positions that will minimize the possibility of pressure necrosis. Sheepskin or air-mattress pads should be used to reduce the incidence of decubiti. Intravenous lines should be changed at intervals of no longer than 3 days. Central lines are frequently left in place for far longer than is necessary. The information they provide is of critical importance for stabilizing acutely ill patients; however, once the physiologic data have been collected, appropriate therapy has been started, and a response has been observed, continued collection of this information adds little to patient care. The risk of catheter-induced complications is significant.[184,185,186,187] Handwashing should be done before and after contact with the patient or any support equipment, so as to minimize the risk of nosocomial infection. Meticulous airway care is needed, as discussed in Chapter 2.

Specific Therapy

The potential mechanisms of injury to the vascular endothelium and alveolar epithelium described above suggest a theoretical rationale for several medications in the treatment of ARDS (Table 6–7). These specific forms of therapy are directed at the cause of the increased permeability. It is important to restate that the mechanism or mechanisms of injury in ARDS are currently too poorly understood to recommend using any of these agents. None have been tested in controlled clinical trials, and most have not been given to patients with ARDS.

Corticosteroids have a variety of actions that suggest they may be beneficial in ARDS (Table 6–7). They are frequently recommended for fat emboli[188,189,190] and aspiration pneumonia.[191] However, no well-designed clinical trials have been done to support or refute their use. One apparently controlled study found that steroids reduced the mortality from sepsis,[167] and another found a marked reduction in alveolocapillary permeability after steroids were given to patients with ARDS secondary to sepsis.[192] These agents have been evaluated in oleic acid and acid-

Table 6–7. Medications That Might Alter the Pathophysiology of ARDS

Corticosteroids
Anti-inflammatory effects
Decreased histamine release
Decreased fibrosis
Decreased injury-associated edema
Decreased arachidonic acid derivatives
Nonsteroidal antiinflammatory agents (aspirin, indomethacin, imidazole)
Decreased platelet aggregation
Decreased TXA_2 formation
Antihistamine (both H1 and H2 blockers)
Decreased effect of histamine on vascular permeability
Heparin
Decreased platelet consumption
Decreased fibrinogen consumption
Decreased pulmonary vascular thrombo-emboli
Antiplatelet agents (dypiridamole, sulfinpyrazone)
Decreased platelet aggregation
Superoxide inhibitors
Decreased effect of OH^-, O_2

aspiration models of ARDS, with favorable results being reported.[193,194] The dose, duration, and frequency of administration of steroids in animal models of ARDS have not been studied, although a few large doses generally have been used.

SEQUELAE

Normal Permeability

When pulmonary edema occurs secondary to an increased Pmv, the acute response to therapy is similar regardless of the specific cause. With conventional management consisting of oxygen, morphine, and other measures designed to increase cardiac output and reduce pulmonary and left ventricular end-diastolic blood volumes, the Pmv generally can be abruptly reduced relieving the acute decompensation. When left ventricular failure is the cause of the increased Pmv, over 90 percent of patients will do well. Intubation rarely is required unless the patient is apneic on presentation.[44] Even when hypercapnia is present, morphine sulfate appears to be safe, and can probably be used without concern for suppressing ventilatory drives. Both respiratory and metabolic acidemia improve within minutes to a few hours after morphine sulfate therapy is begun.[193]

The long-term prognosis for patients presenting with acute pulmonary edema from any of the causes listed in Table 6–1 varies widely, depending upon the underlying condition responsible and the treatment rendered.

Table 6–8. Recovery Following ARDS[202a]

Functional Abnormality	Patients Studied	Patients Abnormal N	%
Airflow obstruction	58	14	24
Exercise desaturation	37	11	30
Diffusing capacity	58	21	36

Increased Permeability

The mortality from ARDS is approximately 50 percent.[169] However, because ARDS is a syndrome that may occur in response to a variety of injuries, these data may not accurately predict the prognosis for a specific patient. For example, when ARDS develops in the setting of sepsis, the mortality is increased to as much as 90 percent.[195,196] In near-drowning, 90 percent of patients survive.[197]

The prognosis in ARDS may relate to PEEP responsiveness. Late in the course of ARDS, patients whose PaO_2 improves rapidly (within 30 min) after a 10 cmH_2O increase in PEEP have a better survival rate (48 percent) than those in whom the improvement either takes longer (30 to 180 min) or does not occur at all (21 percent).[198] The pathologic findings in the study that disclosed these results correlated with the physiologic response observed, since nonresponders had more severe edema and hemorrhagic exudate than did rapid responders; slow responders had more fibrosis. While the use of PEEP has not been shown to influence mortality in ARDS,[195,199,200,201] patients who are PEEP responsive seem to have a lower mortality.[198,202]

The long-term prognosis for those patients surviving an episode of ARDS seems good, although only small numbers of patients have been studied. In each follow-up series reported, surviving patients either have been asymptomatic or only mildly dyspneic when exercising. Pulmonary function tests have shown only mild airflow limitation, primarily located in the small airways, which has been difficult to separate from the effects of smoking (Table 6–8). Mild restrictive disease also has been noted.[157,202a,203,204,205] The resting arterial blood gases in surving patients are generally normal,[157,202a,203,204,205] but some patients have a reduced carbon monoxide diffusion capacity, and develop hypoxemia with exercise. Airflow limitation may develop during recovery from ARDS,[205] but the other pulmonary function abnormalities seem to improve with time.[204] Additional prognostic information may be obtained if a pathologic specimen is available for examination. An intact basal lamina suggests that cellular reorganization will proceed normally with return of the normal anatomy of the lung.[206]

ACKNOWLEDGMENTS

The author's research discussed here was supported by National Institutes of Health Training Grant HL-05819, Pulmonary SCOR Grant HL-14152, HL-20690, and Veterans Administration General Research Funds. Critical review of the manuscript by Drs. E. Pavlin and J. Caldwell is much appreciated, as are the many educational discussions with Dr. T. Hyers concerning the pathophysiology of ARDS, and the excellent secretarial assistance of Ms. Diane Johnson.

REFERENCES

1. Staub NC: Proposed pulmonary space nomenclature. In Central Hemodynamics and Gas Exchange, Appendix III, ed. Giuntini C, Turin, Minerva Medica 465–467, 1971.
2. Staub NC: Pulmonary edema. Physiol Rev 54:678, 1974.
3. Staub NC: Lung fluid and solute exchange. In Lung Water and Solute Exchange, ed. Staub NC New York, Marcel Dekker, 3–16, 1978.
4. Ashaugh DG, Bigelow DB, Petty TL, Levine BE: Acute respiratory distress in adults. Lancet 2:319, 1967.
5. Murray JF: The adult respiratory distress syndrome (may it rest in peace). Am Rev Resp Dis 111:716, 1975.
6. Petty TL: The adult respiratory distress syndrome (Confessions of a "lumper"). Am Rev Resp Dis 111:713, 1975.
7. Sarnoff SJ, Sarnoff LC: Neurohemodynamics of pulmonary edema. II. Role of the sympathetic pathways in the elevation of pulmonary and systemic vascular pressures following the intracisternal injection of fibrin. Circulation 6:51, 1969.
8. Theodore J. Robin ED: Speculations on neurogenic pulmonary edema (NPE). Am Rev Resp Dis 113:405, 1976.
9. Pietra GG, Szidon JP, Fishman AP: Leaky pulmonary vessels. Trans Assoc Am Physicians 85:369, 1972.
10. Schneeberger EE, Karnovsky, MJ: The influence of intravascular fluid volume of the permeability of newborn and adult mouse lungs to ultrastructural protein tracers. J Cell Biol 49:319, 1971.
11. Shirley HH Jr, Wolfram CG, Wasserman K, Mayerson HS: Capillary permeability to macromolecules. Stretched pore phenomenon. Am J Physiol 190:189, 1957.
12. Wray NP, Nicotra MB: Pathogenesis of neurogenic pulmonary edema. Am Rev Resp Dis 118:783, 1978.
13. Fred HL, Schmidt AM, Bates T, Hecht HH: Acute pulmonary edema of altitude: Clinical and physiologic observations. Circulation 25:929, 1962.
14. Hultgren HN, Lopez CE, Lundbert E, et al: Physiologic studies of pulmonary edema at high altitude. Circulation 29:393, 1964.
15. Penaloza D, Sine F: Circulatory dynamics during high altitude pulmonary edema. Am J Cardiol 23:369, 1969.
16. Viswanathan R, Jain SK, Subramanian S, et al: Pulmonary edema of high altitude. II. Clinical, aerohemodynamic, and biochemical studies in a group with history of pulmonary edema of high altitude. Am Rev Resp Dis 100:334, 1969.
17. Albert RK, Lakshminarayan S, Huang TW, Butler J: Fluid leaks from extra-alveolar vessels in living dog lungs. J Appl Physiol 44:759, 1978.
18. Hultgren HN, Wilson R: Blood gas abnormalities and optimum therapy in high altitude pulmonary edema. Clin Res 29:99A, 1981.
19. Flick MR, Perel A, Kagelor W, Staub NC: White blood cells contribute to increased lung vascular permeability after microemboli. (Abstr). Fed Proc 38:1265, 1979.

20. Hackett PH, Creagh CE, Grover RF, et al: High-altitude pulmonary edema in persons without the right pulmonary artery. Engl J Med 302:1070, 1980.
21. Hyers TM, Martinez A, Grover RF, Reeves JT: Hypoxic exercise-induced lung injury in rats. (Abst). Fed Proc 37:292, 1978.
22. Sladen A, Laver MB, Pontoppidan H: Pulmonary complications and water retention in prolonged mechanical ventilation. N Engl J Med 279:448, 1968.
23. Webb HH, Tierney DF: Experimental pulmonary edema due to intermittent positive pressure ventilation with high inflation pressures. Protection by positive end-expiratory pressures. Am Rev Resp Dis 110:556, 1974.
24. Demling RH, Edmunds LH: Effect of continuous positive airway pressure on extravascular lung water. J Appl Physiol 38:907, 1975.
25. Thornton D, Ponhold H, Butler J, et al: Effects of pattern of ventilation on pulmonary metabolism and mechanics. Anesthesiology 42:4, 1975.
26. Wagaruddin M, Bernstein A: Reexpansion pulmonary edema. Thorax 30:54, 1975.
27. Pavlin J, Cheney FW Jr: Unilateral pulmonary edema in rabbits after reexpansion of collapsed lung. J Appl Physiol 46:31, 1979.
28. Ziskind MM, Weill H, George RA: Acute pulmonary edema following the treatment of spontaneous pneumothorax with excessive negative intrapleural pressure. Am Rev Resp Dis 92:632, 1965.
29. Fraser RG, Pare JAP: Diagnosis of diseases of the chest. 2nd Ed, Vol 2, Philadelphia, WB Saunders, 1272, 1978.
30. Jackson FN, Rowland V, Corssen G: Laryngospasm-induced pulmonary edema. Chest 78:819, 1980.
31. Stalcup SA, Mellins RB: Mechanical forces producing pulmonary edema in acute asthma. N Engl J Med 297:592, 1977.
32. Guyton AC, Lindsey AW: Effect of elevated left atrial pressure and decreased plasma protein concentration on the development of pulmonary edema. Circ Res 7:649, 1959.
33. Hendin AS, Greenspan RH: Ventilatory pumping of human pulmonary lymphatic vessels. Radiology 108:553, 1973.
34. Carrington CB, Cugell DW, Gaensler EA, et al: Lymphangioleiomyomatosis. Am Rev Resp Dis 116:977, 1977.
35. Foldi M: Diseases of the Lymphatics and Lymph Circulation. Springfield, IL Charles C Thomas, 1969.
36. Buford TH, Burbank B: Traumatic wet lung. Observations of certain physiologic fundamentals of thoracic trauma. J Thorac Surg 14:415, 1945.
37. Eiseman B, Ashbaugh DG (eds.): Pulmonary effects of nonthoracic trauma. J Trauma 8:623, 1968.
38. McLean APH, Duff JH, MacLean L: Lung lesions associated with septic shock. J Trauma 8:891, 1968.
39. Duberstein JL, Kaufman DM: A clinical study of an epidemic of heroin intoxication and heroin-induced pulmonary edema. Am J Med 51:704, 1971.
40. Louria DB, Hensle T, Rose J: The major medication complications of heroin addiction. Ann Intern Med 67:1, 1967.
41. Steinberg AD, Karliner JS: The clinical spectrum of heroin pulmonary edema. Arch Intern Med 122:122, 1968.
42. Modell JH, Moya F: Effects of volume of aspirated fluid during chlorinated fresh water drowning. Anesthesiology 27:662, 1966.

43. Modell JH: Effects of fluid volume in seawater drowning. Ann Intern Med 67:68, 1967.
44. Fulop M, Horowitz M, Aberman A, et al: Lactic acidosis in pulmonary edema due to left ventricular failure. Ann Intern Med 79:180, 1973.
45. Aberman A, Fulop M: The metabolic and respiratory acidosis of acute pulmonary edema. Ann Intern Med 76:173, 1972.
46. Joffe N: The adult respiratory distress syndrome. Am J Roentgenol 122:719, 1974.
47. Ostendorf P, Birzle H, Vogel W, Mittermayer C: Pulmonary radiographic abnormalities in shock. Roentgen-clinical-pathological correlation. Radiology 115:257, 1975.
48. Webster JR, McCabe MM, Karp M: Recognition and management of smoke inhalation. JAMA 201:287, 1967.
49. Staub NC, Hitoshi N, Pearce ML: Pulmonary edema in dogs, especially the sequence of fluid accumulation in lungs. J Appl Physiol 22:227, 1967.
50. Zapol WM, Snider MT, Schneider RC, et al: Pulmonary hypertension in severe acute respiratory failure. In Artificial Lungs for Acute Respiratory Failure, eds. Zapol WM, Qvist J, New York Academic Press, 435, 1976.
51. Fein A, Grossman RF, Jones JG, et al: The value of edema fluid protein measurement in patients with pulmonary edema. Am J Med 67:32, 1979.
52. Gelb AF, Klein E: Hemodynamic and alveolar protein studies in noncardiac pulmonary edema. Am Rev Resp Dis 114:831, 1976.
53. Robin ED, Carey LC, Grenvik A, et al: Capillary leak syndrome with pulmonary edema. Arch Intern Med 130:66, 1972.
54. Bachofen M, Bachofen H, Weibel ER: Lung edema in the adult respiratory distress syndrome. In Pulmonary Edema, eds. Fishman AP, Renkin EM, Bethesda, American Physiological Society, 241–252, 1979.
55. Anderson RR, Holliday RL, Driedger AA, et al: Documentation of pulmonary capillary permeability in the ARDS accompanying human sepsis. Am Rev Resp Dis 119:869, 1979.
56. Hinshaw HC, Murray JF: Diseases of the Chest. Philadelphia, WB Saunders, 629–652, 1980.
57. Macklin CC: Evidences of increase in the capacity of the pulmonary arteries and veins of dogs, cats, and rabbits during inflation of freshly excised lung. Rev Can Biol 5:199, 1946.
58. Permutt S, Howell JBL, Proctor DF, Riley RL: Effect of lung inflation on static pressure-volume characteristics of pulmonary vessels. J Appl Physiol 16:64, 1961.
59. Glazier JB, Hughes JMB, Maloney JE, West JB: Measurements of capillary dimensions and blood volume in rapidly frozen lungs. J Appl Physiol 26:65, 1969.
60. Bruderman I, Somers K, Hamilton WK, et al: Effect of surface tension on circulation in the excised lungs of dogs. J Appl Physiol 19:707, 1964.
61. Lloyd TC, Wright GW: Pulmonary vascular resistance and vascular transmural gradient. J Appl Physiol 15:241, 1960.
62. Rosenzweig, DY, Hughes JMB, Glazier JB: Effects of transpulmonary and vascular pressures on pulmonary blood volume in isolated lung. J Appl Physiol 28:553, 1970.
63. Gil J, Bachofen H, Geher P, Weibel ER: Alveolar volume-surface area relation in air- and-saline-filled lungs fixed by vascular perfusion. J Appl Physiol 47:990, 1979.
64. Mead J, Takishima T, Leith D: Stress distribution in lungs: A model of pulmonary elasticity. J Appl Physiol 28:596, 1970.

65. Weibel ER, Bachofen H: Structural design of the alveolar septum and fluid exchange. In Pulmonary Edema, eds. Fishman AP, Renkin EM, Bethesda, American Physiological Society 1–20, 1979.
66. Howell BJL, Permutt S, Proctor DF, Riley RL: Effect of inflation of the lung on different parts of pulmonary vascular bed. J Appl Physiol 16:71, 1961.
67. Benjamin JJ, Murtagh PS, Proctor DF, et al: Pulmonary vascular interdependence in excised dog lobes. J Appl Physiol 37:887, 1974.
68. Gee M, Williams DO: Effect of lung inflation on perivascular cuff fluid in isolated dog lung lobes. Microvasc Res 17:192, 1979.
69. Goshy M, Lai-Fook SJ, Hyatt RE: Perivascular pressure measurements by wick-catheter technique in isolated dog lobes. J Appl Physiol 46:950, 1979.
70. Lai-Fook SJ: A continuum mechanics analysis of pulmonary vascular interdependence in isolated dog lobes. J Appl Physiol 46:419, 1979.
71. Smith JC, Mitzner W: Analysis of pulmonary vascular interdependence in excised dog lobes. J Appl Physiol 48:450, 1980.
72. Permutt S: Mechanical influences on water accumulation in the lungs. In Pulmonary Edema, eds. Fishman AP, Renkin EM, Bethesda, MD, American Physiological Society, 175–194, 1979.
73. Albert RK, Lakshminarayan S, Kirk W, Butler J: Lung inflation can cause pulmonary edema in zone I of in-situ dog lungs. J Appl Physiol 49:815, 1980.
74. Iliff LD: Extra-alveolar vessels and edema development in excised dog lungs. Circ Res 28:524, 1971.
75. Mitzner W, Robotham JL: Distribution of interstitial compliance and filtration coefficient in canine lung. Lymphology 12:140, 1979.
76. Whayne TR, Jr, Severinghaus JW: Experimental hypoxic pulmonary edema in the rat. J Appl Physiol 25:729, 1968.
77. Smith HC, Gould VF, Cheney FW, Butler J: Pathogenesis of hemodynamic pulmonary edema in excised dog lungs. J Appl Physiol 37:904, 1974.
78. Albert RK, Lakshminarayan S, Charan NB, et al: Relative contribution of alveolar and extra-alveolar vessels to hydrostatic pulmonary edema. (Abst). Clin Res 28:56A, 1980.
79. Albert RK, Lakshminarayan S, Kirk W, Butler J: Extra-alveolar vessels leak in oleic-acid edema. (Abst). Clin Res 29:66A, 1981.
80. Bhattacharya J, Staub NC: Direct measurement of microvascular pressures in the isolated, perfused dog lung. Science 210:327, 1980.
81. Gaar KA Jr, Taylor AE, Owens LJ, Guyton AC: Pulmonary capillary pressure and filtration coefficient in the isolated perfused lung. Am J Physiol 213:910, 1967.
82. Albert RK, Lakshminarayan S, Charan NB, et al: Lung expansion increases the extra-alveolar vascular recoil in living dog lungs (Abst). Fed Proc 39:485, 1980.
83. Inoue H, Inoue C, Hildebrandt J: Vascular and airway pressures, and interstitial edema affect peribronchial fluid pressure. J Appl Physiol 48:177, 1980.
84. Erdmann AJ, Vaughan TR, Brigham KL, et al: Effect of increased vascular pressure on lung fluid balance in unanesthetized sheep. Circ Res 37:271, 1975.
85. Brigham KL, Woolverton WC, Blake LH, Staub NC: Increased sheep lung vascular permeability caused by *Pseudomonas* bacteremia. J Clin Invest 54:792, 1974.
86. Pattle RE: Properties, function and origin of the alveolar lining layer. Nature 175:1125, 1955.

87. Clements JA: Pulmonary edema and permeability of alveolar membranes. Arch Environ Health 2:280, 1961.
88. Guyton AC, Granger HJ, Taylor AE: Interstitial fluid pressure. Physiol Rev 51:527, 1971.
89. Albert RK, Lakshminarayan S, Hildebrandt J, Kirk W: Increased surface tension favors pulmonary edema formation in anesthetized dogs' lungs. J Clin Invest 63:1015, 1979.
90. Farrel PM, Avery ME: Hyaline membrane disease. Am Rev Resp Dis 111:657, 1975.
91. Henry JN, McArdle AH, Bounous G, et al: The effect of experimental hemorrhagic shock on pulmonary alveolar surfactant. J Trauma 7:691, 1967.
92. Petty TL, Reiss OK, Paul GW, et al: Characteristics of pulmonary surfactant in adult respiratory distress syndrome associated with trauma and shock. Am Rev Resp Dis 115:531, 1977.
93. Luterman A, Horovitz JH, Carrico CJ, et al: Withdrawal from positive end-expiratory pressure. Surgery 83:328, 1978.
94. Cottrell TS, Levine OR, Senior RM, et al: Electron Microscopic alterations at the alveolar level in pulmonary edema. Circ Res 21:783, 1967.
95. Busch C, Jokobsson S, Dahlgren S, et al: Determination of fibrin trapping in the lungs of patients developing the microembolism syndrome. Acta Chir Scand 137:599, 1971.
96. Hill JD, Ratliff JL, Parrott JCW, et al: Pulmonary pathology in acute respiratory insufficiency: Lung biopsy as a diagnostic tool. J Thorac Cardiovasc Surg 71:64, 1976.
97. Orell SR: Lung pathology in respiratory distress following shock in the adult. Acta Pathol Microbiol Scand 79(A):65, 1971.
98. Saldeen T: The microembolism syndrome. Microvasc Res 11:227, 1976.
99. Hechtman HB, Lonergan EA, Shepro D: Platelet and leukocyte lung interactions in patients with respiratory failure. Surgery 83:155, 1978.
100. Schneider RC, Carvalho A, Bloom S, et al: Platelet kinetics in severe acute respiratory failure (ARF). (Abst) Am Rev Resp Dis 113:135, 1976.
101. White MK, Shepro D, Hechtman HB: Pulmonary function and platelet-lung interaction. J Appl Physiol 34:697, 1973.
102. Vaage J: Intravascular platelet aggregation and acute respiratory insufficiency. Circ Shock 4:279, 1977.
103. Busch C, Lindquist O, Saldeen T: Respiratory insufficiency in the dog induced by pulmonary microembolism and inhibition of fibrinolysis. Effect of defibrinogenation, leucopenia and thrombocytopenia. Acta Chir Scand 140:255, 1974.
104. Curreri PW, Wilterdink ME, Baxter CR: Characterization of elevated fibrin split-products following thermal injury. Ann Surg 181:157, 1975.
105. Luterman A, Manwarina D, Curreri PW: The role of fibrinogen degradation products in the pathogenesis of the respiratory distress syndrome. Surgery 82:703, 1977.
106. Manwaring D, Thorning D, Curreri PW: Mechanism of acute pulmonary dysfunction induced by fibrinogen degradation product D. Surgery 84:49, 1978.
107. Binder AS, Staub NC: Increased lung vascular permeability after microemboli does not depend on fibrin deposition. (Abstr). Am Rev Resp Dis 117:311, 1978.
108. Hyers, TM: Pathogenesis of the adult respiratory distress syndrome. Sem Resp Med. 2:104, 1981.
109. Saba TM, Blumenstock FA, Scovill WA, Bernard H: Cryoprecipitate reversal of

opsonic σ_2-surface binding glycoprotein deficiency in septic surgical and trauma patients. Science 201:622, 1978.
110. Saba TM, Jaffe E: Plasma fibronectin (opsonic glycoprotein): Its synthesis by vascular endothelial cells and role in cardiopulmonary integrity after trauma as related to reticuloendothelial function. Am J Med 68:577, 1980.
111. Scovill WA, Saba TM, Blumenstock FA, et al: Opsonic σ_2-surface binding glycoprotein therapy during sepsis. Ann Surg 188:521, 1978.
112. Scovill WA, Annest SJ, Saba TM, et al: Cardiovascular hemodynamics after opsonic alpha-2-surface binding glycoprotein therapy in injured patients. Surgery 86:284, 1979.
113. Mosher DF, Williams EM: Fibronectin concentration is decreased in plasma of severely ill patients with disseminated intravascular coagulation. J Lab Clin Med 91:729, 1978.
114. Craddock PR, Hammerschmidt D, White JG, et al: Complement (C5a)-induced granulocyte aggregation in-vitro. A possible mechanism of complement-mediated leukostasis and leukopenia. J Clin Invest 60:260, 1977.
115. Goldstein IM, Cala D, Radin A, et al: Evidence of complement metabolism in acute pancreatitis. Am J Med Sci 275:257, 1978.
116. Hosea S, Brown E, Hammer C, Frank M: Role of complement activation in a model of adult respiratory distress syndrome. J Clin Invest 66:375, 1980.
117. Goldstein IM, Roos D, Weissman G, Kaplan HB: Influence of corticosteroids on human polymorphonuclear leukocyte function in-vitro. Reduction of lysosomal enzyme release and superoxide production. Inflammation 1:305, 1976.
118. Lee CT, Fein AM, Lippmann M, et al: Elastolytic activity in pulmonary lavage fluid from patients with adult respiratory distress syndrome. N Engl J Med 304:192, 1981.
119. McGuire CA: Role of leukocytes in the lung after endotoxin administration. Adv Exp Med Biol 23:77, 1971.
120. Fredovick I: The biology of oxygen radicals. Science 201:875, 1978.
121. Sacks T, Moldow CF, Craddock PR, et al: Oxygen radicals mediate endothelial cell damage by complement stimulated granulocytes. An in-vitro model of immune vascular damage. J Clin Invest 61:1161, 1978.
122. Flick MR, Perel A, Staub NC: Increased lung vascular permeability after microemboli in unanesthetized sheep requires circulating leukocytes. Physiologist 22:39, 1979.
123. Heflin AC, Brigham KL: Granulocyte depletion prevents increased lung vascular permeability after endotoxemia in sheep. Clin Res 27:399A, 1979.
124. Johnson A, Malik AB: Effect of granulocytopenia on extravascular lung water content after microembolization. Am Rev Resp Dis 122:561, 1980.
125. Guenter CA: Role of leukocytes in the lung after endotoxin administration. Adv Exp Med Biol 23:77, 1971.
126. Hurley JV: Substances promoting leukocyte emigration. Ann NY Acad Sci 116:918, 1964.
127. Millen JE, Glauser FL, Smeltzer D, et al: The role of leukocytes in ethchlorvynol-induced pulmonary edema. Chest 73:75, 1978.
128. Pingleton WW, Coalson JJ, Guenter CA: Significance of leukocytes in endotoxin shock. Exp Mol Pathol 22:183, 1975.
129. Bloom R, Taveira AM, Silva DA, Bracey A: Reversible respiratory failure due to intravascular leukostasis in chronic myelogenous leukemia. Am J Med 67:679, 1979.

130. Ward HN: Pulmonary infiltrates associated with leukoagglutinin transfusion reactions. Ann Intern Med 73:689, 1970.
131. Henson PM, McCarthy K, Larson GL, et al: Complement fragments, alveolar macrophages and alveolitis. Am J Pathol 97:93, 1979.
132. Cook JA, Wise WC, Haluska PV: Elevated thromboxane levels in the rat during endotoxic shock. J Clin Invest 65:227, 1980.
133. Goetzel EJ: Mediators of immediate hypersensitivity derived from arachidonic acid. N Engl J Med 303:822, 1980.
134. Williams TJ, Jose PJ: Mediation of increased vascular permeability after complement activation. J Exp Med 153:136, 1981.
135. Warlow C, Terry G, Kenmure ACF, et al: A double-blind trial of low doses of subcutaneous heparin in the prevention of deep vein thrombosis after myocardial infarction. Lancet 2:934, 1973.
136. Gallus AS, Hirsh J, Tuttle RJ, et al: Small subcutaneous doses of heparin in prevention of venous thrombosis. N Engl J Med 288:545, 1973.
137. Dikshil K, Vyden J, Forrester JS, et al: Renal and extra-renal hemodynamic effects of furosemide in congestive heart failure after acute myocardial infarction. N Engl J Med 288:1087, 1973.
138. Kim YI, Noble RJ, Zipes DP: Dissociation of the inotropic effect of digitalis from its effect on atrioventricular conduction. Am J Cardiol 36:459, 1975.
139. Beller GA, Smith TW, Abelman WH, et al: Digitalis intoxication. A prospective clinical study with serum level correlations. N Engl J Med 284:989, 1971.
140. Evered DC, Chapman C: Plasma digoxin concentrations and digoxin toxicity in hospital patients. Br Heart J 33:540, 1971.
141. Forrester JS, Waters DD: Hospital treatment of congestive heart failure. Am J Med 65:173, 1978.
142. Robin ED, Cross CE, Zelis R: Pulmonary edema. N Engl J Med 288:292, 1973.
143. Zelis R, Mason DT, Braunwald E: A comparison of the effects of vasodilator stimuli on peripheral resistance vessels in normal subjects and in patients with congestive heart failure. J Clin Invest 47:960, 1968.
144. Zelis RF, Mason DT, Spann JF Jr, et al: The effects of morphine on the venous bed in man: Demonstration of a biphasic response. Am J Cardiol 25:136, 1971.
145. Mahajan VK, Simon M, Huber GL: Reexpansion pulmonary edema. Chest 75:192, 1979.
146. Braunwald E, Frahm CJ: Studies on Starling's law of the heart. IV. Observations on the hemodynamic functions of the left atrium in man. Circulation 24:633, 1961.
147. Tooker J, Huseby J, Butler J: The effect of Swan-Ganz catheter height on the wedge pressure-left atrial pressure relationship in edema during positive pressure ventilation. Am Rev Resp Dis 117:721, 1978.
148. Benumof JL, Saidman LJ, Arkin DB, Diamant M: Where pulmonary arterial catheters go: Intrathoracic distribution. Anesthesiology 46:336, 1977.
149. Sackner MA, Landa J, Hirsch J, Zapata A: Pulmonary effects of oxygen breathing. Ann Int Med 82:40, 1975.
150. Singer MM, Wright F, Stanley LK, et al: Oxygen toxicity in man. A prospective study in patients after open-heart surgery. N Engl J Med 283:1473, 1970.
151. Van de Water JM, Kagley KS, Miller IT, et al: Response of the lung to six to twelve hours of 100% oxygen in normal man. N Engl J Med 283:621, 1970.

152. Deneke SM, Fanburg BL: Normobaric oxygen toxicity of the lung. N Engl J Med 303:76, 1980.
153. Clark JM, Lambertson CJ: Pulmonary oxygen toxicity: A review. Pharmacol Rev 23:37, 1971.
154. Ayers LN, Tierney DF, Imagawa D: Shortened survival of mice with influenza when given oxygen at one atmosphere. Am Rev Resp Dis 107:955, 1970.
155. Fisher HK, Clements JA, Wright RR: Enhancement of oxygen toxicity by the herbicide paraquat. Am Rev Resp Dis 107:246, 1973.
156. Tierney DF, Ayers L, Kasauyama RS: Altered sensitivity to oxygen toxicity. Am Rev Resp Dis 115:595, 1977.
157. Ashbaugh DG, Petty TL, Bigelow DB, Harris TM: Continuous positive-pressure breathing (CPPB) in the adult respiratory distress syndrome. J Thorac Cardiovasc Surg 57:31, 1969.
158. Kumar A, Falke KJ, Geffin B, et al: Continuous positive-pressure ventilation in acute respiratory failure: Effects on hemodynamics and lung function. N Engl J Med 283:1430, 1970.
159. Sugerman HJ, Olofsson KB, Pollock TW, et al: Continuous positive end-expiratory pressure ventilation (PEEP) for the treatment of diffuse interstitial pulmonary edema. J Trauma 12:263, 1972.
160. Schmidt GR, O'Neill WW, Kotb K, et al: Continuous positive airway pressure in the prophylaxis of the adult respiratory distress syndrome. Surg Gynecol Obstet 143:613, 1976.
161. Weigelt JA, Mitchell RA, Snyder WH: Early positive end-expiratory pressure in the adult respiratory distress syndrome. Arch Surg 114:497, 1979.
162. Suter PM, Fairley HB, Isenberg MD: Optimum end-expiratory airway pressure in patients with acute pulmonary failure. N Engl J Med 292:284, 1975.
163. Downs JB, Klein EE Jr, Modell JH: The effect of incremental PEEP on PaO_2 in patients with respiratory failure. Anesth Analg 52:210, 1973.
164. Dueck R, Wagner PD, West JB: Effects of positive end-expiratory pressure on gas exchange in dogs with normal and edematous lungs. Anesthesiology 47:359, 1977.
165. Kirby RR, Downs JB, Civetta JM, et al: High level end-expiratory pressure (PEEP) in acute respiratory insufficiency. Chest 67:156, 1975.
166. Kirby RR, Perry JC, Calderwood HW: Cardiorespiratory effects of high pressure end-expiratory pressure. Anesthesiology 43:533, 1975.
166a. Gallagher TJ, Civetta JM, Kirby RR: Terminology update: Optimal PEEP. Crit Care Med 6:323, 1978.
167. Schumer WC: Steroids in the treatment of clinical septic shock. Ann Surg 184:333, 1976.
168. Coffey RL, Albert RK, Robertson HT: Components of dead space in oleic acid edema. (Abstr). Fed Proc 40:537, 1981.
169. Hopewell PC, Murray JF: The adult respiratory distress syndrome. In Respiratory Emergencies, eds. Shibel EM, Moser KM, St. Louis, CV Mosby, 101–128, 1977.
170. Danek SJ, Lynch JP, Weg JG, Dantzker DR: The dependence of oxygen uptake on oxygen delivery in the adult respiratory distress syndrome. Am Rev Resp Dis 122:387, 1980.
171. De la Torre FJ, Tomasa A, Klamburg J, et al: Incidence of pneumothorax and pneumomediastinum in patients with aspiration pneumonia requiring ventilatory support. Chest 72:141, 1977.

172. Kumar A, Pontoppidan H, Falke K, et al: Pulmonary barotrauma during mechanical ventilation. Crit Care Med 1:181, 1973.
173. Steier M, Ching N, Roberts EB, et al: Pneumothorax complicating continuous ventilatory support. J Thorac Cardiovasc Surg 67:17, 1974.
174. Cassidy SS, Robertson CH Jr, Pierce AK, Johnson RL Jr: Cardiovascular effects of positive end-expiratory pressure in dogs. J Appl Physiol 44:743, 1978.
175. Jardin F, Farcot JC, Boisante L, et al: Influence of positive end-expiratory pressure on left ventricular performance. N Engl J Med 304:387, 1981.
176. Scharf SM, Caldini P, Ingram RH Jr: Cardiovascular effects of increasing airway pressure in the dog. Am J Physiol 232:H35, 1977.
177. Cassidy SS, Gaffney F, Johnson RL Jr: A perspective on PEEP. N Engl J Med 304:421, 1981.
178. Qvist J, Pontoppidan H, Wilson RS, et al: Hemodynamic responses to mechanical ventilation with PEEP. Anesthesiology 42:45, 1975.
179. Hemmer M, Suter PM: Treatment of cardiac and renal effects of PEEP with dopamine in patients with acute respiratory failure. Anesthesiology 50:399, 1979.
180. Prewitt RM, Oppenheimer L, Sutherland JB, Wood LDH: Acute effects of nitroprusside (NP) on hemodynamics and oxygen exchange in patients with hypoxemic respiratory failure (HRF). (Abstr). Am Rev Resp Dis 121:1795, 1980.
181. Kamanek DJ, Shannon DC: Adverse effect of positive end-expiratory pressure on pulmonary perfusion and arterial oxygenation. Am Rev Resp Dis 112:457, 1975.
182. Prewitt RM, McCarthy J, Wood LDH: Treatment of acute low pressure pulmonary edema in dogs. J Clin Invest 67:409, 1981.
183. Gorin AB, Weidner WJ, Demling RH, Staub NC: Noninvasive measurement of pulmonary transvascular protein flux in normal man. J Clin Invest 66:869, 1980.
184. Foote GA, Schabel SI, Hodges M: Pulmonary complications of the flow-directed balloon-tipped catheter. N Engl J Med 290:927, 1974.
185. Goodman DJ, Rider AK, Billingham ME, Schroeder JS: Thrombolic complications with the indwelling balloon-tipped pulmonary arterial catheter. N Engl J Med 291:777, 1974.
186. O'Toole JD, Wurtzbacher JJ, Wearner NE, Jain AC: Pulmonary-valve injury and insufficiency during pulmonary artery catheterization. N Engl J Med 301:1167, 1979.
187. Pape LA, Haffajee CI, Markis JE, et al: Fata l pulmonary hemorrhage after use of the flow-directed balloon-tipped catheter. Ann Intern Med 90:344, 1979.
188. Ashbaugh DG, Petty TL: The use of corticosteroids in the treatment of respiratory failure associated with massive fat embolism. Surg Gynecol Obstet 123:493, 1966.
189. Fischer JE, Turner RH, Herndon JH, Riseborough EJ: Massive steroid therapy in severe fat embolism. Surg Gynecol Obstet 132:667, 1971.
190. Wertzberger JJ, Peltier IF: Fat embolism: The effect of corticosteroids on experimental fat embolism in the rat. Surgery 64:143, 1968.
191. Wynne JW, Modell JH: Respiratory aspiration of stomach contents. Ann Intern Med 87:466, 1977.
192. Sibbald WJ, Anderson RR, Reid B, et al: Alveolocapillary permeability in human septic ARDS. Chest 79:133, 1981.
193. Grossman RF, Aberman A: Emergency management of acute pulmonary edema. Ann Intern Med 84:488, 1976.
194. Toung TJK, Bordos D, Benson DW, et al: Aspiration pneumonia: Experimental evaluation of albumin and steroid therapy. Ann Surg 183:179, 1976.

195. Cotev S, Perel A, Katzenelson R, et al: The effect of PEEP on oxygenating capacity in acute respiratory failure with sepsis. Crit Care Med 4:186, 1976.
196. Kaplan RL, Sahn SA, Petty TL: The incidence of the adult respiratory distress syndrome in gram-negative sepsis. Arch Intern Med 139:867, 1979.
197. Modell JH, Graves SA, Ketover A: Clinical course of 91 consecutive near drowning victims. Chest 70:231, 1976.
198. Lamy M, Fallat RJ, Koeniger E, et al: Pathologic features and mechanisms of hypoxemia in adult respiratory distress syndrome. Am Rev Resp Dis 114:267, 1976.
199. Bone RC: Treatment of adult respiratory distress syndrome with diuretics, dialysis, and positive end-expiratory pressure. Crit Care Med 6:136, 1978.
200. Leftwich EI, Witorsch RJ, Witorsch P: Positive end-expiratory pressure in refractory hypoxemia. A critical evaluation. Ann Intern Med 79:187, 1973.
201. McMahon SM, Halprin GM, Sieker HO: Positive end-expiratory airway pressure in severe arterial hypoxemia. Am Rev Resp Dis 108:526, 1973.
202. Springer RR, Stevens: The influence of PEEP on survival of patients in respiratory failure. A retrospective analysis. Am J Med 66:196, 1979.
202a. Lakshminarayan S, Hudson LD: Pulmonary function following the adult respiratory distress syndrome. Chest 74:489, 1978.
203. Douglas ME, Downs JB: Pulmonary function following severe acute respiratory failure and high levels of positive end-expiratory pressure. Chest 71:18, 1977.
204. Lakshminarayan S, Stanford RE, Petty TL: Prognosis after recovery from adult respiratory distress syndrome. Am Rev Resp Dis 113:7, 1976.
205. Simpson DL, Goodman M, Spector SL, et al: Long-term followup and bronchial reactivity testing in survivors of the adult respiratory distress syndrome. Am Rev Resp Dis 117:449, 1978.
206. Vracko R: Basal lamina scaffold: Anatomy and significance for maintenance of orderly tissue structure. Am J Pathol 77:314, 1974.

7

Massive Pulmonary Embolism

Thomas M. Hyers, M.D.

INTRODUCTION

Massive pulmonary embolism can be defined as the presence of emboli sufficient to occlude 50 percent of the segmental vasculature, or an equivalent amount of clot in the proximal vasculature.[1,2,3] This quantification can be done with an objective method,[4] or can be done subjectively by counting the visualized segmental pulmonary arteries and enumerating those that are occluded. Quantification of an equivalent amount of proximal clot is more difficult, but the term generally implies occlusion of at least two lobar arteries.

Massive pulmonary embolism is a common occurrence. In large, angiographically diagnosed series, it accounts for approximately one-half of all cases of embolism.[1,2,3] Massive pulmonary embolism occurs more often in hospitalized patients than in outpatients, and is more often associated with syncope and an increased component of the second heart sound. In contrast, submassive pulmonary embolism is more likely to present with pleuritic pain, hemoptysis, and a peripheral wedge-shaped infiltrate on a chest radiograph.[5] The great majority of massive pulmonary emboli are known to originate from thigh and iliac venous thrombi which in turn have propagated from a nidus in veins of the calf. These emboli probably travel in large segments to the right side of the heart, where mixing occurs and fragmentation results in the embolization of smaller fragments to the lung. The mortality in properly treated massive pulmonary embolism is similar to that seen with submassive pulmonary embolism.[1] However, undiagnosed or untreated massive pulmonary embolism is frequently a lethal process, and it is incumbent upon clinicians who suspect this diagnosis to initiate a workup that either results in a diagnosis or a definitive exclusion of the condition.

Pulmonary embolism remains the direct cause of death of thousands of people in the United States annually. Recently, it has been stated that the condition is being overdiagnosed because of the too frequent utilization of lung scans in the

Table 7–1. Risk Factors for Venous Thromboembolism

Stasis: Immobilization, venous disease, congestive heart failure, obesity
Trauma: Burns, surgery, childbirth, fractures
Estrogens, exogenous
Malignancy: Primarily adenocarcinoma of the viscera and lungs
Advanced age
Previous episode of venous thromboembolism

diagnostic workup.[6] While this assertion may be true, careful autopsy and clinical studies continue to indicate the underdiagnosis of pulmonary embolism.[7–10] When the diagnosis is made and proper therapy is begun, the death rate is low (less than 10 percent), and the prognosis generally is good.[11] In contrast, the death rate in untreated pulmonary embolism is appallingly high.[12–14] Recent years have seen new trends emerge in the diagnosis, treatment, and prevention of pulmonary embolism. Much of this new information will be discussed briefly in this chapter, and one of the most exciting developments—the use of thrombolytic therapy for acute, massive pulmonary embolism and deep venous thrombosis—will be described in detail.

SCREENING FOR PULMONARY EMBOLISM

In screening patients who have symptoms or physical findings suggestive of pulmonary embolism, it is useful to consider predisposing factors (Table 7–1). Although the epidemiology of venous thromboembolism is not as well understood as that of coronary artery disease, certain predisposing factors have been identified. These include stasis, trauma, estrogen use, and certain malignancies.[8,9,15,16] The combination of surgery (trauma) and immobility (stasis) is an extremely potent stimulus to venous thromboembolism. For this reason, nearly all of the prophylactic trials utilizing low-dose, subcutaneous herapin or dextran 70 have been done with patients undergoing elective abdominal surgery.

The clinical diagnosis of pulmonary embolism is highly inaccurate. However, after an accurate diagnosis has been made, some estimation of the extent of the embolism can be made retrospectively from the history and the physical examination. In this regard, a large study showed that while the symptom of dyspnea was present in nearly all patients regardless of the size of the embolus, pleuritic chest pain and hemoptysis were associated more frequently with submassive pulmonary embolism, whereas syncope and an increased component of the second heart sound were more frequently associated with massive pulmonary embolism.[5] In screening for pulmonary embolism, a careful history and physical examination should be done, and an arterial blood gas determination, electrocardiogram (ECG), and chest radiograph should then be obtained. The ECG is most useful for ruling out intrinsic cardiac problems; no electrocardiographic pattern is specific for pulmonary embolism. The initial chest radiograph is normal in approximately one-half of patients with pulmonary embolism, but a few radiographic signs can be helpful. These include a local area of oligemia (Westermark's sign),[17] or the enlargement of a hilar artery due to distention by pressure behind a thrombus. These findings are infrequent, but occasionally are present with massive central embolism. A peripheral, wedge-shaped density on the chest radiograph (Hampton's sign)[18] is seen infrequently, and is associated with submassive embolism and infarction. The most common radiographic findings in pulmonary embolism are pleural effusion and loss of lung volume, both of which are nonspecific. An arterial blood gas determination is useful in screening for pulmonary embolism, since approximately 90 percent of affected individuals will have hypoxemia; the alveolar-to-arterial oxygen gradient will be abnormally increased. Persons with an embolism will also usually show evidence of hyperventilation and mild respiratory alkalemia. However, it should be remembered that approximately 10 percent of individuals with proven pulmonary embolism will have normal arterial blood gases or only show evidence of acute hyperventilation. Hypoxemia is a nonspecific finding and cannot be used to make the diagnosis.

The most useful and readily available screening test for pulmonary embolism is the perfusion lung scan. Since this is a visual representation of pulmonary blood distribution, it will display absent or decreased perfusion in the affected areas. Only 1 to 2 percent of individuals with proven pulmonary embolism will have a normal perfusion lung scan.[1,19,20] Thus, a normal perfusion lung scan essentially rules out a pulmonary embolus; an abnormal perfusion lung scan calls for more definitive diagnositc procedures: (1) the ventilation lung scan; and (2) the pulmonary angiogram.

Ventilation-Perfusion Lung Scanning

The hallmark of a pulmonary embolus in a pulmonary ventilation-perfusion study is a well-defined segmental or multisegmental perfusion defect that ventilates in a relatively normal fashion. Such a study is said to show dissociation between ventilation and perfusion. Any area that ventilates will correspond radiographically to aerated lung. Because the combination of decreased perfusion and normal ventilation is indicative of a pulmonary artery lesion but not specific for a thrombotic pulmonary embolus, ventilation-perfusion scans are usually interpreted in terms of probabilities rather than certainties.[21] A ventilation-perfusion study without abnormalities is, of course, interpreted as normal. If there are matching ventilation-perfusion defects with no clear-cut areas of dissociation, the interpretation is a low probability of pulmonary embolism. If there are areas suggestive of dissociation, with relative preservation of ventilation in areas where perfusion defects are not segmental or the ventilation study was not performed in the optimum projection, the interpretation is a moderate probability of pulmonary embolism, and a pulmonary angiogram is indicated to obtain a more definitive diagnosis. If there are well-defined segmental or multisegmental perfusion defects that ventilate, the interpretation is a high probability of pulmonary embolism. If there are segmental densities radiographically, these areas will show both perfusion and ventilation defects, and may represent pulmonary embolism with infarction or any of the other causes of radiographic pulmonary densities. In this case the region of the density is interpreted as indeterminate. The indeterminate interpretation is only applied to the region of radiographic density, and not to all of the lung fields. The indeterminate interpretation is therefore often used in conjunction with one of the other interpretations. If there are typical findings of pulmonary embolism in an aerated portion of lung, it is often assumed that the associated radiographic density with an indeterminate etiology is the result of an embolus with infarction. With the indeterminate pattern, if the scan findings in aerated portions of the lung are normal or are those of low-probability or moderate-probability embolism, an angiogram is suggested. Depending on patient selection, 20 to 50 percent of patients with pulmonary embolism will fall into the lung scan categories of moderate probability or indeterminate.[22–24]

The use of ventilation-perfusion lung scanning in the diagnosis of pulmonary embolism remains controversial.[6] In highly selected patients with previously normal lungs who have angiographically documented pulmonary embolism, a segmental or multiple segmental perfusion defect with intact ventilation appears to be diagnostic.[25,26] Such a pattern is shown in Figure 7–1. Unfortunately, many patients who suffer pulmonary embolism have pre-existing lung disease. In this setting the ventilation-perfusion scan patterns become more difficult to interpret: there are often ventilation abnormalities, and perfusion defects frequently are diffuse and subsegmental. In this regard, false-positive ventilation-perfusion lung scans have been reported in a number of conditions. These include chronic obstructive pulmonary disease (COPD),[27,28] pneumonia,[28,29] bronchogenic carcinoma,[30,31] intravenous drug abuse,[32,33] following lung irradiation,[34,35] vasculitis,[36,37] and with previous pulmonary embolism[1,38] False-negative lung scans have been reported with high frequency in the past in cases of congestive heart failure,[39,40] but a recent study suggests that congestive heart failure does not cause false-negative scans.[20]

Critics of ventilation-perfusion lung scanning also correctly point out that pulmonary embolism is associated with two types of ventilation-perfusion abnormality. The first, which occurs at the site where the thromboembolus lodges, involves an area that is poorly perfused but retains relatively more ventilation than perfusion. This is the cause of the ventilation-perfusion mismatch that is the hallmark for the lung-scan diagnosis of pulmonary embolism. This first ventilation-perfusion abnormality consists essentially of respiratory dead space, and can be responsible for an elevated PCO_2 in massive pulmonary embolism.[41] The second ventilation-perfusion abnormality involves areas of lung, contiguous to the embolized portion, in which perfusion is still intact but ventilation is impaired. The abnormality in these areas is similar to a physiologic shunt, and is responsible for the hypoxemia so often associated with pulmonary embolism. Such poor-ventilation areas contiguous to the embolized portion of the lung are commonplace and make the interpretation of ventilation scans difficult.

Unfortunately, more heat than light has been shed on the subject of ventilation-perfusion lung scanning in the last several years. What is sorely needed is a rigid prospective trial comparing lung scanning and pulmonary angiography in the

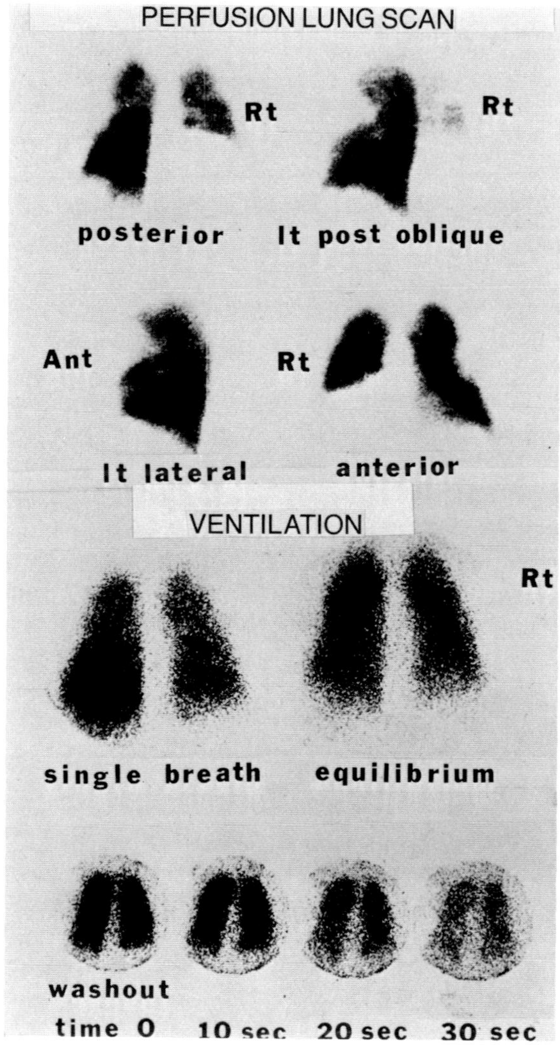

Figure 7–1. This ventilation-perfusion lung scan shows the most specific pattern for pulmonary embolism. The perfusion study (upper two panels) shows lobar loss of perfusion to the right middle and lower lobes and segmental loss to the anterior segment of the left upper lobe. The ventilation study shows uniform uptake and equilibrium of ventilation, and a normal washout over 30 seconds. The chest radiograph was normal with the exception of a slightly elevated right hemidiaphragm. Interpretation: Segmental and lobar perfusion defects with normal ventilation, indicating the high probability of pulmonary embolism in a compatible clinical setting.

diagnosis of pulmonary embolism. All patients who enter such a trial would undergo both studies, and both studies would be analyzed independently. If such a trial were done carefully, employing a wide cross-section of patients suspected of having pulmonary embolism, the role of ventilation-perfusion lung scanning would be much clearer. Recently, attempts to address this question have been published.[22,23]

Despite the current controversy, pulmonary ventilation-perfusion scanning is usually done when there is clinical suspicion of pulmonary embolism. Furthermore, since pulmonary emboli may resolve over a period of several days, it is considered important to obtain the pulmonary ventilation-perfusion study as early as possible after the onset of symptoms. The ventilation study is done first, since the radiation energy from ^{133}Xe gas is lower than the radiation energy from the ^{99M}Tc microspheres used in most perfusion studies.[42,43] The complete ventilation study with xenon gas usually is done only in the posterior projection, since it demonstrates the greatest percentage of ventilation defects of all the projections. The ventilation study is done in three parts: a single-breath image; an equilibrium image; and a series of washout images. The single-breath image is recorded following the deep inspiration of a bolus of ^{133}Xe. The radioactivity in this image is distributed predominantly according to normal ventilation. The equilibrium image is recorded following 3 minutes of rebreathing of xenon and oxygen in a closed system. The distribution of radioactivity in this image reflects areas of both normal and low ventilation. The washout images are obtained while the patient is expiring air containing xenon, and inspiring nonradioactive room air. In these images the relative distribution of radioactivity is again determined by the distribution of normal ventilation, but, in contrast to the single-breath image, areas of normal ventilation are shown as areas of decreased activity, while areas of poor ventilation are shown as areas of relatively increased activity. The perfusion study is done in most instances with the intravenous injection of ^{99M}Tc microspheres. These albumin particles are distributed according to blood flow and, being larger than the capillaries, are extracted by the pulmonary capillary bed with 100 percent efficiency. Once the particles are extracted by the pulmonary capillary bed, the radioactivity on the particles provides a static image of the distribution of pulmonary arterial perfusion. Images are then recorded in the anterior and posterior and in both lateral and both posterior oblique positions.

The ventilation-perfusion lung scan is safe and relatively easy to perform. ^{99M}Tc-labeled microspheres do not substantially aggravate the hypoxemia associated with pulmonary embolism, and the incidence of adverse reactions to this radionuclide is low. However, the current interpretative strategy for ventilation-perfusion lung scanning must be qualified in several ways. First, as stated earlier, perfusion defects that ventilate may be occasionally caused by lesions other than pulmonary emboli. Second, the perfusion-ventilation dissociation caused by some emboli may never resolve, making it difficult to be certain of the age of the embolus if prior ventilation studies are unavailable. Third, if the patient is studied several days following the symptomatic event, sufficient resolution of the embolus may have occurred to change the findings from those of a high-probability interpretation to those of moderate or low probability. Fourth, an assumption is always made that emboli smaller than those necessary to occlude segmental or larger arteries are not clinically important. One reason for this assumption is that ventilation of subsegmental perfusion defects is difficult to evaluate with the spatial resolution of standard ventilation imaging methods. The complications of chronic and recurrent pulmonary embolism will be discussed later in this chapter.

Follow-up ventilation-perfusion studies done 7 to 10 days after the initial studies are sometimes useful in increasing the certainty of diagnosis, at least in retrospect. Since most acute pulmonary emboli will show some resolution in 7 to 10 days, a partial or complete resolution of the initial findings raises the probability of acute pulmonary embolism. The absence of change over a 7- to 10-day period lowers the probability of acute pulmonary embolism and, in some cases, supports the idea that the findings are secondary to an old pulmonary embolus.

A number of newer techniques for the visualization of pulmonary emboli are in the experimental stage, but have not yet found widespread application. Ventilation imaging after the perfusion study can be accomplished with ^{127}Xe or ^{81M}Kr or by the inhalation of indium-labeled aerosols.[42–44] These radionuclides all have higher energies than ^{99M}Tc. When the ventilation study is performed secondarily, it can therefore be done in the projection that best demonstrates the perfusion defect, or it can be omitted when the perfusion scan is normal. A more novel approach is to identify the area of involvement as an area of increased activity with inhaled ^{15}O-labeled carbon dioxide.[45] Normally, carbon dioxide diffuses through the alveolar wall and is circulated in the blood and expired. In areas of pulmonary embolism with minimal blood flow, the presence of carbon dioxide radioactivity is prolonged. Unfortunately, an on-site medical cyclotron is required for the production of ^{15}O.

Pulmonary Angiography

The pulmonary angiogram remains the single best diagnositc test both for identifying and defining the extent of pulmonary embolism. The radiographic evaluation of pulmonary embolism begins with a chest radiograph and the ventilation-perfusion lung scan. In the proper clinical setting, a normal ventilation scan with segmental or multisegmental defects on the perfusion scan leads to a high-probability interpretation of pulmonary embolism, and a pulmonary angiogram is not necessary. Conversely, when the perfusion lung scan is normal, the diagnosis of pulmonary embolism is essentially ruled ut. However, when the ventilation-perfusion lung scan is interpreted as indicating a moderate probability of pulmonary embolism, or is indeterminate, a further investigation for a confident diagnosis of pulmonary embolism is needed (Table 7–2). The technique for such a confident diagnosis in this setting remains the pulmonary angiogram.

Pulmonary angiography is safer than it was 10 years ago because perforation of the heart is virtually impossible with the new pigtail catheter, in contrast to the blunt-tipped catheter used previously by both cardiologists and radiologists. There was formerly also an increased risk of bradycardia and ventricular standstill

Table 7–2. Indications for Pulmonary Angiography

Patients with indeterminate lung scans (a radiographic abnormality that matches the area of perfusion scan abnormality).
Patients with moderate probability of pulmonary embolism by lung scan.
All patients in whom surgical intervention is contemplated (pulmonary embolectomy, inferior vena caval interruption).

when injections were made into the main pulmonary artery in patients who had pulmonary hypertension. This complication has been reduced with selective injections, and patients can now be referred for pulmonary angiography to exclude embolism. who have high pulmonary artery pressures (even above a mean pressure of 40 mmHg). The current dominant risk is an arrhythmia during the study, but even this is unusual, and occurs in less than 5 percent of cases. Most angiographic studies are now performed with the pigtail catheter placed in the femoral vein. If femoral vein thrombosis or caval thrombi are present, a cutdown is done on an upper-extremity vein. Pulmonary angiography usually takes 60 to 90 minutes, with the patient experiencing little discomfort even during the injection. Most of the practitioners who perform pulmonary angiography suggest that it be done within 72 hours of the acute symptomatic event. A few perform the study as late as 3 to 7 days following the onset of symptoms, although there is probably a slight risk of missing an embolus with this delay. Unlike the lung-scan perfusion defect, which may take months to disappear, a small embolus actually may dissolve during the first week.

The diagnosis of pulmonary embolism depends on specific angiographic findings. Nonspecific findings, including slow flow to an area of the lung, slow clearance of contrast material, or the pruning of vessels are indirect signs, and cannot be used to make a confident diagnosis of pulmonary embolism. The only specific findings are a filling defect demonstrated within a vessel, or the complete blockage or cutoff of a vessel (Fig. 7–2). When a pulmonary angiogram is performed with appropriate projections, including magnification views when necessary, a negative study carries great significance.[46] If the study has been done early in the course of the suspected embolism and is normal, no further anticoagulant therapy should be given, and other diagnoses should be entertained. When intraluminal filling defects or cutoffs are seen on the pulmonary angiogram, one can diagnose pulmonary embolism and appropriate therapy can be given.

It has recently been contended that too much reliance has been put on ventilation-perfusion lung scanning in the diagnosis of pulmonary embolism.[6] It appears from current studies that approximately 20 to 50 percent of patients who have a pulmonary embolism will have either an indeterminate or a moderate-probability lung scan.[22,23] These are the patients who benefit from pulmonary angiography because a confident diagnosis can be made and anticoagulation therapy can be promptly and effectively instituted. Fortunately, it now appears that more pulmonary angiograms are being performed in the diagnosis of patients in these groups.

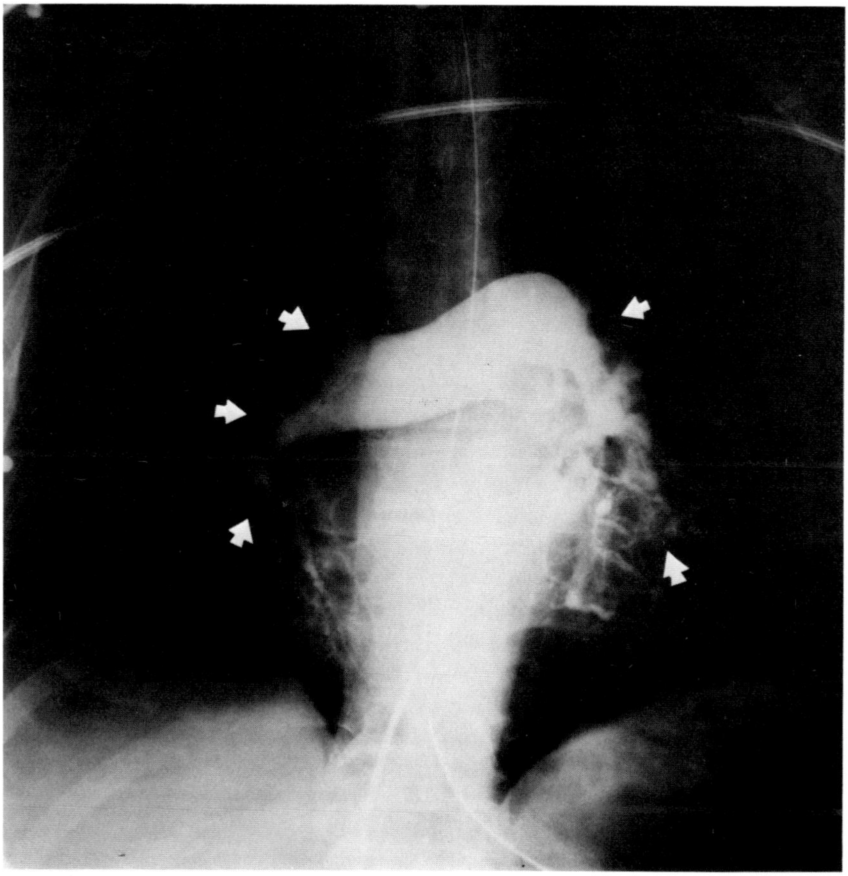

Figure 7–2. This pulmonary arteriogram performed with a main pulmonary artery injection shows massive pulmonary embolism. Both upper lobe vessels are occluded and there are filling defects in vessels to both lower lobes as well as in the intermediate vessel on the right. This patient was in shock. He was treated successfully with thrombolytic therapy followed by heparin.

Several groups have lately reported the utilization of the flow-directed balloon catheter to perform pulmonary angiography on subsegmented arteries.[47] However, while subsegmental angiography may become useful for finding small, peripheral emboli, it will have limited application as a general diagnostic technique, since only a small portion of the pulmonary vasculature can be visualized with each injection. The use of a fiberoptic transvenous catheter for the direct visualization of pulmonary emboli in dogs has also been recently reported.[48] The published photographs of these emboli were not clear, and it remains to be seen what utility, if any, this technique will have in humans.

PATHOGENIC MECHANISMS IN MASSIVE PULMONARY EMBOLISM

In massive pulmonary embolism in humans and animals, there is an immediate increase in the pulmonary artery mean pressure, associated with a normal or low cardiac output. This combination results in an increase in the total pulmonary vascular resistance that is directly proportional to the increase in pulmonary artery mean pressure.[49,50] It is generally believed that in acute pulmonary embolism, the normal right ventricle begins to fail when an afterload that is proportionate to approximately 40 mmHg of pulmonary artery mean pressure is exceeded, and it has been stated that higher pressures rarely are seen in the absence of prior cardiopulmonary disease.[51] There also is a reasonable correlation between the degree of obstruction on an angiogram or the perfusion defect on a lung scan and the pulmonary artery mean pressure.[1] Such a statement means that there is a clear relationship between the extent of embolism and the resultant hemodynamic abormalities. In the past, some emphasis was focused on humoral events that were thought to follow pulmonary embolism and contribute to the hemodynamic and airway abnormalities observed.[52–55] It was hypothesized that a fresh fibrin clot contained active thrombin, which caused the adherence of platelets with the subsequent release of the bioactive amines serotonin and histamine.[54] These amines were shown to increase the pulmonary hypertension and airway resistance in experimental animals.[53] These and similar studies were used as a rationale for the use, in humans, of heparin initially in unusually large doses for the treatment of pulmonary embolism, in an attempt to block the hypothesized platelet–thrombin interaction. In fact, most of these studies were conducted in animals, particularly rabbits and cats, whose platelets have a greatly increased histamine and serotonin content relative to human platelets. When dogs were studied the effect was less marked.[55] Thus, some of the humoral mediators that contribute to worsened hemodynamics and airway physiology in animals are not present in similar concentration in human platelets. Furthermore, many of the animal studies utilized microemboli (less than 1 mm diameter), whereas human pulmonary emboli are usually much larger.[56] In the final analysis, the secondary airway and hemodynamic events that have been observed in animals are not seen clinically in humans. Although there is probably some secondary bronchoconstriction in human pulmonary embolism, wheezing is rare, and when present is usually found in patients with underlying airway disease or congestive heart failure.[57] In addition, the exceptionally high levels of heparin (greater than 100,000 units/day) that have been recommended for the treatment of the platelet–thrombin "problem" have resulted in unacceptable hemorrhagic complications; and this level of heparin is not recommended for the treatment of either acute or chronic pulmonary embolism.

Once a massive pulmonary embolism occurs, the right ventricle can respond to the acutely increased afterload in one of two ways. Most often the right ventricle will maintain cardiac output in such a way that the total pulmonary resistance is increased but blood flow continues. The resultant hemodynamic and airway abnormalities associated with this state include areas of respiratory dead-space in the locale of the embolus, in which alveolar units are aerated but not perfused, and also areas having a physiologic, shunt-like effect contiguous to the embolized segment or lobe, in which the alveoli are perfused but not ventilated. In rare instances in which high cardiac outputs have been associated with massive pulmonary embolism, focal-overperfusion pulmonary edema has apparently resulted in areas with a patent vasculature.[58]

If the right ventricle fails and the cardiac output falls, the right ventricular end-diastolic pressure rises precipitously and the patient dies of acute cor pulmonale. These events can occur quickly, with the bedisde observer hearing only a loud right-sided gallop sound prior to the patient's cardiopulmonary arrest. In this state there is often little time for therapy, and the clinician can only institute vigorous cardiopulmonary resuscitation in the hope that external compression may fragment the large central embolus and result in better perfusion and right-sided cardiac output.[59]

In summary, it must be emphasized that in humans, increases in total pulmonary vascular resistance are related directly to the massivity of the embolus. In contrast, airway abnormalities and hypoxemia can be seen with emboli of all sizes.[60] Because the hemodynamic abnormalities that result from an embolus are life-threatening, therapy must therefore be aimed either at immediately arresting the embolic process or mechanically or enzymatically removing the embolus from the lung.

PROPHYLAXIS OF PULMONARY EMBOLISM

As early as 1950, Detakats[61] suggested that it took less heparin to prevent a pulmonary thromboembolism than to treat it. Sharonoff[62,63] later presented uncontrolled data to support this idea. Subsequently, controlled studies on the incidence of deep venous thrombosis of the lower extremities using ^{125}I-fibrinogen, indicated a prophylactic effect of low-dose, subcutaneous heparin in general abdominal and thoracic surgery patients,[64,65] and in gynecologic surgery patients.[66] Early in these studies it became apparent that the preventive effect of low-dose, subcutaneous heparin was not as great in individuals undergoing hip surgery.[67,68] One study of general-surgery patients suggested that low-dose heparin therapy begun in the perioperative period was more effective than full-dose anticoagulation with a coumarin derivative,[69] probably because most venous thrombosis occurs perioperatively and full-dose coumarin anticoagulation does not become effective until at least 2 to 3 days following the initiation of therapy. Subsequently, two large, multi-center trials have shown that 5000 units of heparin injected subcutaneously every 8 or 12 hours for 7 to 8 days significantly reduces the incidence of fatal postoperative pulmonary embolism in patients undergoing elective abdominal surgery.[70,71] These studies were performed with calcium heparin, whereas until now, sodium heparin has been the only preparation available in this country. This distinction is important, because calcium heparin has different absorption characteristics from sodium heparin when given subcutaneously.[72]

However, calcium heparin is now available in this country. With regard to the prophylaxis of venous thromboembolism, recent trials indicate that dextran-70 given in the perioperative period has a preventive benefit that is similar to that of low-dose subcutaneous heparin.[73,74]

The problem of effective prophylaxis in patients undergoing hip surgery remains. A number of studies have indicated an effect of low-dose subcutaneous heparin in this group, provided that the therapy is started within 12 hours of hospitalization for hip trauma, and that the heparin is given subcutaneously, in 5000-unit doses, every 8 hours.[75,76] However, other studies have indicated no significant effect of heparin. It may be that the tissue damage is so extensive in hip trauma, with the subsequent release of both procoagulants and heparin-neutralizing substances—and especially platelet factor 4—that low-dose heparin will not be effective in this setting.[78] These factors, added to the immobility necessitated by hip surgery, constitute a substantial predisposition to venous thromboembolism. In addition, most orthopedists in this country and abroad do not think that low-dose heparin is at all effective in massive hip trauma or surgery, somewhat in contradiction to the published data. This feeling, coupled with the reasonable concern that a small wound hematoma can jeopardize total hip replacement, has made the use of prophylactic heparin infrequent in hip surgery. Localized bleeding also can cause major complications in neurosurgical and ophthalmologic procedures, and low-dose heparin prophylaxis is consequently usually not used in these settings. Another surgical situation in which low-dose heparin does not seem to be effective is open prostatic surgery.[79,80]

Recently, a number of mechanical procedures have been developed to stimulate venous return in immobilized lower extremities. These include devices that compress the leg muscles mechanically[81,82] or stimulate muscle contraction[83,84] to prevent stasis and speed venous return. These techniques may prove of benefit in certain high-risk patients. However, at this time, none of these technques has undergone the rigorous testing applied to low-dose, subcutaneous heparin and dextran 70 therapy, and the mechanical techniques must therefore be considered experimental.[85]

TREATMENT OF PULMONARY EMBOLISM

Prior to the institution of heparin therapy for venous thromboembolism, the death rate from pulmonary embolism varied from approximately 18 to 32 percent.[11-13] Earlier reports indicated an even higher death rate in untreated pulmonary embolism. A landmark study by Barritt and Jordan[13] in 1960 indicated that heparin therapy followed by an oral anticoagulant could be expected to lower the death rate in pulmonary embolism from approximately 25 to 5 percent. This has been the only randomized, controlled study indicating an effect of heparin on established pulmonary embolism. However, subsequent studies utilizing a heparin-treated group alone have supported this markedly lower death rate.[15,16] It is interesting to note that astute observers had indicated, some 25 years before Barritt and Jordan's study, that heparin could be expected to lower the mortality in pulmonary embolism by the amount indicated by Barritt and Jordan.[86]

Heparin inhibits the major clotting enzymes, thrombin and factor X, by potentiating antithrombin III, a plasma protein that combines with and inactivates clotting enzymes. Heparin resistance can be said to occur when a seemingly adequate amount of heparin fails to adequately prolong the clotting assay used to monitor therapy. The most common cause of such resistance is antithrombin III deficiency, which is seen congenitally, in severe liver disease, and in severe ongoing thrombotic processes.[87,88]

An adequate amount of heparin must be administered to achieve an antithrombotic state in established pulmonary embolism. Clinically it appears that an activated partial thromboplastin time (APTT), or similar test, of at least one and one-half times the control time is necessary to indicate this state.[89] For coumarin derivatives, it appears that a prothrombin time of at least one and one-half times the control time is necessary.[90] It is important to monitor anticoagulant therapy with a standardized clotting test to document that the level of anticoagulation is adequate. While anticoagulant requirements probably are highest in the first 2 to 3 days following an acute thromboembolic event, individual patient requirements are variable enough to require the periodic monitoring of anticoagulation.[91,92]

Recently, two prospective, well-controlled trials have shown that continuous intravenous heparin, in a dosage sufficient to prolong the APTT to greater than one and one-half times the control value, causes less bleeding than intermittent bolus heparin, while equally preventing recurrent pulmonary embolism.[93,94] A single study appears to contradict the last-noted finding.[95] Here the authors found an unusually high incidence of recurrent venous thromboembolism with continuous intravenous heparin. However, these investigators used smaller amounts of heparin than usual, and some of their patients may not have been anticoagulated adequately. In contrast, unusually high doses of heparin result in excessive bleeding.[96]

Coumarin Derivatives

These agents include a number of chemicals that act to inhibit the vitamin K-dependent clotting proteins (factors II, VII, IX and X). Their molecular mechanism appears to involve inhibition of the gamma carboxylation of glutamic acid residues in the protein backbones of the clotting factors. Thus, the proteins are produced, but are biologically inactive.[97] Other vitamin K-dependent enzymes have been identified in both blood and in tissue, but the coincidental suppression of these enzymes by coumarin derivatives given to prevent clotting has not caused evident clinical problems. Coumarin derivatives require 6 to 7 consecutive days of administration to achieve their full antithrombotic effect, whether or not an initial loading dose is given.[98] They are given orally and are suitable for outpatient therapy; when used properly, they allow long-term anticoagulation for patients with thrombotic problems. It is important to monitor the prothrombin times during the course of coumarin administration in order to insure that the patient is anticoagulated adequately (a prothrombin time of approximately twice the control value), but that the patient is not predisposed to a bleeding diathesis because of an inordinately prolonged prothrombin time.

The duration of full anticoagulation in established pulmonary embolism remains controversial. The study by O'Sullivan indicated that 1 month of full-dose anticoagulation may be adequate in most patients with pulmonary embolism,[99] and a recent study appears to confirm this point.[100] However, other studies have indicated that 2 weeks of full-dose anticoagulation is probably inadequate.[90,101] In this regard, a recent study has shown that a regimen of 10 days of full-dose heparin (5000 units three times a day) followed by low-dose, subcutaneous heparin is not adequate for the treatment of most deep venous thrombosis because of a resultant excessive incidence of recurrent thrombosis and pulmonary embolism.[102] Thus, the recommendation by one reviewer that such a regimen is adequate for most pulmonary embolism probably is incorrect.[103] At this time it appears that in the ambulatory patient with no continuing predisposition to embolism, the minimal period of full-dose anticoagulation therapy for venous thromboembolic disease is 4 weeks. This duration usually necessitates a regimen of heparin followed by an oral agent. If the oral agent is begun with the institution of intravenous heparin, the patient is usually adequately anticoagulated with the oral agent within 7 to 10 days of the thromboembolic event, and can be discharged home if his or her condition so indicates. The patient can then be followed with weekly measurement of the prothrombin time, and the oral agent can be discontinued at the discretion of the physician (Table 7–3). Obviously some patients with a continuing predisposition to venous thromboembolism will need full-dose anticoagulation for a longer period of time than 4 weeks.

Table 7–3. Recommendations for Anticoagulation

Intravenous heparin 5000–10,000 units bolus followed by 1000–1500 units per hour to prolong the activated partial thromboplastin time (or similar test) to 2 to 2½ times control.
Monitor platelets by peripheral smear or counts every 2–3 days.
Start daily maintenance dose of coumarin derivative concurrent with heparin and allow 6–7 days for full antithrombotic effect.
Stop heparin after 7–10 days when prothrombin time is consistently 2 times control.
Full anticoagulation for at least 6 weeks.

Surgical Intervention

Vena Caval Interruption (Clip, Ligation, Filter, Umbrella)

This procedure is done less frequently now that knowledge of the use of anticoagulants has improved; however, occasionally a patient who is on an adequate anticoagulation regimen will suffer recurrent pulmonary embolism. Such an event constitutes an indication for vena caval interruption. Vena caval interruption also should be performed adjunctively in the infrequent case in which pulmonary embolectomy is deemed necessary. It is important to interrupt the cava in this setting because surgery makes anticoagulation a contraindication in these patients for several days. One must remember, however, that vena caval interruption is a stopgap measure; collateral circulation, endocardial mural thrombosis, or the migration of an umbrella can lead to recurrent pulmonary embolism if adequate anticoagulation therapy is not re-started within 10 days. In recent years, interest has turned toward transvenously implantable filters that do not require general anesthesia and major surgery. The two most widely known such devices are the Mobin-Uddin umbrella filter[104] and the Kim-Ray Greenfield filter.[105] Both filters appear to retard the formation of large collaterals resulting from total vena caval obstruction; unfortunately, both are associated with other complications, as recent reports attest.[106,107]

Pulmonary Embolectomy

Pulmonary embolectomy is indicated in massive pulmonary embolism (more than 50 percent vascular occlusion) associated with shock and a deteriorating clinical course despite medical therapy. In the past, the procedure has been associated with a high mortality rate.[108] However, recent studies indicate a more acceptable mortality rate of 25 percent in selected patients.[109–111] In patients with massive pulmonary embolism involving 60 to 70 percent of the pulmonary vasculature, pulmonary embolectomy appears to be the only effective treatment.[2] However, it must be emphasized that strictly controlled trials of thrombolytic therapy and pulmonary embolectomy have not been performed in such cases.

Thrombolytic Therapy

An exciting new development in the treatment of pulmonary embolism is the release for clinical use of two agents, which can dissolve clots, in contrast to heparin, which only blocks clot propagation. These agents can be considered an alternative to surgical pulmonary embolectomy, and one might refer to them as medical embolectomy agents. Both agents are enzymes and activate the plasma enzyme plasminogen, which degrades fibrin clots, fibrinogen, and several other clotting factors. One of the two, urokinase, is a human protein purified either from pooled human urine or from cultured human embryo kidney cells.[112] The molecular weight of cell-culture-derived urokinase is approximately 34,000 daltons, and it acts by cleaving the proenzyme plasminogen into the active enzyme plasmin. The other embolectomy agent, streptokinase, is a protein obtained from cultures of group C beta hemolytic streptococci. Its molecular weight is 47,000 daltons, and it acts by combining with plasminogen to form a complex which in turn activates adjacent plasminogen. Streptokinase is antigenic, and it is recommended that its repeat use, if necessary, not be made within 6 months of prior administration. In addition, there is some pyrogenicity associated with streptokinase, and occasionally patients will have a mild fever, although this is not an important problem with the currently available preparations. Streptokinase also is simple to administer. It is available for use in pulmonary embolism, deep venous thrombosis of the upper

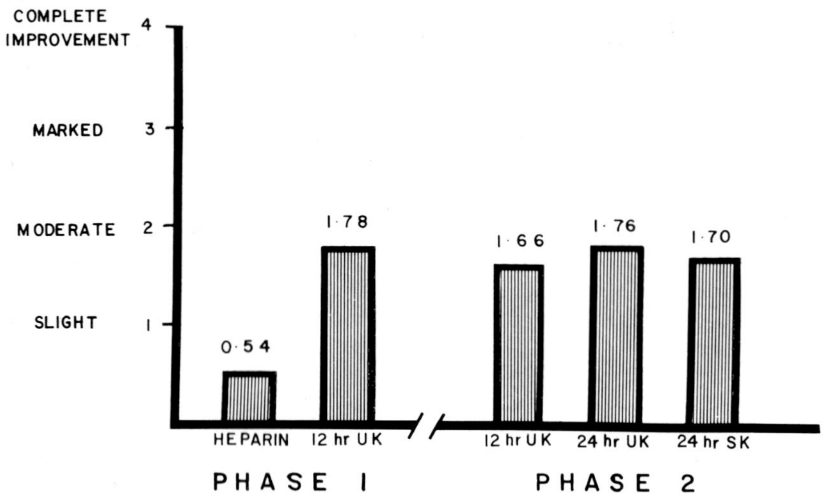

Figure 7–3. Arteriographic severity change at 24 hours, reflecting both clot lysis and improvement in perfusion, is shown for heparin and 12-hour urokinase (phase 1); and 12-hour urokinase, 24-hour urokinase, and 24-hour streptokinase (phase 2). Each group represents 60-80 patients studied. All thrombolytic regimens achieved similar resolution (nearly "moderate"), and each was significantly greater than that seen with heparin (less than "slight").

leg, and peripheral arterial embolism. Urokinase is available for use in pulmonary embolism.

Both agents have similar thrombolytic effects as judged by national clinical trials in pulmonary embolism.[113,114] These trials were conducted over approximately 6 years by the National Heart, Lung, and Blood Institute of the National Institutes of Health. In the first phase of the trials, which involved 160 patients, a 12-hour infusion of urokinase followed by heparin was judged to be significantly more effective in resolving pulmonary thromboemboli at 24 hours than was heparin alone.[113] The comparative pulmonary angiographic evidence of clot lysis is shown in Figure 7–3. As can be seen, the clot resolution obtained with urokinase followed by heparin was approximately three times that seen with heparin alone when the angiogram was repeated 24 hours later and compared with the pretreatment angiogram.

In a second phase of the trials, infusions of urokinase for 12 and 24 hours and infusions of streptokinase for 24 hours were compared.[114] As can be seen in Figure 7–3, the thrombolytic effect documented by angiography was similar in the patient groups treated in all three ways, and corresponded to that seen with 12-hour urokinase infusion in the first phase of the trial. Many individuals have asked an obvious question concerning the minimal duration of thrombolytic therapy: If 12 hours of urokinase is as effective as 24 hours, would a much shorter infusion be equally effective? Unfortunately, the appropriate studies to provide an answer to this question have not yet been done, and in pulmonary embolism urokinase is

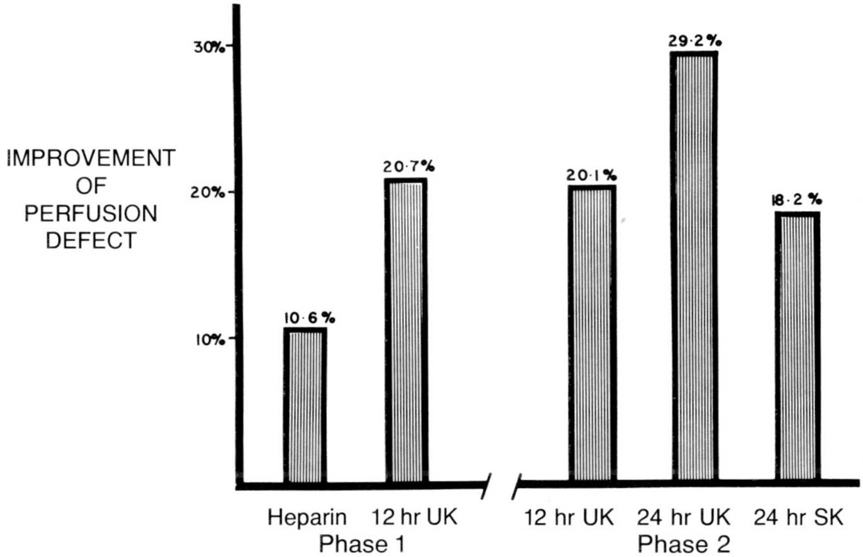

Figure 7–4. Lung scan resolution, expressed as percent improvement in perfusion defect, is shown for all treatment regimens in both phases of the trial. Thombolytic regimens averaged from 20 to 30 percent resolution of the initial perfusion defect, significantly greater than the 10.6 percent average resolution seen with heparin treatment alone. Each group contained from 50 to 80 patients.

recommended for 12-hour infusion, and streptokinase for 24-hour infusion.

Lung scan studies have also shown a significant improvement in pulmonary perfusion following thrombolytic therapy when compared with heparin therapy alone at 24 hours (Fig. 7–4). It should be noted, however, that by 14 days after beginning therapy, the perfusion lung scan was similar in groups treated with heparin alone or treated with urokinase or streptokinase followed by heparin. Thus it appears that the superior effect of the thrombolytic agent occurs acutely at a time when the hemodynamic and respiratory compromise is greatest, and that within a few days, natural mechanisms tend to return the pulmonary perfusion lung scan to a more normal pattern, regardless of whether the patient received urokinase or streptokinase followed by heparin, or heparin alone. However, recent evidence suggests that despite equal resolution of lung scans in the late follow-up period, patients treated initially with a thrombolytic agent appear to have an improved pulmonary capillary blood volume as measured by the diffusing capacity of carbon monoxide.[115]

The foregoing trials also revealed that thrombolyttherapy significantly improved pulmonary artery and right heart hemodynamics over the first 24 hours (Fig. 7–5). With thrombolytic therapy, the pulmonary artery mean pressure fell significantly, returning on the average to an almost normal level. In contrast, with heparin therapy alone, the pulmonary artery mean pressure still was elevated significantly after 24 hours, indicating a lesser degree of reversion toward normal

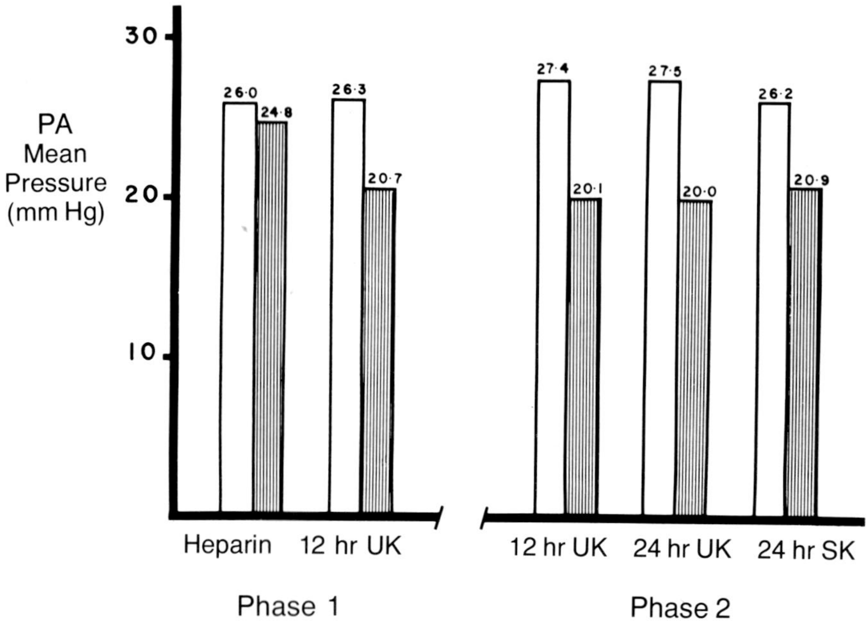

Figure 7–5. Pulmonary artery mean pressures pre-therapy (white bars) and at 24 hours (line bars) are shown for all treatment regimens in both phases of the trial. Thrombolytic regimens yielded from 5 to 7 mmHg average reduction in pulmonary artery mean pressure, whereas heparin alone resulted in an average 1.2 mmHg reduction. Each group was made up of 50 to 70 patients.

of the hemodynamic abnormalities precipitated by a pulmonary embolism. When the pulmonary artery mean pressure was combined with flow data in these trials, streptokinase or urokinase therapy achieved a significant reduction in total pulmonary resistance when compared to heparin alone.

To date, no study in pulmonary embolism has shown a survival benefit provided by a thrombolytic agent followed by heparin over heparin alone. This fact is not startling when one considers that the mortality in large series of heparin-treated pulmonary embolism is low (less than 10 percent), thus making a survival effect extremely difficult to demonstrate without studying literally thousands of patients. Nevertheless, the striking effect of thrombolytic agents on angiographic resolution and hemodynamic improvement in the critical acute period of embolism suggests that they have a role in the treatment of acute massive pulmonary embolism. On the basis of the data accumulated to date, thrombolytic therapy is thought to be most effective in acute massive pulmonary embolism, in pulmonary embolism accompanied by unstable hemodynamics, and when surgical pulmonary embolectomy is being considered as a life-saving measure.

The only significant complication associated with the use of urokinase or streptokinase is bleeding, which also is a problem associated with anticoagulants. The initial NIH trials showed a high risk of bleeding with either thrombolytic therapy

Table 7–4. Contraindications to Thrombolytic Therapy

Surgery or parturition within 10 days.
Recent stroke or brain trauma within 2 months.
Any active bleeding diathesis or clotting factor deficiency.
Severe hypertension.
Renal or hepatic failure.
Bacterial endocarditis, active ulcer disease or other condition associated with hemorrhagic tendency.

or anticoagulant therapy alone, probably because of the extensive invasive procedures required to document thrombolysis in these patients. This risk subsequently has been reduced as invasive procedures have been minimized, and the bleeding risk with a thombolytic agent is now probably not significantly higher than the risk with anticoagulants alone.[116] Bleeding can be minimized by careful attention to hemostasis and the avoidance of invasive procedures. The contraindications to thrombolytic therapy are similar to those associated with anticoagulant therapy (Table 7–4).

The individual who might be expected to respond best to a thrombolytic agent is one who is acutely ill, with an acute, massive pulmonary embolism, but who does not have any contraindication to thrombolytic therapy (Table 7–4). In such cases, both urokinase and streptokinase offer a reasonable alternative to surgical pulmonary embolectomy, a difficult procedure fraught with complications and a high mortality. Either urokinase or streptokinase can return the pulmonary vasculature to a more normal state more rapidly than can heparin alone. It is important to emphasize that these agents be used early in the course of pulmonary embolism, and that the diagnosis be secure because of the risk of bleeding. Heparin should not be given concurrently with thrombolytic agents, but should be administered during the diagnostic work-up of a patient with suspected pulmonary embolism, and should be restarted following the use of thrombolytic therapy to minimize re-thrombosis.

In general, the decision to treat with thrombolytic agents should be based on a firm diagnosis utilizing either a positive pulmonary angiogram or a high-probability ventilation-perfusion lung scan (Table 7–5). If there are no contraindications to thrombolytic therapy (Table 7–4), heparin infusion is discontinued and a clotting test is done to determine that the hemostatic system has returned toward normal. Usually, either a thrombin time or an activated partial thromboplastin time that is no more than 10 seconds longer than the control time is sufficient. The loading dose of the thrombolytic agent is given according to the manufacturer's instructions, and this is followed by the maintenance dose given via a constant intravenous infusion. The laboratory monitoring of thrombolytic therapy is optional, since several studies have shown little correlation between in vivo thrombolysis and in vitro fibrinolysis[112]. Most authorities recommend a single test within 4 to 6 hours of the initiation of thrombolytic therapy to indicate induction of the "lytic state"[116,117] (Table 7–6).

Table 7–5. Checklist for Use of Urokinase or Streptokinase

Positive diagnosis (usually angiographic) of acute massive pulmonary embolism or hemodynamically unstable pulmonary embolism.
No contraindication to thrombolytic therapy.
Stop heparin and measure clotting test (See Table 7–6).
Determine loading and maintenance doses and reconstitute according to manufacturer's instructions.
Administer the thrombolytic agent intravenously by constant infusion apparatus.
Administer heparin following thrombolytic agent when clotting test has returned toward normal (see Table 7–6).

Table 7–6. Laboratory Monitoring of Thrombolytic Therapy

Pre-therapy: Thrombin time or PTT should be no more than 10 seconds longer than control to document dissipation of heparin effect.
During therapy: Monitoring optional; prolonged clotting test, high fibrin degradation products or low fibrinogen may be used to demonstrate "lytic state."
Post-therapy: Document dissipation of fibrinolytic effect before restarting heparin, using same criteria as before thrombolytic therapy.

LONG-TIME SEQUELAE OF MASSIVE PULMONARY EMBOLISM

In the past it was thought that heparin was adequate therapy for all pulmonary emboli, and that if the patient survived the acute period the outlook was uniformly good, provided that recurrent pulmonary embolization could be halted. This view ignored reports that after pulmonary embolism, some patients developed chronic pulmonary hypertension, particularly with exercise, regardless of the duration or intensity of anticoagulation.[118,119] More recently, studies have shown that seemingly adequately anticoagulated patients have defects in their pulmonary microvascular circulation that persist for up to a year after the embolic episode, even in the absence of clinical episodes of recurrence. That early thrombolytic therapy may block these chronic effects has been suggested.[115] However, the study in which this suggestion was made must be regarded as preliminary; at present, the evidence that thrombolytic therapy offers an advantage over conventional anticoagulation in regard to the chronic sequelae of massive pulmonary embolism needs confirmation.

Some massive pulmonary emboli resolve to only a slight extent, if at all, despite seemingly adequate anticoagulation. In other patients, recurrent pulmonary embolism appears to overwhelm the body's capacity for resolution. Either sequence of events can lead to chronic, severe pulmonary hypertension and cor pulmonale (Fig. 7–6). The frequency of these events has been exceedingly difficult to ascertain, particularly when embolization involves smaller-than-segmental arteries. Open lung biopsy with careful microscopic examination of the pulmonary vasculature can be useful for documenting recurrent pulmonary embolization.[120] Once

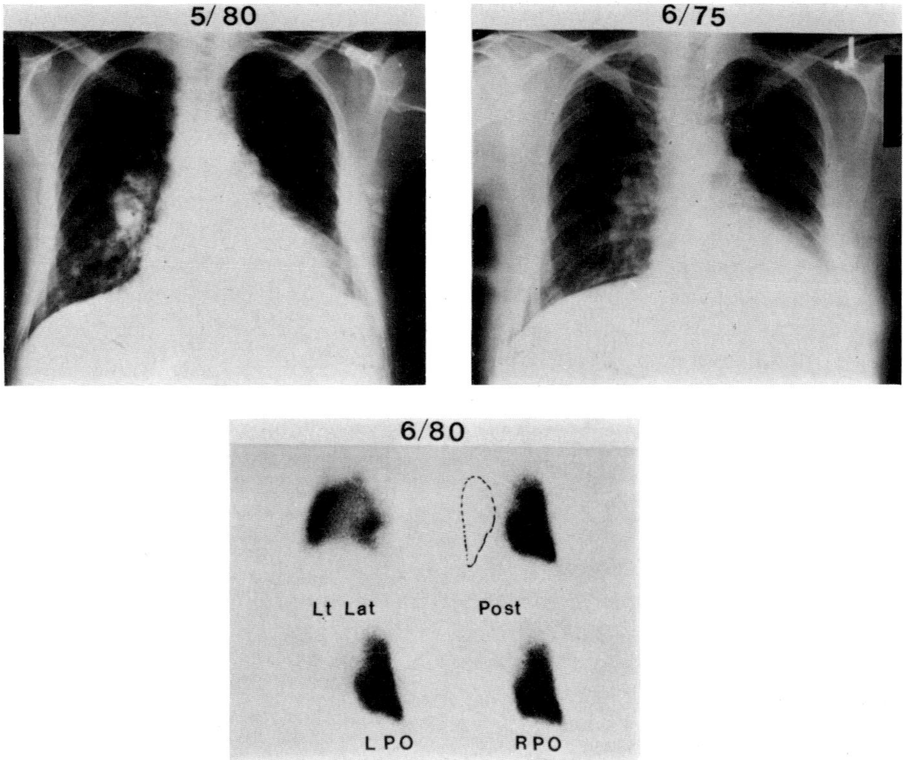

Figure 7–6. Two chest radiographs spanning 5 years in a patient with recurrent, chronic pulmonary embolism. The perfusion lung scan performed in 1980 shows no perfusion to the left lung. Despite heparin therapy the patient developed pulmonary hypertension and died of cor pulmonale. At autopsy, asymmetric intimal changes indicative of recurrent pulmonary embolism were found in all of the lobar arteries on the left and in several segmental arteries on the right.

intimal fibrosis and pulmonary hypertension develop, anticoagulant therapy and vena caval interruption offer little benefit.

The usual approach to the treatment of chronic pulmonary embolism is surgical removal of the embolus, utilizing cardiopulmonary bypass procedures.[121–123] The operation has a high mortality (25 to 30 percent), but appears to give a good result in survivors. One pathophysiologic response of the pulmonary circulation to chronic pulmonary embolism is hypertrophy of the bronchial arterial system, to correct for decreased perfusion via the pulmonary artery. In this regard, angiography of the bronchial arteries has been recommended prior to surgical embolectomy for chronic pulmonary embolism because it permits the surgeon to detect those areas that are most involved prior to surgery.[124,125] So-called back-bleeding from the bronchial artery into the pulmonary artery at the time of embolus removal has been reported to be a good sign of intact circulation to an involved area of the lung. An unusual complication of surgical embolectomy is localized areas of hemorrhagic pulmonary edema, apparently resulting from the acutely increased perfusion at the time of embolectomy. At present, it is unclear if transvenous catheter embolectomy, currently under evaluation in acute embolism, has a place in the treatment of chronic pulmonary embolism.[126] It is unlikely that this technique will find wide application, because chronic emboli are more firmly anchored to the pulmonary artery wall and are removed less easily.

The cardiopulmonary sequelae of repeated pulmonary embolism might be reduced by the more complete initial resolution of deep venous thrombosis. A recent controlled study has indicated that early streptokinase treatment of proximal deep venous thrombosis markedly reduces the long-term incidence of the postphlebitic syndrome.[127] The series was too small to glean any effect of lytic therapy on the pulmonary circulation. Long-term controlled studies in documented pulmonary embolism will be necessary to answer this question.

ACKNOWLEDGMENT

This work was supported by the Medical Research Service of the Veterans Administration and by NIH Grant No. HL 31867.

REFERENCES

1. The Urokinase Pulmonary Embolism Trial: A national cooperative study. Circulation (Suppl) 47:1–100, 1973.
2. Tibbutt DA, Davies JA, Anderson JA, et al: Comparison by control clinical trial of streptokinase and heparin in the treatment of life-threatening pulmonary embolism. Br Med J 1:343, 1974.
3. Ly B, Arnesen H, Eie H: A controlled clinical tiral of streptokinase and heparin in the treatment of major pulmonary embolism. Acta Med Scand 203:465, 1978.
4. Walsh PN, Greenspan RH, Simon M, et al: An angiographic severity index for pulmonary embolism. Circulation (Suppl) 1973.
5. Bell WR, Simon TL, DeMetz DL: The clinical features of massive and submassive pulmonary embolism. Am J Med 62:355, 1977.
6. Robin ED: Overdiagnosis and overtreatment of pulmonary embolism: the emperor may have no clothes. Ann Intern Med 87:775, 1977.
7. Sigel B, Justin JR, Gibson RJ, et al: Risk assessment of pulmonary embolism by multivariate analysis. Arch Surg 114:188, 1979.
8. Foster CS, Genton E, Henderson M et al (eds): Epidemiology of venous thrombosis. Milbank Mem Fund Q (Suppl) 50:1, 1972.
9. Havig O: Deep vein thrombosis in pulmonary embolism: an autopsy study with multiple regression analysis of possible risk factors. Acta Chir Scand (Suppl) 479: 1, 1977.
10. Coon WW: Epidemiology of venous thromboembolism. Ann Surg 186:149, 1977.
11. Alpert JS, Smith R, Carlson J, et al: Mortality in patients treated for pulmonary embolism. JAMA 236:1477, 1976.

12. Barker NW, Nygaard KK, Walter W, et al: A statistical study of postoperative venous thrombosis in pulmonary embolism. III. Time of occurrence during the postoperative period. Proc Staff Meet May Clin 16:17, 1941.
13. Barritt DW, Jordan SC: Anticoagulant drugs in the treatment of pulmonary embolism. Lancet 1:1309, 1960.
14. Zilliacus H: On specific treatment of thrombosis in pulmonary embolism with anticoagulants, with particular refrence to posthrombotic sequelae. Acta Med Scand (Suppl) 171:446,
15. Jick H, Slone D, Borda IT: Efficacy and toxicity of heparin in relation to age and sex. N Engl J Med 279:284, 1968.
16. Kernohan RJ, Todd C: Heparin therapy in thromboembolic disease. Lancet 1:621, 1966.
17. Westermark N: On the roentgen diagnosis of lung embolism. Acta Radiol 19:357, 1938.
18. Hampton AO, Castleman B: Correlation of postmorten chest teleroentgenograms with autopsy findings. With special reference to pulmonary embolism and infarction. Am J Roentgenol 43:305, 1940.
19. Secker-Walker RH, Siegel BA: The use of nuclear medicine in the diagnosis of lung disease. Radiol Clin North Am 11:215, 1973.
20. Bogren HG, Berman DS, Vismara VS, et al: Lung ventilation-perfusion scintigraphy in pulmonary embolism. Acta Radiol 19:933, 1978.
21. Wagner HN Jr, Strauss HW: Radioactive tracers in the differential diagnosis of pulmonary embolism. Prog Cardiovasc Dis 17:271, 1975.
22. Cheely R, McCarney WH, Perry IR, et al: The role of noninvasive tests versus pulmonary angiography in the diagnosis of pulmonary embolism. Am J Med 70:17, 1981.
23. Taplin V, Chopra SK: Lung perfusion-inhalation scintigraphy in obstructive airways disease in pulmonary embolism. Radio Clin North Am 16:491, 1978.
24. Menzoian JO, Williams LF: Is pulmonary angiography essential for the diagnosis of acute pulmonary embolism) Am J Surg 137:543, 1979.
25. McNeil BJ: A diagnositc strategy using ventilation-perfusion lung scans in patients suspect of pulmonary embolism. J Nucl Med 17:613, 1976.
26. Biello BR, Mattar AG, Osei-Wusu A, et al: Interpretation of indeterminate lung scintigrams. Radiology 133:189, 1979.
27. Simon H: Ventilation perfusion mismatch lung scan without pulmonary emboli. Clin Nucl Med 2:124, 1977.
28. Williams O, Lyall J, Vernon M, et al: Ventilation perfusion lung scanning for pulmonary emboli. Br Med J 1:600, 1974.
29. Li DK, Seltzer SE, McNeil BJ: Ventilation perfusion mismatches unassociated with pulmonary embolism. J Nucl Med 19:1331, 1978.
30. Secker-Walker RH, Alderson PO, Wilhelm J, et al: Ventilation perfusion scanning in carcinoma of the bronchus. Chest 65:660, 1974.
31. Fletcher JW, James AE, Holman BL: Regional lung function and cancer. In Progress in Nuclear Medicine, Regional Pulmonary Function in Health and Disease, Vol 3, Baltimore, University Park Press 135, 1973.
32. Soin JS, McKusick KA, Wagner HN Jr: Regional Lung function abnormalities in narcotics addicts. JAMA 224:1717, 1973.
33. Thomashow D, Summer WR, Soin J, et al: Lung disease in reformed drug addicts. Diagnostic and physiologic correlations. Johns Hopkins Med J 141:1, 1977.

34. Bateman NT, Croft DN: False positive lung scans and radiotherapy. Br Med J 1:807, 1976.
35. Prato FS, Kurdyak R, Saibil EA, et al: Physiologic and radiographic assessment during the development of pulmonary radiation fibrosis. Radiology 122:389, 1977.
36. Moser KM, Guisan M, Cuomo A, et al: Differentiation of pulmonary vascular from parenchymal diseases by ventilation perfusion scintiphotography. Ann Intern Med 75:597, 1971.
37. Potchen EJ, Adelstein FJ, Hoffer P, et al (eds.): Nuclear Radiology Syllabus. Chicago, American College of Radiology 240–246, 1974.
38. Paraskos JA, Adelstein SJ, Smith RE, et al: Late prognosis of acute pulmonary embolism. N Engl J Med 289:55, 1973.
39. Gilday DL, James AE: Lung scan patterns in pulmonary embolism versus those in congestive heart failure and emphysema. Am J Roentgenol 115:739, 1972.
40. Moses DC, Silver TM, Bookstein JJ: The complementary roles of chest radiography, lung scanning and selective pulmonary angiography in the diagnosis of pulmonary embolism. Circulation 49:179, 1974.
41. Haynes JB, Iseman MD: Massive Pulmonary embolism presenting with hypercapnea and minimal intrapulmonary shunting. Rocky Mt Med J 76:135, 1979.
42. Schor RA, Shames DM, Webber PM, et al: Regional ventilation studies with Kr-81 M and Xe-133: a comparative analysis. J Nucl Med 19:348, 1978.
43. Atkins HL, Suskind H, Klopper JF, et al: A clinical comparison of Xe-127 and Xe-133 for ventilation studies. J Nucl Med 18:653, 1977.
44. Coates G, Nahmias C: Xenon 127, a comparison with Xenon-133 for ventilation studies. J Nucl Med 18:221, 1977.
45. Nickols AB, Cochavi S, Hales CA, et al: Scintigraphic detection of pulmonary emboli by serial position imaging of inhaled 0-15 labelled carbon dioxide. N Engl J Med 299:279, 1978.
46. Novelline RA, Baltarowich OH, Athanasoulis CA, et al: The clinical course of patients with suspected pulmonary embolism and a negative pulmonary angiogram. Radiology 126:561, 1978.
47. Stein PD: Wedge arteriography for the identification of pulmonary emboli in small vessels. Am Heart J 82:618, 1971.
48. Moser KM, Shure D, Harrell JH, et al: Angioscopic visualization of pulmonary emboli. Chest 77:198, 1980.
49. McIntyre KM, Sasahara AA: The hemodynamic response to pulmonary embolism in patients without prior cardiopulmonary disease. Am J Cardiol 28:288, 1971.
50. Miller GAH, Sutton GC: Acute massive pulmonary embolism: Clinical and hemodynamic findings in 23 patients studied by cardiac catheterization in pulmonary arteriography. Br Heart J 32:518, 1970.
51. McIntyre KM, Sasahara AA: Determinants of right ventricular functions and hemodynamics after pulmonary embolism. Chest 65:534, 1974.
52. Nelson JR, Smith JR: Pathologic physiology of pulmonary embolism. Physiologic discussion of the vascular reaction following pulmonary arterial obstruction by emboli of varying size. Am Heart J 58:916, 1959.
53. Comroe JH Jr, VanLingen B, Stroud RC, et al: Reflex and direct cardiopulmonary effects of 5-OH-tryptamine (serotonin): Their possible role in pulmonary embolism and coronary thrombosis. Am J Physiol 173:379, 1953.

54. Thomas DP, Gurewich V, Ashford TP: Platelet adherence to thromboemboli in relation to the pathogenesis and treatment of pulmonary embolism. N Engl J Med 274:953, 1966.
55. Sanders R, Waalkes PT, Gilbert JW, et al: Serotonin (5-hydroxy-tryptamine) in pulmonary thromboembolism. Surg Gynecol Obstet 109:455, 1959.
56. Stein M, Levy SE: Reflex and humoral responses to pulmonary embolism. Prog Cardiovasc Dis 17:167, 1974.
57. Windebank WJ, Boyd A, Moran F: Pulmonary thromboembolism presenting as asthma. Br Med J 1:90, 1973.
58. Hyers TM, Fowler AA, Wicks AB: Focal pulmonary edema after massive pulmonary embolism. Am Rev Resp Dis 123:232, 1981.
59. Heimbecker RO, Keon WJ, Richards KU: Massive pulmonary embolism: A new look at surgical management. Arch Surg 107:740, 1973.
60. Jardin F, Gurdjian F, Desfonds P: Hemodynamic factors influencing arterial hypoxemia in massive pulmonary embolism with circulatory failure. Circulation 59:909, 1979.
61. DeTakats G: Anticoagulants in Surgery. JAMA. 142:527, 1950.
62. Sharnoff JG: Results in the prophylaxis of postoperative thromboembolism. Surg Gynecol Obstet 123:303, 1966.
63. Sharnoff JG, DeBlasio G: Prevention of fatal postoperative thromboembolism by heparin prophylaxis. Lancet 2:1006, 1970.
64. Gordon-Smith IC, Grundy DJ, LeQuesne LP: Controlled trial of two regimens of subcutaneous heparin in prevention of postoperative deep vein thrombosis. Lancet 1:1133, 1972.
65. Nicolaides AN, DuPont PA, Desai S: Small doses of subcutaneous sodium heparin in preventing deep vein thrombosis after major surgery. Lancet 2:890, 1973.
66. Ballard RM, Bradley-Watson PJ, Johnstone FD: Low doses of subcutaneous heparin in the prevention of deep venous thrombosis after gynecological surgery. J Obstet Gynecol Br Commw 80:469, 1973.
67. Hume M, Kuriakase, TX, Zuch L, et al: I-125 fibrinogen and the prevention of venous thrombosis. Arch Surg 107:803, 1973.
68. Kakkar VV, Corrigan T, Spindler J: Efficacy of low doses of heparin in prevention of deep vein thrombosis after major surgery, a double blind randomized trial. Lancet 2:101, 1972.
69. Van Vroonhoven TJMV, Van Zijl J, Muller H: Low dose subcutaneous heparin versus oral anticoagulants in the prevention of postoperative deep venous thrombosis. Lancet 1:375, 1974.
70. The International Multicentre Trial: Prevention of fatal postoperative pulmonary embolism by low doses of heparin. Lancet 2:45, 1975.
71. Kiil J, Kiil J, Axelsen F, et al: Prophylaxis against postoperative pulmonary embolism in deep vein thrombosis by low dose heparin. Lancet 1:1115, 1978.
72. Johnson EA, Kirkwood TBL, Stirling Y, et al: Four heparin preparations: Anti-Xa potentiating effect of heparin after subcutaneous injection. Thromb Haemost 35:586, 1977.
73. Kline A, Hughes LE, Campbell H, et al: Dextran-70 in prophylaxis of thromboembolic diseases after surgery: Clinically oriented randomized double blind trial. Br Med J 2:109, 1975.

74. Gruber UF, Saldeen T, Brokop T: Incidences of fatal postoperative pulmonary embolism after prophylaxis with Dextran-70 and low dose heparin: An international multicentre trial. Br Med J 280:69, 1980.
75. Sagar S, Stamatakis JD, Higgins AF: Efficacy of low dose heparin in the prevention of extensive deep venous thrombosis in patients undergoing total hip replacement (arthroplasty). Lancet 1:1151, 1976.
76. Mannucci PM, Citterio LE, Panajotopoulos N: Low dose heparin in deep vein thrombosis after total hip replacement. Thromb Haemost 36:157, 1976.
77. Harris WH, Salzman EW, Athansoulis C, et al: Comparison of warfarin, low molecular weight dextran, aspirin and subcutaneous heparin in prevention of venous thromboembolism after total hip replacement. J Bone Joint Surg 56a:1552, 1974.
78. Walsh PN: Platelets, heparin and blood coagulation. In Heparin Chemistry and Clinical Usage, eds. Kakkar VV, Thomas DP, London, Academic Press, 125, 1976.
79. Williams HT: Prevention of postoperative deep venous thrombosis with perioperative subcutaneous heparin. Lancet 2:950, 1971.
80. Rosenberg IL, Evans M, Pollock AV: Prophylaxis of postoperative leg vein thrombosis by low dose subcutaneous heparin or perioperative calf muscle stimulation: a controlled clinical trial. Br Med J 1:649, 1955.
81. Cotton LT, Roberts VC: The prevention of deep vein thrombosis, with particular reference to mechanical methods of prevention. Surgery 81:228, 1977.
82. Barnes AB: External pneumatic compression for prevention of deep vein thrombosis and pulmonary emboli. Am J Obstet Gynecol 133:226, 1979.
83. Doran FSA, Drury M, Sivyer A: A Simple way to correct the venous stasis which occurs in the lower limbs during surgical operations. Br J Surg 511:486, 1964.
84. Nicolaides AN Kakkar VV, Steele ES, et al: Optimal electrical stimulus for prevention of deep vein thrombosis. Br Med J 3:756, 1972.
85. Salzman EW: Physical methods for prevention of venous thrombosis. Surgery 81:123, 1977.
86. Jorpes JE: Heparin in the Treatment of Thrombosis: An Account of its Chemistry, Physiology and Application in Medicine. 2nd Ed, London, Oxford University Press, 1946.
87. Rosenberg RD: Chemistry of the hemostatic mechanism and its relation to the action of heparin. Fed Proc 36:10, 1977.
88. Marciniak E, Gockerman JP: Heparin induced decrease in circulating antithrombin III. Lancet 2:581, 1977.
89. Basu D, Gallus A, Hirsh J, et al: A prospective study of the value of monitoring heparin treatment with the activated partial thromboplastin time. N Engl J Med 287:325, 1972.
90. Coon WW, Willis PW, Symons MJ: Assessment of anticoagulant therapy of pulmonary thromboembolism. Ann Surg 170:559, 1969.
91. Simon TL, Hyers TM, Gaston JP, et al: Heparin pharmacokinetics: Increased requirements in pulmonary embolism. Br J Haematol 39:111, 1978.
92. Hirsh J, van Aken WG, Gallus AS: Heparin kinetics in venous thrombosis and pulmonary embolism. Circulation 53:691, 1976.
93. Salzman EW, Shapiro RM, Deykin D, et al: Management of heparin therapy: Controlled prospective trial. N Engl J Med 292:1042, 1975.
94. Glazier RL, Crowell EB: Randomized prospective trial of continuous versus intermittent heparin therapy. JAMA 236:1365, 1976.

95. Bynum LJ, Wilson JE III: Continuous vs. intermittent heparin in pulmonary embolism. Clin Res 24:32A, 1976.
96. Mant MJ, O'Brien BD, Thong KL, et al: Haemorrhagic complications of heparin therapy. Lancet 1:1133, 1977.
97. Stenflo J: Vitamin K, prothrombin and gamma-carboxyglutamic acid. N Engl J Med 296:624, 1977.
98. O'Reilly RA, Aggler PM: Studies on coumarin anticoagulant drugs: initiation of warfarin therapy without a loading dose. Circulation 38:169, 1968.
99. O'Sullivan EF: Duration of anticoagulant therapy in venous thromboembolism. Med J Aust 2:1104, 1972.
100. Bynum LJ, Wilson JE III: Los dose heparin therapy in the long-term management of venous thromboembolism. Am J Med 67:553, 1979.
101. Coon WW, Willis PW III: Recurrence of venous thromboembolism. Surgery 73:823, 1973.
102. Hull R, Delmore T, Genton E, et al: Warfarin sodium versus low-dose heparin in the long term treatment of venous thrombosis. N Engl J Med 301:855, 1979.
103. Moser, KM: Pulmonary embolism. Am Rev Resp Dis 115:829, 1977.
104. Mobin-Uddin K, Utley JR, Bryant LR: The inferior vena cava umbrella filter. Prog Cardiovasc Dis 17:391, 1975.
105. Greenfield LJ, Zocco JJ, Wilk JD, et al: Clinical experience with the Kim-Ray Greenfield vena caval filter. Ann Surg 185:692, 1977.
106. Adelson J, Steer ML, Glotzer DJ, et al: Thromboembolism after insertion of the Mobin-Uddin caval filter. Surgery 87:184, 1980.
107. Phillips MR, Widrich WC, Johnson WC: Perforation of the inferior vena cava by the Kim-Ray Greenfield filter. Surgery 87:233, 1980.
108. Sautter RD, Myers WO, Ray JF, et al: Pulmonary embolectomy: Review and current status. Prog Cardiovasc Dis 17:371, 1975.
109. Paneth M, Miller GAH: Massive pulmonary embolism: The role of pulmonary embolectomy. Am Heart J 91:133, 1976.
110. Eisenmann B, Kretz JG, Heitz A: Massive pulmonary embolism. A series of 59 successful emergency pulmonary embolectomies. In Progress in Respiratory Research. Pulmonary Embolism, ed. Widimsky J, Basel, S Karger, 151, 1980.
111. Saylam A, Melo JQ, Ahmad A, et al: Pulmonary embolectomy. West J Med 128:377, 1978.
112. Marder VJ, Donahue JF, Bell WR, et al: Changes in the plasma fibrinolytic system during urokinase therapy: Comparison of tissue culture urokinase with urinary source urokinase in patients with pulmonary embolism. J Lab Clin Med 92:721, 1978.
113. Urokinase pulmonary embolism trial: Phase I Results. JAMA 214:2163, 1970.
114. Urokinase-streptokinase embolism trial: Phase II Results. JAMA 229:1606, 1974.
115. Sharma GVRK, Burleson VA, Sasahara AA, et al: Effect of thrombolytic therapy on pulmonary capillary blood volume in patients with pulmonary embolism. N Engl J Med 303:842, 1980.
116. Marder VJ: The use of thrombolytic agents: Choice of patient, drug administration, laboratory monitoring. Ann Intern Med 90:802, 1979.
117. Thrombolytic therapy in thrombosis. National Institutes of Health Consensus Development Conference Summary 3:1, 1980.
118. Desoyza NDB, Murphy ML: Persistent post-embolic pulmonary hypertension. Chest 62:665, 1972.

119. Kober G, Becker HJ, Preussler W, Hemodynamics in the acute and late phase after non-fulminanet pulmonary embolism. In Progress in Respiration Research. Pulmonary Embolism, ed. Widemsky J, Basel, S Karger, 49, 1980.
120. Wagenvoort CA: Lung biopsies in the evaluation of pulmonary vascular disease. Chest 77:614, 1980.
121. Moser KM, Houk VN, Jones RC, et al: Chronic massive obstruction of the pulmonary arteries. Analysis of 4 operative cases. Circulation 32:377, 1965.
122. Cabrol C, Cabrol A, Acar J, et al: Surgical correction of chronic post-embolic obstruction of the pulmonary arteries. J Thorac Cardiovasc Surg 76:620, 1978.
123. Sabiston DC, Wolfe WG, Oldham NH, et al: Surgical management of chronic pulmonary embolism. Ann Surg 185:699, 1977.
124. Mills SR, Jackson DC, Sullivan DC: Angiographic evaluation of chronic embolism. Radiology 136:301, 1980.
125. Viamonte M, Parks RE, Smoak VM: Guided catheterization of the bronchial arteries. Radiology 85:205, 1965.
126. Greenfield LJ, Zocco JJ: Intraluminal management of acute massive pulmonary thromboembolism. J Thorac Cardiovasc Surg 77:402, 1979.
127. Elliott MS, Immelman EJ, Jeffery P, et al: A comparative randomized trial of heparin versus streptokinase in the treatment of acute proximal venous thrombosis: An interim report of a prospective trial. Br J Surg 66:838, 1979.

8

Massive Hemoptysis

Roger C. Bone, M.D.

INTRODUCTION

Hemoptysis is defined as the coughing up of blood. The term is not quantitative, since it may refer to blood streaked mucus or cupfuls of blood. Fortunately, although massive pulmonary hemorrhage is life-threatening and associated with a high mortality,[1,2] massive hemoptysis is rare, occurring in only 1 to 4 percent of patients with hemoptysis[3,4]; it has been arbitrarily defined as the expectoration of greater than 600 ml of blood in 24 hours, and is associated with as high as an 80 percent mortality.[5,6] Importantly, the obtunded or debilitated patient may develop respiratory failure with much less hemoptysis; mortality in such cases usually results from asphyxiation rather than exsanguination. Patients with hemoptysis require diagnosis, identification of the bleeding site, and expedient institution of effective therapy if asphyxiation is to be avoided.[6]

The major causes of massive hemoptysis are listed in Table 8–1. The anatomic source of bleeding varies with the cause of the hemoptysis. In chronic fibrocavitary disorders, bleeding arises from the erosion or rupture of bronchopulmonary anastomoses or enlarged bronchial arteries. In tuberculosis, bleeding can result from vessel-wall invasion and the production of an aneurysm, with subsequent rupture.

Table 8–1. Causes of Massive Hemoptysis

Tuberculosis
Mycetoma
Lung cancer
Bronchial adenoma
Bronchiectasis
Lung abscess
Cystic fibrosis
Congenital heart disease
Broncholith
Pulmonary contusion

MAJOR CAUSES OF MASSIVE HEMOPTYSIS

Tuberculosis

Tuberculosis is one of the major causes of hemoptysis. It is a less common cause of massive hemoptysis than previously because of more effective drug treatment.[6] Hemoptysis is more often seen in patients with smear-positive tubercular infections than in those with inactive disease. However, in inactive disease, inflammation in areas of tissue destruction and scarring can lead to the aneurysmal dilatation of small bronchial and pulmonary arteries which are left unsupported by surrounding tissue, producing a Rasmussen's aneurysm.[7]

Pulmonary Mycosis

Fungal colonization of a pulmonary cyst or cavity (mycetoma) is another important cause of massive hemoptysis. The most common organism producing mycetomas is *Aspergillus.* The mycetoma most commonly forms within an inactive tuberculous cavity, but has been described with histoplasmosis cavities and sarcoid cysts. Other fungal species, such as *Candida,* can produce fungus balls. Cultures are often positive with an *Aspergillus* mycetoma, and precipitating antibodies are found in nearly all cases. The chest radiograph often shows a crescent sign, and a lateral decubitus view may show a shift of the fungus ball within the cavity.

A pulmonary mycosis should be considered as a cause for hemoptysis in any indeterminate lung lesion with negative cultures for tubercle bacilli. Hemoptysis occurs in 15 percent of primary coccidioidal infections and in 50 percent of patients with chronic coccidioidal cavities. Hemoptysis also can occur with histoplasmosis, cryptococcosis, and blastomycosis. Sputum cultures for fungi are advisable in patients with undiagnosed lung lesions and hemoptysis.

Neoplasms

Lung cancer causes hemoptysis when it erodes into airways, obstructs bronchi resulting in distal pneumonia or abscess, or when it ulcerates the mucosa. When hemoptysis occurs, either extensive disease involving a large airway or a large, necrotic parenchymal lesion is usually present. This causes the erosion of bronchial vessels and leads to profuse bleeding. Metastatic disease in the chest infrequently causes bleeding. Two uncommon metastatic lesions associated with hemoptysis include choriocarcinoma and osteogenic sarcoma. Bronchial adenomas are the most common benign tumors responsible for massive hemoptysis.

Additional Causes

Any process in the airways or lung parenchyma which produces chronic suppuration can cause massive hemoptysis. Examples include bronchiectasis, lung abscess, and cystic fibrosis. Major hemorrhage occurs in about 5 percent of patients with lung abscess and is an indication for early resection. Hemorrhage can occur into the cavity without immediately causing hemoptysis, and may thus be initially undetected. Radiologic evidence of intracavitary bleeding includes: (1) a rising air-fluid level; (2) a rounded intracavitary mass; (3) a radiodensity that replaces intracavitary gas; and (4) repeated emptying and refilling of the cavity. These signs indicate the site of hemorrhage and allow resection of the bleeding segment to be planned more confidently.

Vascular conditions that can be associated with massive hemoptysis include arteriovenous malformation, congenital or acquired aortic aneurysm, and conditions causing pulmonary venous obstruction. Although it is uncommon, patients with pulmonary embolism and infarction can present with massive hemoptysis. We reported two patients who had massive hemoptysis associated with the institution of heparin therapy for pulmonary infarction.[8]

Other, less common causes of massive hemoptysis include pulmonary contusion, mitral valve disease, congenital heart disease, broncholithiasis, foreign body penetration, Goodpasture's syndrome, pulmonary endometriosis, idiopathic pulmonary hemosiderosis, aortic aneurysm with rupture into a major bronchus, and coagulopathy secondary to the use of anticoagulant medication.

DIAGNOSTIC METHODS

History

Important historic points in diagnosis of the cause of hemoptysis include the character and quantity of blood expectorated, the duration of the symptoms, and the presence of underlying lung disease. For example, minimal hemoptysis is more typical of bronchogenic carcinoma and chronic bronchitis, whereas massive hemoptysis has been more frequently associated with tuberculosis and bronchiectasis. The pattern of hemoptysis is also important. Brief episodes occurring over several years are more suggestive of bronchiectasis. The patient's occupational and cigarette smoking history (lung cancer), prior respiratory symptoms (acute bronchitis), drug history (anticoagulants), and history of any bleeding disorder are also important.

Hematemesis, the vomiting of blood, may be confused with hemoptysis. Several distinguishing characteristics of hemoptysis and hematemesis will aid in differentiation of the two[9] (Table 8–2). Major differential points are that true hemoptysis contains frothy blood which is bright red in color and alkaline. Hematemesis usually does not produce bright red blood and is acid in reaction. Also, hemoptysis is followed by blood-streaking in the sputum for several days. When these findings are not present, the history of hemoptysis should be questioned.

Frequently the patient will be able to localize the bleeding area and will have chosen to lie on that side to avoid paroxysms of coughing. For reasons discussed later, the accurate localization of the site of bleeding is important.[6]

Table 8–2. Differential Features of Hemoptysis and Hematemesis

Hemoptysis	Hematemesis
Respiratory distress and hypoxemia often present.	Lack of respiratory distress or blood gas abnormality.
History of respiratory disease is often present.	History of gastrointestinal disease or alcoholism may be present.
Hemoptysis often preceded by cough.	Hematemesis often preceded by nausea and vomiting.
Blood is coughed up, not vomited.	Blood is vomited.
Portion of blood usually frothy.	Blood is not frothy.
Blood is usually bright red in color and alkaline.	Blood is dark red in color and acid.
Continued blood-tinged sputum which lasts several days.	Blood-tinged sputum usually absent.
Blood is mixed with sputum.	Blood may contain food particles.
Melena usually not present.	Melena usually present.
Anemia usually not present.	Laboratory findings of blood loss often present before hematemesis.

Adapted from Lyons HA: Differential diagnosis of hemoptysis and its treatment. Chest 72:601, 1977.

Physical Examination

Careful examination of the upper respiratory tract is important in establishing whether the bleeding has originated from sources other than the lungs and bronchi. One should examine the mouth for lacerations or tumors, first removing dentures to look for a bleeding site. A mirror examination of the larynx is indicated to rule out pharyngeal causes for hemoptysis. Physical examination may provide confirmatory evidence of the presence of chronic lung disease such, as finger clubbing or adventitious breath sounds. Determination of the state of consciousness, presence of orthostatic changes in blood pressure and pulse, and evidence of chest trauma or rib fracture should also be made. Chest examination may reveal localizing signs of bronchial breathing or crackles over the area of hemorrhage. Wheezes and ronchi may localize bleeding airways narrowed by blood clots.

Laboratory Studies

The initial laboratory evaluation of a patient with hemoptysis should include a hemogram, platelet count, prothrombin time, partial thromboplastin time, and arterial blood gas determination. A blood-urea nitrogen (BUN), creatinine, electrolytes, and sputum examination (acid-fast smear, culture, and cytologic examination) should also be done.

Chest Roentgenogram

A posteroanterior and lateral chest radiograph should be obtained on every patient with hemoptysis, regardless of the clinical setting. This will often localize the pathology. The chest radiograph may reveal a cavitary or mass lesion, a fungus ball, or an air-fluid level. Often the chest roentgenogram reveals extensive bilateral disease, or in some cases an alveolar filling process representing intra-alveolar hemorrhage.[6] Signs of obstructive lung disease (hyperinflation, increased bronchial markings, and decreased vascular markings) may have significance when considering the patient for surgery.

SPECIAL DIAGNOSTIC STUDIES

Bronchoscopy

The most important step in the management and diagnosis of a patient with pulmonary hemorrhage is the precise localization of the bleeding site by bronchoscopy. In addition, bronchoscopy allows inspection of the tracheobronchial tree. An examination of bronchial washings also may yield vital diagnostic information (malignant cells or acid-fast organisms).[10,11]

Both the fiberoptic and rigid bronchoscopes are useful for the evaluation of patients with massive hemoptysis. The fiberoptic bronchoscope allows greater visualization of the peripheral airways (up to the fifth- to sixth-order bronchi). This examination should be done when hemoptysis is active so that the bronchoscopist can follow the trail of blood directly to the affected segmental or subsegmental bronchus. The rigid bronchoscope allows greater suction capability and more visibility in the briskly hemorrhaging patient, and can also be used as an airway for ventilation. If hemorrhage contributes to respiratory failure, the patient can be intubated and ventilated, and the fiberoptic bronchoscope can be introduced through an endotracheal tube. With the use of a special adapter, the fiberoptic bronchoscope can be passed through an 8.0-mm endotracheal tube.

Bronchial Arteriography

Bronchial arteriography may be useful in localizing a tortuous or dilated vessel from which bleeding may be occurring. Actual visualization of a "bleeding blush" is rare.

The bronchial arteries have some variation in their origin. Approximately 90 percent of patients have one of four types of bronchial circulation as follows: type 1, with two bronchial arteries on the left and one on the right; type 2, with one bronchial artery on the left and one on the right; type 3, with two bronchial arteries on the left and two on the right; and type 4, with one bronchial artery on the left and two on the right.[12] Vascular interconnections exist between the intercostal and bronchial arteries.[13] Importantly, the anterior and posterior radicular branches may originate from the intercostals to supply radiculomedullary branches to the spinal cord. Thus, in an occasional case, transverse myelitis can occur following bronchial embolization.

Table 8–3. Management of Massive Hemoptysis

Oxygen
Suction machine at bedside
Laryngoscope, endotracheal tube at bedside
Intubation (if necessary)
Typing and cross-matching of six units of blood
Localization of bleeding site
Options

Surgical resection	Bronchial artery embolization	Fogarty catheter in bleeding segment

Aortography, Tomography, and Computed Axial Tomography

If an aortic aneurysm is suspected in a case of hemoptysis, aortography may assist in the diagnosis of aorto-bronchial communications. Tomography or computed axial tomography (CAT) may assist in the deliniation of cavitary lesions. Bleeding associated with diffuse alveolar filling in a chest radiograph should suggest a coagulopathy or immunologic disorder such as Goodpasture's syndrome.

Bronchography

If massive hemoptysis has subsided and the etiology is still undetermined, bronchography may be done to seek evidence of bronchiectasis.

TREATMENT

The treatment of hemoptysis depends on the severity and etiology of the bleeding and the status of the patient (Table 8–3). Three immediate goals of treatment are:

1. To prevent asphyxiation.
2. To stop the bleeding.
3. To treat the primary cause of the bleeding.

Patients with massive hemoptysis rarely exsanguinate; the most common cause of death is asphyxiation. Thus, protection of the upper airway is a vital part of the initial management of such cases. Since massive hemoptysis rarely ceases spontaneously and if there are no contraindications to surgery, the patient should be taken to the operating room as soon as possible. In submassive hemoptysis or in patients who have an absolute contraindication to surgery, other measures should be employed or considered.

If coughing is troublesome or precipitates additional bleeding, therapy should include sedation and bed-rest, avoidance of excessive chest manipulation (chest percussion and spirometry), and cough supression (codeine or morphine). If

Table 8–4. Precautions for Bronchial Embolization Therapy of Massive Hemoptysis

1. Frequent anatomic anomalies of bronchial circulation
2. Spinal artery arising from bronchial artery or intercostal trunk
3. Catheter well-introduced into artery to prevent migration of emboli into aorta
4. Bronchoscopy prior to procedure to delineate area of bleeding

sedatives are used, small doses are recommended, since these drugs may depress consciousness and allow aspiration of blood into the contralateral lung. If the bleeding is massive or submassive and there is minimal respiratory reserve, an emergency situation exists. Arterial blood gases should be monitored and hypoxemia corrected with supplemental oxygen. An arterial oxygen tension of 50 to 60 mmHg with supplemental oxygen is a reasonable therapeutic goal. Patients with hypercapnia and respiratory acidemia from massive hemoptysis should be intubated and treated with mechanical ventilation. Following intubation, suctioning should be done, which may partially or completely reverse the respiratory failure. If marked blood loss has occurred, as manifested by orthostasis or a decreased hematocrit, transfusions should be given. The patient should be positioned with the suspected bleeding site dependent so as to minimize aspiration of blood into the contralateral lung.

After the patient is hemodynamically stable and acidosis and hypoxemia are corrected, bronchoscopy should be performed to localize the bleeding site. Suctioning and lavage should be done to remove clotted material, and temporary measures may be tried to halt the bleeding, such as ice saline lavage and epinephrine (1:20,000 dilution). If the patient is judged to be an operative candidate, gauze packing, done through a rigid bronchoscope, may also be done.

Alternatively, one or more occlusive, balloon-tipped catheters (No. 4 French-Fogarty) may be placed through either the rigid or fiberoptic bronchoscope to prevent the aspiration of blood into nonhemorrhaging areas. The precautions and techniques for this procedure are outlined in Tables 8–4 and 8–5. The catheter is wedged into the appropriate segment or subsegment under direct vision.[14,15] This technique may be helpful not only diagnostically but also therapeutically; the catheters used have been left in place for hours to days to tamponade the bleeding. Saw et al.[14] reported 10 patients with massive hemoptysis who were treated by tamponading the involved segment with a balloon-tipped catheter placed during fiberoptic bronchoscopy. Notably the source of bleeding in 9 of the 10 patients was in an upper lobe, where it would have been inaccessible to a rigid bronchoscope. Lavage was done first, to sufficiently cleanse the bronchial tree of blood in order to permit visualization of the bleeding segment; in one case, a rigid bronchoscope was used for the preliminary evacuation of blood. When the bleeding segment had been identified, a Fogarty balloon-tipped catheter was placed in the involved segment and the balloon inflated. The catheter was left in place for 24 hours, the balloon was deflated, and if bleeding did not recur the catheter was removed. This method of treatment was successful in all 10 cases, and there was no mortality or morbidity. A similar method employing the rigid bronchoscope

Table 8–5. Technique of Bronchial Embolization Therapy for Massive Hemoptysis

1. Seldinger technique, femoral route
2. Viamonte shape No. 4 or No. 5 polyethylene or Teflon catheter
3. Selective catheterization of bronchial artery
4. Injection 2–3 cc contrast material
5. Gelfoam, 2 mm width, soaked in saline for 5 minutes, inserted into syringe with small amount of saline
6. Saline and Gelfoam pressure-injected by hand into catheter
7. Depending upon size of bronchial artery, 4–8 Gelfoam strips injected
8. Repeat angiogram to verify obstruction

has also been used. However, since the upper lobes are not accessible with the rigid bronchoscope, a catheter that is to be placed in these lobes must be placed with a fiberoptic bronchoscope. Nevertheless, in cases of massive hemoptysis, it is probably preferable to use the rigid bronchoscope in those areas of the lung that can be approached with this. If the patient is an operative candidate, the treatment of choice for life-threatening pulmonary hemorrhage is surgical excision of the bleeding area. Obviously, inadequate cardiopulmonary reserve and coexistent contralateral disease may contraindicate resection.

In an emergency situation, an endotracheal tube can be placed in the mainstem bronchus of the non-bleeding lung. After ventilation is established through the endotracheal tube, one can proceed with surgical resection. Alternatively, if time and the patient's clinical status permit, a double-lumen endotracheal tube such as a Carlens tube or a Robertshaw tube may be placed, to allow the independent management of each lung. Importantly, these tubes require experienced personnel for their placement.

Unfortunately, many patients with massive hemoptysis have such contraindications to resectional surgery as an inadequate cardiopulmonary reserve, coagulopathy, disseminated terminal malignancy, Goodpasture's syndrome, or a bleeding site that has not been localized. If a balloon-tip catheter does not achieve tamponade or prevent aspiration of blood into the contralateral lung, bronchial arteriography and embolization of the bleeding vessels should be considered.

Bronchial arteriography and embolization can be an effective and expedient alternative to resectional surgery in certain situations. There is considerable evidence that bronchial embolization produces effective control of bleeding. Bronchial arteriography should be done prior to bronchial embolization to make certain that no communication exists between the bronchial and anterior spinal arteries. Recent improvements in angiographic technique have minimized the potential complication of spinal artery occlusion during arteriography.[16] The following case history shows the type of result that can be achieved with bronchial embolization.

A 41-year-old female was treated for tuberculosis in the early 1970s. On August 22, 1977, she presented with a 5-day history of hemoptysis. On the day of admission she coughed up one cup of bright-red blood. She was admitted to the intensive care unit but refused bronchoscopy for the localization of her bleeding.

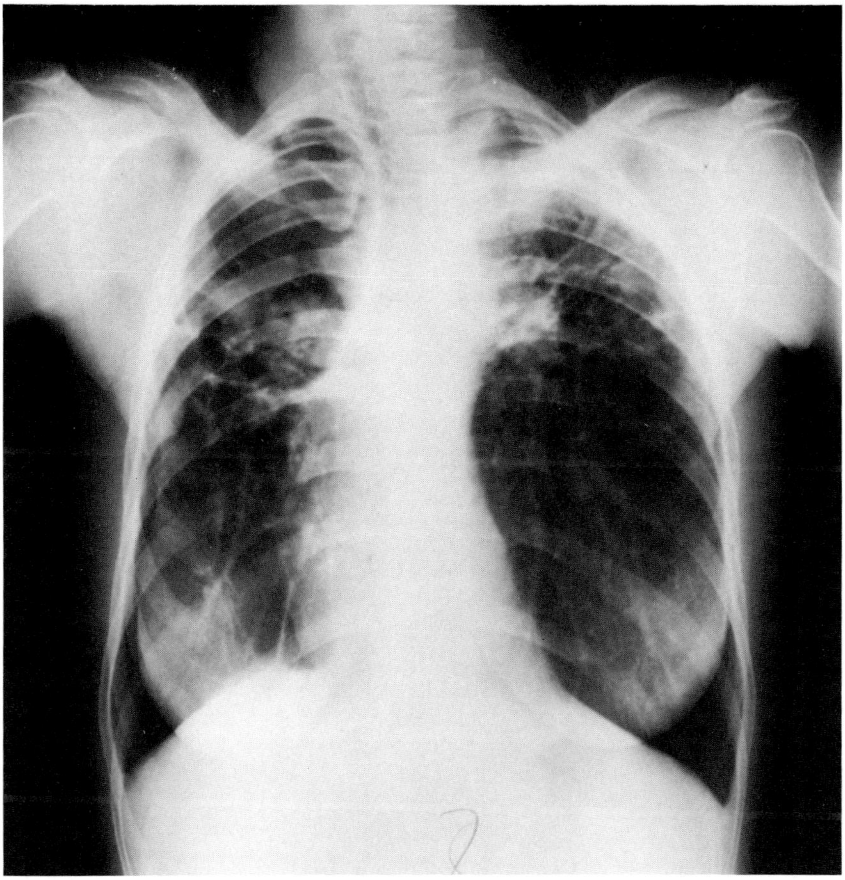

Figure 8–1. Admission chest radiograph. Destructive changes in the upper lobes bilaterally and a "fungus ball" on the right near the right hilus (see text for discussion).

Laboratory data showed negative bacterial cultures and acid-fast smears, a hematocrit of 38 vol percent, positive aspergillus precipitins, and an FEV_1 of 1.00 liter. The PaO_2 was 46 mmHg and the $PaCO_2$ was 48 mmHg. The chest radiograph showed destructive changes in the upper lobes bilaterally and a "fungus ball" on the right, near the right hilus (Fig. 8–1). The hemoptysis subsided spontaneously and the patient was discharged on oral iron therapy. On June 21, 1978 she presented with a 5-day history of hemoptysis. On the day of admission she had an estimated 700 ml of hemoptysis. A chest radiograph showed an air-fluid level on the right and opacification of the left upper lobe, presumably from bleeding (Fig. 8–2A and B). The hematocrit was 25 vol percent. Fiberoptic bronchoscopy showed fresh blood in the left upper lobe. Bronchial arteriography was done and showed a

(Text continues on p. 238.)

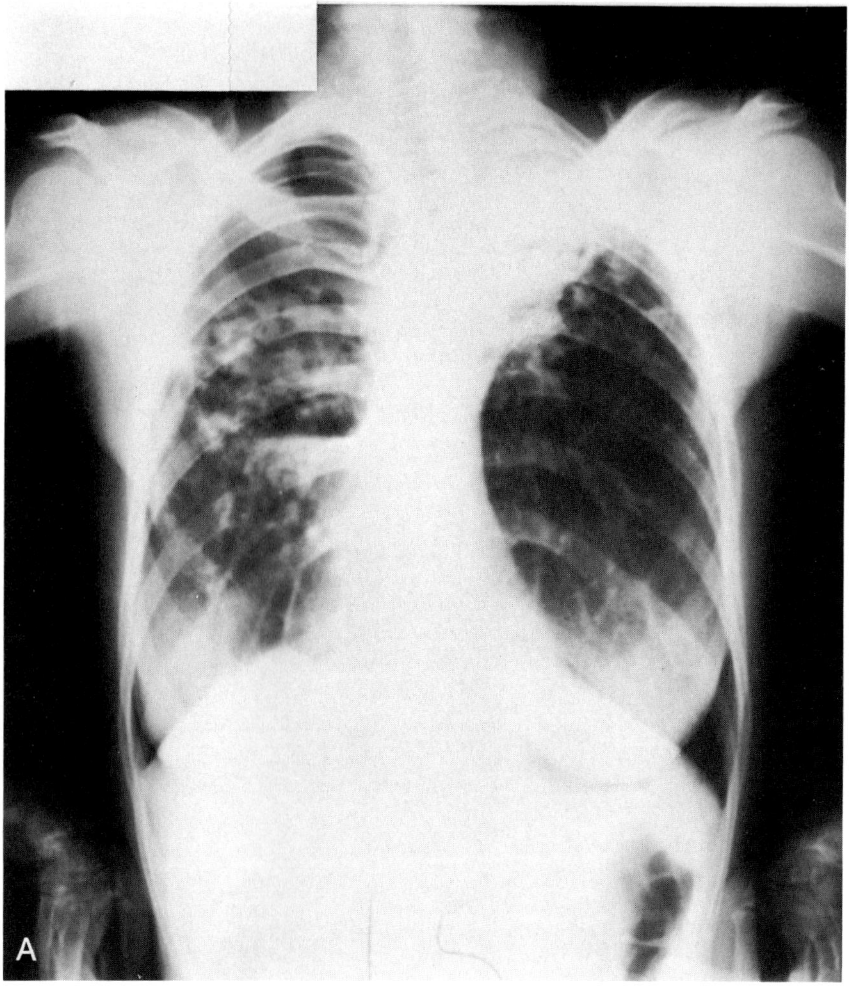

Figure 8–2. (A) Massive hemoptysis. Admission chest radiograph on 6/21/78. An air-fluid level is present on the right as well as opacification of the left upper lobe presumably from bleeding.

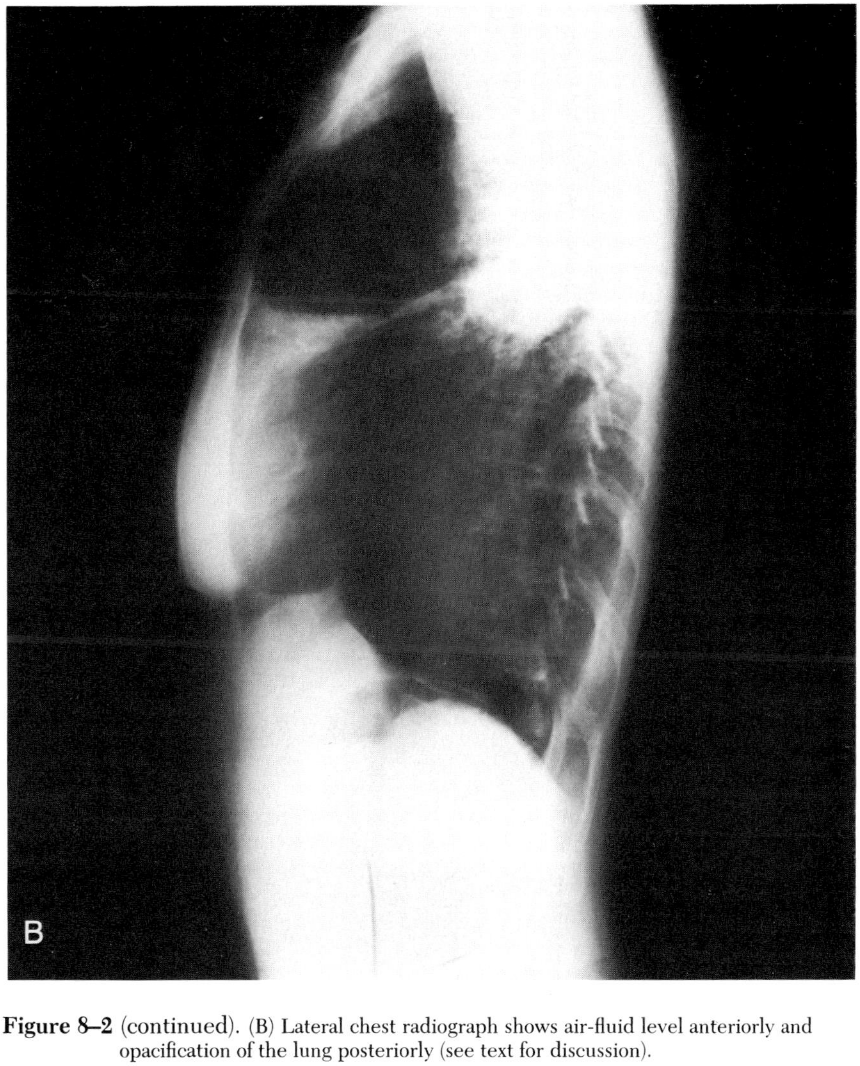

Figure 8–2 (continued). (B) Lateral chest radiograph shows air-fluid level anteriorly and opacification of the lung posteriorly (see text for discussion).

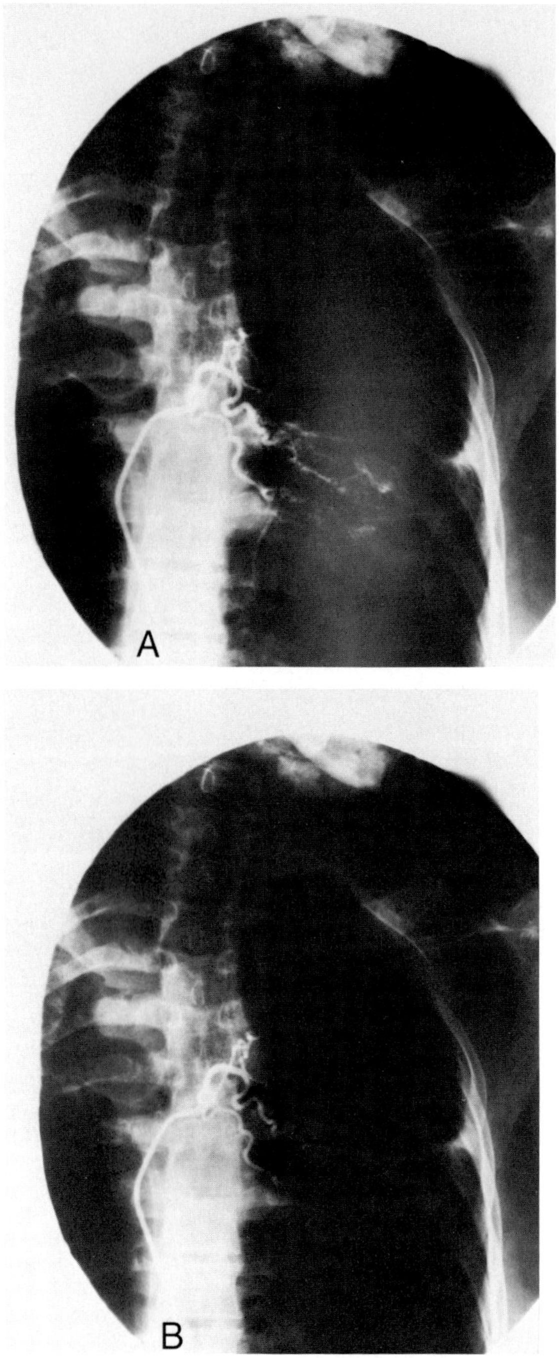

Figure 8–3. (A) Bronchial artery arteriogram prior to Gelfoam embolization. (B) Bronchial artery arteriogram after three Gelfoam emboli.

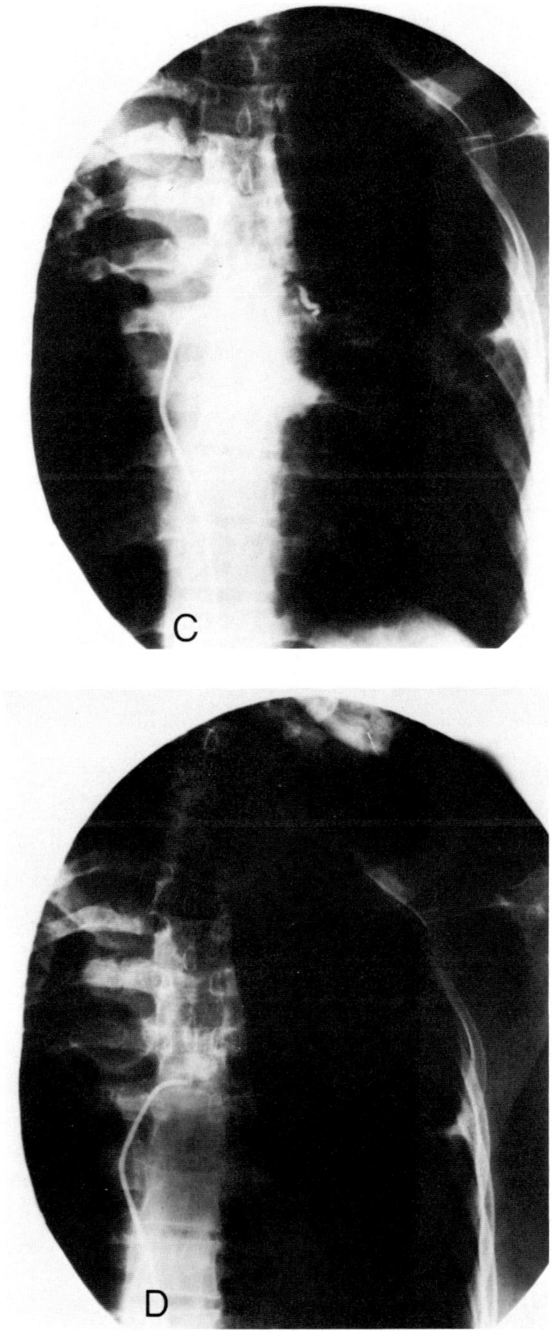

Figure 8–3 (continued). (C) Bronchial artery arteriogram after six Gelfoam emboli. (D) Bronchial artery arteriogram after nine Gelfoam emboli (see text for discussion).

tortous bronchial artery. Figure 8–3A shows the bronchial artery prior to Gelfoam embolization. Figure 8–3B shows the bronchial artery after three Gelfoam emboli were created. Figure 8–3C shows the artery after six Gelfoam emboli had been created. Figure 8–3D shows bronchial artery arteriography after nine Gelfoam emboli. The hemoptysis stopped, with only blood streaking of the sputum over the next 2 days. During a 1 year follow-up, there has been no recurrence of the patient's hemoptysis.

REFERENCES

1. Zavorella C, Jaffe A, Tellez G, et al: Pulmonary arteriovenous fistula: A review. Vasc Surg 9:244, 1975.
2. Crocco JA, Rooney JS, Fankushen OS, et al: Massive hemoptysis. Arch Intern Med 121:495, 1968.
3. Pursel SE, Lindeskog GE: Hemoptysis. Am Rev Resp Dis 84:329, 1961.
4. Johnston RN, Lockhart W, Ritchie RT, et al: Hemoptysis. Br Med J 1:592, 1960.
5. Gourin A, Garzon AA: Operative treatment of massive hemoptysis. Ann Thorac Surg 18:52, 1974.
6. Adams FV: Respiratory tract hemorrhage: guide to emergency management. Hosp Med 66:77, 1978.
7. Rasmussen V: On hemoptysis, especially when fatal, in its anatomical and clinical aspects. (Translated from the Hospitals-Tidende, 11th year, No. 9–13, Copenhagen, 1868, by William Daniel Moore.) Edinburgh Med J 14:385, 1968.
8. Bone RC, Jay SJ, Reynolds RC, et al: Massive pulmonary hemorrhage an uncommon complication of heparin therapy. Amer J Med Sci 272:197, 1977.
9. Lyons, HA: Differential diagnosis of hemoptysis and its treatment. Chest 72:601, 1977.
10. Bone RC: Fiberoptic Bronchoscopy. In Annual Review of Allergy, ed. Frasier CA, Chicago, Year Book Medical Publishers, 1977.
11. Wilson FJ, Bone RC, Hiller FC: Fiberoptic Bronchoscopy. In Annual Review of Allergy, ed. Frasier CA, Chicago, Year Book Medical Publishers, 1979.
12. Wholey MH, Chanorro HA, Rao G, et al: Bronchial artery embolization for massive hemoptysis. JAMA 236:2501, 1976.
13. Pinet F, Froment JC: Angiography of the thoracic systemic arteries. Radiol Clin North Am 16:441, 1978.
14. Saw EC, Gottlieb LS, Yokoyama T, et al: Flexible fiberoptic bronchoscopy and endobronchial tamponade in the management of massive hemoptysis. Chest 70:589, 1976.
15. Gottlieb LS, Hillberg R: Endobronchial tamponade therapy for intractable hemoptysis. Chest 67:482, 1975.
16. Ishikara T, Knowe H, Kobayoski K, et al: Selective bronchial arteriography and hemoptysis in nonmalignant lung disease. Chest 66:633, 1974.
17. Reny J, Arnaud A, Fordou H, et al: Treatment of hemoptysis by embolization of bronchial arteries. Radiology 122:33, 1977.
18. Phioleau WH, Vujic I, Parker EF: Control of hemoptysis by bronchial artery embolization. Chest 78:878, 1980.

9

Pneumothorax

Steven A. Sahn, M.D.

INTRODUCTION

Pneumothorax literally means air in the chest. Actually the term refers to the presence of air in the pleural space. Normally, as will be discussed in detail below under pathophysiology, the pleural space is free of air due primarily to the low partial pressures of gases in the venous blood. Air can enter the pleural space either from the lung or directly from the atmosphere.

Before proceeding, several definitions are in order so that the reader can clearly understand the type of pneumothorax that is being discussed.

Spontaneous pneumothorax occurs when air enters the pleural space from the lung, either due to an "unknown" cause or as a consequence of a disease process affecting the lungs. There are two types of spontaneous pneumothorax: (1) primary spontaneous pneumothorax, a pneumothorax that occurs in a person who has no evidence of underlying pulmonary disease; and (2) secondary spontaneous pneumothorax, which occurs when air enters the pleural space secondary to clinically manifest disease of the lung. Obviously, those persons who develop a primary spontaneous pneumothorax have clinically inapparent pathology of the lung.

Neonatal spontaneous pneumothorax refers to the occurrence of pneumothorax in the neonate. This is usually designated as a separate category because of the unique circumstances of pneumothorax occurring during the first few days of life.

Traumatic pneumothorax occurs as a result of blunt or penetrating chest trauma. With penetrating chest trauma, air enters the pleural space from the atmosphere, while in nonpenetrating chest trauma air enters the pleural space from the lung.

Iatrogenic pneumothorax occurs as a consequence of a diagnostic or therapeutic procedure. "Pneumothorax" therapy was once an integral part of treatment for tuberculosis; however, in the chemotherapeutic era, it is no longer used. Rarely, air is introduced into the pleural space to better define a pleural lesion. Pneumothorax is a complication of such procedures as thoracentesis or subclavian catheter placement.

HISTORICAL PERSPECTIVE

Paré described subcutaneous emphysema secondary to a rib fracture early in the seventeenth century.[1] Riolan, in 1648, recorded the observation of air coming from the pleural space at the time of thoracentesis.[2] Littre, in 1713, described a patient who developed subcutaneous emphysema following a penetrating wound of the chest.[2] In 1724 Boerhaave provided the first description of esophageal rupture; this is probably the first description of pneumothorax in the absence of chest trauma.[2] Meckel,[3] in 1759, reported the finding of tension pneumothorax at autopsy. It was probably Monro in 1761 who first advocated thoracentesis as the treatment for pneumothorax.[2]

Near the end of the eighteenth century, Bromfield reported the insertion of a cannula through the chest wall to allow the escape of intrapleural air. He also observed that the playing of an oboe by a patient accelerated the expansion of the lung.[2]

Itard[4] coined the term pneumothorax in the early 1800s and proposed the concept that pneumothorax could occur secondary to a disease process in the lung. Laennec[5] provided the first clinical description of the symptoms and physical findings associated with pneumothorax in 1819. In 1823 Davy[6] reported on the gas composition of air evacuated from the pleural space following tension pneumothorax. Devilliers,[7] in 1826, found at autopsy that the source of a spontaneous pneumothorax in a patient was a ruptured bleb. Noble,[8] in 1873, reported the use of a rubber tube to connect the chest cannula used to treat a pneumothorax to an underwater seal and demonstrated the escape of air in a patient with pneumothorax. In 1880 Biach[9] collected 819 cases of pneumothorax, with close to 80 percent of those cases being due to tuberculosis.

Prior to the development of x-ray techniques, the diagnosis of pneumothorax was based on clinical or autopsy findings. In 1901 Martin[10] reported the first case in which pneumothorax was diagnosed by chest radiography. The development of the chest x-ray constituted one of the major advances in the understanding of pneumothorax.

In 1902 Fussell and Riesman[11] reported 2 cases of nontuberculous spontaneous pneumothorax and collected 56 others from the literature in which there was no evidence of tuberculosis. They were the first to suggest that young males were more prone to spontaneous pneumothorax than were other individuals, and that their prognosis was good. In the early twentieth century, Spengler[12] advocated the instillation of chemical irritants into the pleural space for the treatment of spontaneous pneumothorax.

Kjaergaard[13] reported a follow-up study of 51 healthy patients who had spontaneous pneumothorax. This work brought acceptance of the fact that spontaneous pneumothorax resulted from rupture of a subpleural bleb and not from pulmonary tuberculosis. This report also contained the first publication of a radiographically demonstrable lung bleb.

In 1935 Bethune[14] reviewed and investigated the use of mechanical and chemical means for producing pleural symphysis. He thought the results from the use of intrapleural talc were superior to those from other techniques, and the use of this substance became widespread as therapy for spontaneous pneumothorax.

Bigger[15] was one of the first to perform a thoracotomy with resection of a subpleural bleb in a patient with spontaneous pneumothorax. In 1939 Hamman[16] pointed out that pneumomediastinum could be associated with the presence or absence of air in the pleural space. In 1954 Ellis and Carr[17] suggested that parietal pleurectomy might be a procedure beneficial in preventing recurrent spontaneous pneumothorax. In 1956 Gaensler[18] described the technique of parietal pleurectomy and reported its application in nine cases of recurrent spontaneous pneumothorax. Pre- and postoperative studies revealed no significant changes in the ventilatory function of these patients.

INCIDENCE

The exact incidence of primary spontaneous pneumothorax is difficult to assess, since many episodes resolve without coming to the attention of a physician. However, several studies have been able to provide an approximate incidence of this form of pneumothorax. The reported incidence of primary spontaneous pneumothorax has ranged from approximately 2.5 to 18 per 100,000 population.[19] In terms of hospital admissions, the figures range from 0.01 to 0.17 percent of all such admissions.[19] The true incidence of primary spontaneous pneumothorax is somewhat clouded by the large number of reports that deal only with military personnel.

In a postmortem chest radiographic study of 3500 cases in a random autopsy population, 77 (2.2 percent) were found to have pneumothorax;[20] thirty-nine of these 77 cases were under tension. The pulmonary findings at autopsy in the cases of pneumothorax were most commonly pneumonia, chronic obstructive pulmonary disease, and pulmonary infarction. In a review of 210 consecutive patients with spontaneous pneumothorax in a large teaching hospital, approximately one-third had respiratory tract disease which could have been responsible for the pneumothorax.[21]

Chronic obstructive pulmonary disease (COPD) has been claimed to account for about 10 percent of pneumothoraces in older individuals,[22] but other results have suggested a higher incidence of pneumothorax from such disease.[21] However, Dines, Clagett, and Payne[23] found an incidence of pneumothorax of only 0.3 percent in a review of 22,000 patients with chronic obstructive pulmonary disease.

The exact incidence of pneumothorax in patients with cystic fibrosis is unknown; however, Holsclaw[24] reported 93 episodes of pneumothorax in 51 cystic fibrosis patients among approximately 2200 patients seen over a period of 20 years.

Pneumothorax may also occur as a complication of bronchial asthma. Turiaf et al.[25] reported 15 adults with pneumothorax in a population of 2000 asthmatics, an incidence of 0.7 percent. Jorgensen et al.[26] noted 7 (2.6 percent) cases of pneumothorax among 269 children hospitalized with bronchial asthma.

In the past, pulmonary tuberculosis was thought to be the leading cause of

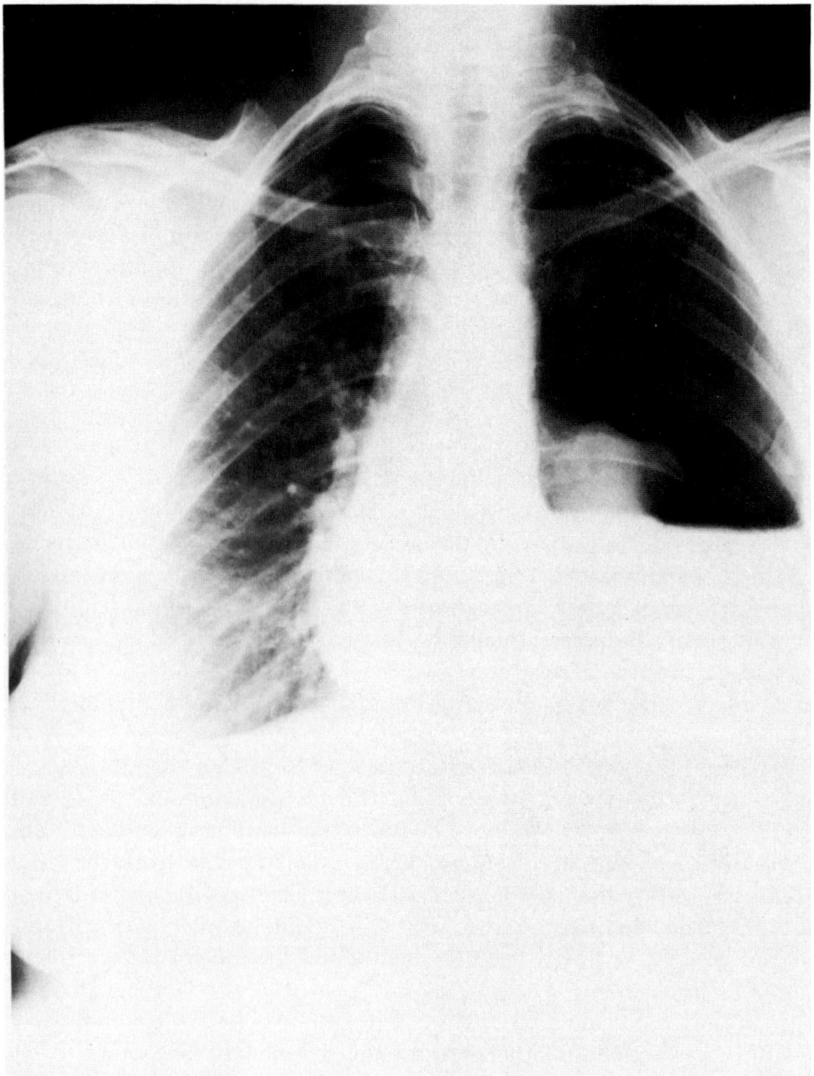

Figure 9–1. Postero-anterior chest radiograph of a 57-year-old female who had a left radical mastectomy 10 years previously. She presented with left chest pain and dyspnea. Note left hydropneumothorax and very dense left lung, suggesting pulmonary disease. At surgery metastases were found in the left lung and pleura.

spontaneous pneumothorax. The incidence of pneumothorax secondary to active tuberculosis is probably about 1.5 percent.[27] The combination of tuberculosis and silicosis probably raises this incidence to close to 5 percent.[28] The hypothesis that there is an increased incidence of spontaneous pneumothorax complicating tuberculosis treated with corticosteroids has not been substantiated.[29]

Pneumothorax secondary to staphylococcal pneumonia is the leading cause of spontaneous pneumothorax in children and infants beyond the neonatal period.[30] In one study, pyopneumothorax occurred in 29 percent of 557 cases of staphylococcal pneumonia in children,[31] and in another study it developed in approximately 5 percent of cases of staphylococcal pneumonia in adults.[32]

Pneumothorax secondary to carcinoma of the lung is rare, as is pneumothorax secondary to pulmonary metastasis (Fig. 9–1). However, a high percentage of cases of pulmonary metastases resulting in pneumothorax are due to sarcoma, particularly osteogenic sarcoma.[33]

The incidence of pneumothorax following diagnostic or therapeutic procedures involving the thorax will vary with the expertise of the operator. Pneumothorax is probably the most common complication of thoracentesis, yet its exact incidence in this procedure has never been determined. It is a relatively common complication of cutting-needle biopsy of the lung, and occurs less frequently with aspiration needle biopsy, the incidence decreasing as the gauge of the needle increases.[34]

ETIOLOGY

The classification and various causes of secondary spontaneous pneumothorax and iatrogenic pneumothorax are listed in Table 9–1.

Spontaneous pneumothorax is a major problem in young adults with cystic fibrosis. Recurrences are common, and occur in about 50 percent of patients, with a large number occurring in the opposite hemithorax.[24] The average age of cystic fibrosis patients who develop their first pneumothorax is approximately 15 years, and these patients tend to have moderate to severe pulmonary involvement before the initial episode. In most cases no specific form of treatment or precipitating cause can be identified as the inciting factor. The episodes of pneumothorax have occurred at rest, while coughing, with exercise, with changes in altitude, and with the use of intermittent positive pressure breathing devices. Pneumothorax probably occurs in cystic fibrosis because of the formation of subpleural blebs as a result of chronic air trapping. These blebs are most commonly seen at the apices of the lung and can reach large proportions.

In persons over the age of 40 years, spontaneous pneumothorax is most commonly due to COPD[35] (Fig. 9–2A and B). Owing to the changes that occur in the lung parenchyma with progressive airways obstruction, thin-walled blebs are formed in a subpleural location and are subject to rupture upon an increase in intra-alveolar pressure. The bullae are formed by progressive destruction of alveolar walls, with an associated loss of lung retractility.[36] Pneumothorax in the setting of COPD may escape clinical recognition, as attested to by the high frequency of unsuspected pneumothorax found at autopsy.[37] Because of the poor pulmonary reserve in most patients with COPD, spontaneous pneumothorax usually causes a sudden worsening of the patients' symptoms. Immediate treatment of pneumothorax in these patients is mandatory, since the pulmonary reserve is limited.

Table 9–1. Classification and Etiology of Pneumothorax

1. Spontaneous
   A. Primary (no clinically apparent lung disease)
   B. Secondary
      (1) Cystic fibrosis
      (2) Chronic obstructive pulmonary disease
      (3) Status asthmaticus
      (4) Infection (staphylococcus, tuberculosis)
      (5) Pulmonary infarction
      (6) Interstitial lung disease (eosinophilic granuloma)
      (7) Malignancy (sarcomas)
      (8) Radiation therapy
      (9) Drugs (cytotoxins)
      (10) Catamenial (endometriosis)
      (11) Marfan's syndrome
      (12) Pregnancy
   C. Neonatal
2. Traumatic
   A. Penetrating
   B. Blunt
3. Iatrogenic
   A. Thoracentesis
   B. Subclavian catheter placement
   C. Mechanical ventilation (especially with PEEP)
   D. Postsurgical
   E. Cardiopulmonary resuscitation
   F. Needle biopsy of lung (especially cutting needle)
   G. Transbronchial and brush biopsy through bronchoscope
   H. Endoscopy
   I. Diagnostic
   J. Intercostal nerve block
   K. Therapeutic (obsolete)

In the mid-1950s and early 1960s, the mortality rate among patients with COPD who developed a spontaneous pneumothorax was about 16 percent.[38] However, a more recent study by George et al.[35] found a lower mortality rate in patients with uncomplicated COPD who developed spontaneous pneumothorax. Factors that can be associated with the development of pneumothorax in COPD are carcinoma of the bronchus with partial obstruction, acute bronchitis with obstructing secretions, and the use of positive pressure breathing devices.

Spontaneous pneumothorax also can occur as complication of bronchial asthma, but usually occurs only with an exacerbation of the disease. Air trapping, with an increased intra-alveolar pressure, enhances the chance of alveolar rupture into the pleural space. Both the use of positive pressure breathing devices and acute bronchitis may be precipitating causes of pneumothorax in this setting. When a patient with bronchial asthma develops status asthmaticus, the chance of pneumothorax increases, especially if the status asthmaticus requires treatment with mechanical ventilation.[39]

Bacterial pneumonia with necrosis or abscess formation is another condition that can lead to spontaneous pneumothorax. *Staphylococcus aureus*, which characteristically produces abscesses and pneumatoceles, is probably the most common cause of infection resulting in pneumothorax.[32] However, other organisms responsible for necrotizing pneumonia, including the Gram-negative aerobes and anaerobic bacteria, can be a cause of spontaneous pneumothorax.

Active pulmonary tuberculosis, which was once thought to be the cause of most cases of spontaneous pneumothorax, must still be considered high on the list of causes of secondary spontaneous pneumothorax. Pleural adhesions resulting from pulmonary tuberculosis commonly cause fixation of the visceral pleura to the chest wall, so that a pneumothorax that occurs may be small and localized. In the era prior to effective anti-tuberculosis chemotherapy, the mortality from spontaneous pneumothorax associated with active tuberculosis was from 30 to 50 percent,[27] and pneumothorax complicating silicotuberculosis was a serious problem.[28] The rupture of a tuberculous focus into the pleural space results in tuberculous pleurisy and often a persistent bronchopleural fistula. Prompt treatment of the pneumothorax under the coverage of effective anti-tuberculosis chemotherapy greatly diminishes the risk of chronic pneumothorax, trapped lung, or a bronchopleural fistula.

Pneumothorax can occur in the setting of interstitial lung disease and has been described with various pneumoconioses,[28,40,41] sarcoidosis,[42] and eosinophilic granuloma.[43] Spontaneous pneumothorax is frequent in eosinophilic granuloma and may be the first indicator of pulmonary disease, occasionally occurring in the absence of demonstrable radiographic lesions.[44] The pneumothorax in sarcoidosis usually develops in the end stage of the disease but may occasionally be a presenting manifestation.

Carcinoma of the lung causes spontaneous pneumothorax rarely, although the latter may be the initial manifestation of the lung tumor.[45] Pneumothorax can result from the tumor eroding the visceral pleura, from rupture of a localized bleb caused by the tumorous obstruction of a bronchus, or from the rupture of an abscess that has developed behind an obstructing bronchial lesion. When carcinoma of the lung is complicated by pneumothorax, the usual radiographic signs of pneumothorax may be obscured. In the case of an endobronchial lesion that completely obstructs the bronchus, the air bronchogram usually seen in the lung collapsed by pneumothorax will be replaced by the image of a collapsed lung of homogeneous density.[46] In addition, when there is bronchial obstruction, the volume of the ipsilateral hemithorax will decrease as the pneumothorax resolves, with an ipsilateral mediastinal shift and hemidiaphragmatic elevation.

Schulman et al.[47] have suggested that intensive cytotoxic chemotherapy may result in spontaneous pneumothorax, owing to the rapid lysis of tumorous metastases producing necrosis with rupture into the pleural space. Obviously, these metastases must be situated in a strategic area of the lung for this to occur. Nor is this type of complication unique to the lung; rapid shrinkage of abdominal lymphoma is known to lead to perforation of the bowel in some patients. Tumors especially prone to such a complication might be those highly responsive to chemotherapy, such as oat-cell carcinomas, germinal tumors, malignant lymphomas, and soft-tissue sarcomas.

Catamenial pneumothorax—recurrent pneumothorax associated with endome-

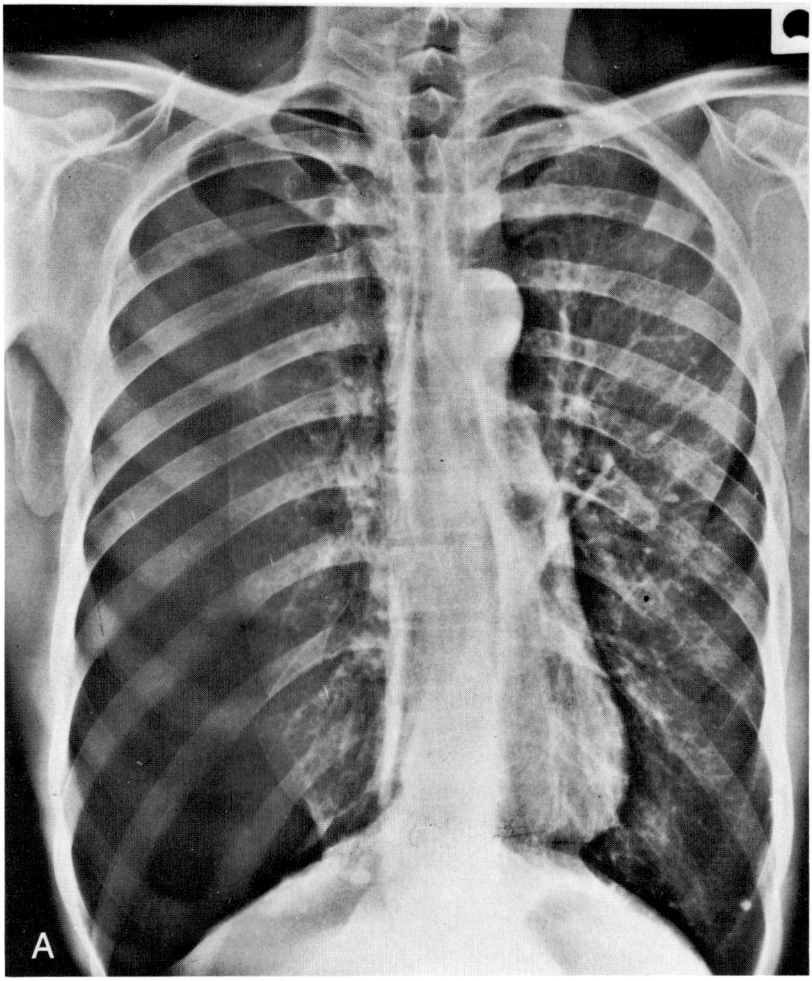

Figure 9–2. (A) Postero-anterior chest radiograph of a 50-year-old male with COPD. Note right pneumothorax under moderate tension, with contralateral mediastinal shift and depressed ipsilateral hemidiaphragm.

triosis—has been reported in over 40 patients.[48] Patients with catamenial pneumothorax are usually parous women over the age of 30 who experience a number of episodes of pneumothorax with menses, but not necessarily with each menstruation. All previously reported cases, with one possible exception, have occurred on the right side; and there has been only one report of bilateral pneumothoraces.[48] Catamenial pneumothoraces may be terminated by ovulation-suppressing drugs, hysterectomy, ovariectomy, and pregnancy. Ovulation is not necessary for the occurrence of catamenial pneumothorax, since this condition has occurred at menstruation in women receiving cyclical therapy.[49] Pleurodesis also has been found to stop catamenial pneumothoraces.

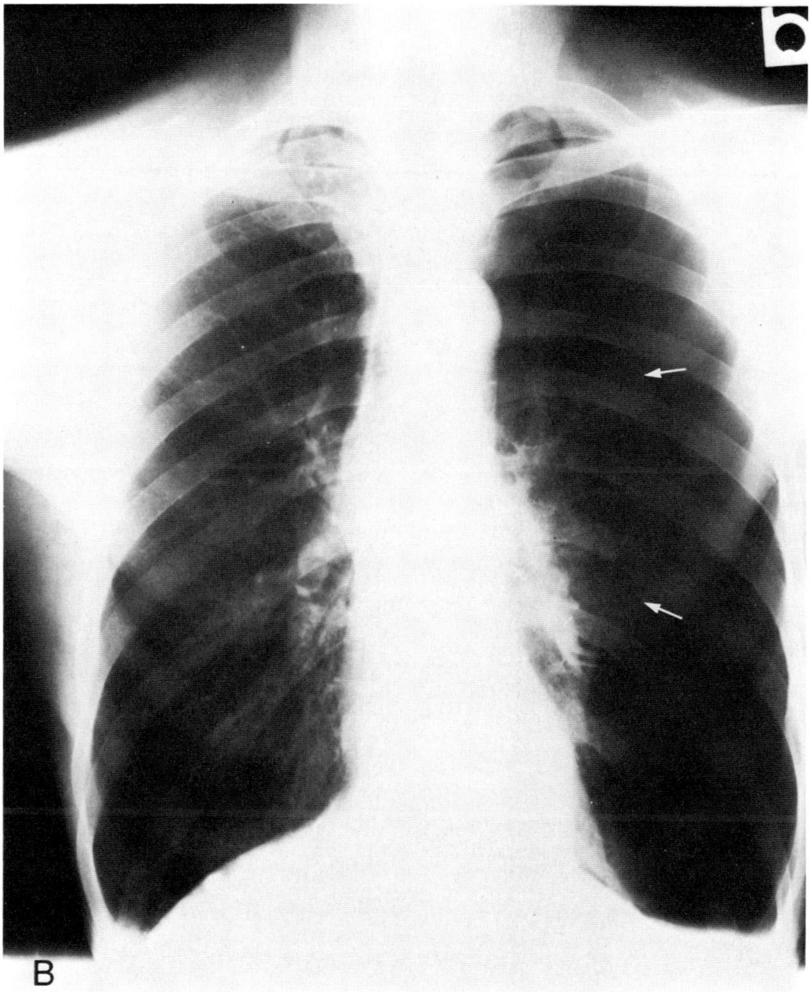

Figure 9–2 (continued). (B) Postero-anterior chest radiograph 2 years later showing a left pneumothorax (arrows) and small amount of pleural fluid. There is a slight contralateral mediastinal shift.

The precise mechanism responsible for catamenial pneumothorax is not clear. The finding of endometrial tissue in the diaphragm or parietal pleura cannot account for this phenomenon, and involvement of lung and visceral pleura has been found in only a minority of cases. Other possible explanations have been movement of air from the peritoneal cavity to the right pleural space through diaphragmatic fenestrations,[50] and possible alveolar damage secondary to vascular and bronchial spasm caused by increased levels of dinoprost tromethamine released from menstrual debris.[51]

Pneumothorax occurs so rarely during pregnancy that only 10 reports of it have been published.[52] In most of the reported cases, the pneumothorax has occurred around term. In all but 2 cases, labor had not started, and in the two exceptions pneumomediastinum preceded the pneumothorax. Fetal hypoxia is a definite threat from pneumothorax in pregnancy, but all reported cases have so far done well because of early recognition and treatment. Spontaneous pneumothorax should be considered in the differential diagnosis of chest pain and dyspnea during pregnancy, delivery, and in the postpartum period.

Neonatal spontaneous pneumothorax is considered separately because of the unique circumstances that exist at delivery and during the initial days of life. At birth, it is necessary that a large gradient exist between the airway and pleural space in order for lung inflation to occur during the first inspiration. This pressure gradient ranges upward from 40 cmH_2O.[53] The diaphragm of the neonate is capable of generating extremely high levels of negative intrathoracic pressure (from -60 to -80 cmH_2O) prior to inflation of the lungs.[54] Consequently the majority of alveoli expand within the first few breaths. Following lung expansion, however, the diaphragm is moved to a lower position, the mechanical advantage of the diaphragm is reduced, and a transpulmonary pressure gradient of approximately 30 cmH_2O is all that the neonate can create. This gradient should not be sufficient to cause alveolar rupture.[53] Yet some alveoli do not expand promptly after birth, leading to local areas of atelectasis. Under these conditions, increased tension with each inspiratory effort is transmitted to certain areas of open alveoli, creating compensatory overinflation. In this setting, alveolar rupture into the pleural space or interstitium of the lung can occur. The magnitude of the transpulmonary pressure during the first few fetal breaths, especially when there are areas of overinflated alveoli, is probably sufficient to cause neonatal spontaneous pneumothorax.[53-55]

Besides resulting from irregular expansion of the lung, focal areas of atelectasis and overinflation also result from the presence of mucus and meconium in the bronchi. Atelectasis was found at autopsy in 28 of 34 neonates with pneumothorax; in 16 of these cases there were areas of atelectasis and overinflation due to bronchial plugging.[56]

Hypoplasia of the lung is another condition that has been associated with a high incidence of spontaneous pneumothorax.[56] This correlation supports the theory that non-uniform expansion of the lung at birth predisposes to alveolar rupture.

Pneumonitis, possibly secondary to bronchial aspiration, hyaline membrane disease, and positive pressure resuscitation have all been implicated in the development of spontaneous neonatal pneumothorax.[56,59] Oztalay and Beard[57] have shown that intermittent positive pressure breathing (IPPB) with oxygen flow rates in the range of 3 to 5 L/min can produce elevation of airway pressure in the neonate to levels greater than 100 cmH_2O.

Pneumothorax complicating chest trauma (see Chapter 11) can obviously occur with penetrating chest wounds but can also occur with blunt chest trauma even in the absence of radiographic evidence of rib fracture. When a rib fracture is present, the likely mechanism of causation of a pneumothorax is laceration of the visceral pleura by the rib fragment; hemopneumothroax is common in this circumstance. When rib fractures do not occur, the etiology of a pneumothorax is either from rupture of a pre-existing subpleural bleb or more likely from rupture of an alveolus due to pulmonary contusion or parenchymal laceration.

Some forms of iatrogenic pneumothorax can essentially be prevented by careful technique. If, for example, a thoracentesis is performed one interspace below the area of physical findings of a pleural effusion, pneumothorax should not occur. The higher incidence of pneumothorax with cutting-needle biopsy of the lung has led in most institutions to the abandonment of this technique in favor of aspiration needle biopsy. There is also a likelihood of pneumothorax occurring with transbronchial and brush biopsy in the setting of opportunistic pneumonia upon attempts to obtain the most distal samples for the diagnosis of *Pneumocystis carinii* pneumonia. Additionally, pneumothorax is an accepted complication of mechanical ventilation, especially with the use of PEEP. This is most likely to occur in the setting of status asthmaticus, chronic obstructive pulmonary disease (COPD), and necrotizing pneumonitis. The risk of pneumothorax in such circumstances can be minimized by using the lowest possible peak cycling pressures and allowing adequate time for the expiratory phase, so that marked overinflation of the lung does not occur.[39]

Rarely, during fiberoptic bronchoscopy with partial occlusion of the large airways, a small amount of positive end expiratory pressure is generated which will increase the risk of pneumothorax. This is particularly true in patients undergoing fiberoptic bronchoscopy who are on mechanical ventilation. Finally, proper technique in cardiopulmonary resuscitation (CPR) should decrease the incidence of rib fractures and rib cartilage dislocations during this procedure, and thus the risk of pneumothorax (see Chapter 1).

PATHOPHYSIOLOGY

This discussion of the pathophysiology of pneumothorax will be concerned with primary spontaneous pneumothorax, which is the most common and most frequently studied form of this entity. Primary spontaneous pneumothorax occurs when a strategically located subpleural bleb or alveolus ruptures into the pleural space. The air-containing, subvisceral pleural bleb is usually less than 2 cm in diameter and is most commonly located in the apex of the lung. The mechanism of the formation of a cyst or subpleural bleb has been ascribed to the passage of air from a ruptured alveolus via the interstitial space and into the fibrous layer beneath the visceral pleura, and its accumulation in this location.[58,59] The reasons for alveolar rupture are unclear. However, Lichter and Gwynne,[60] in a pathologic study of 20 patients who underwent surgery for the treatment of spontaneous pneumothorax, found evidence of post-inflammatory changes in surgical specimens from these patients.

An underlying congenital abnormality related to the anatomy of the thorax in tall, thin individuals may be associated with bleb formation; it has been suggested that in such persons there is a rapid growth rate relative to the growth of the pulmonary vasculature, producing relative ischemia and bleb formation during

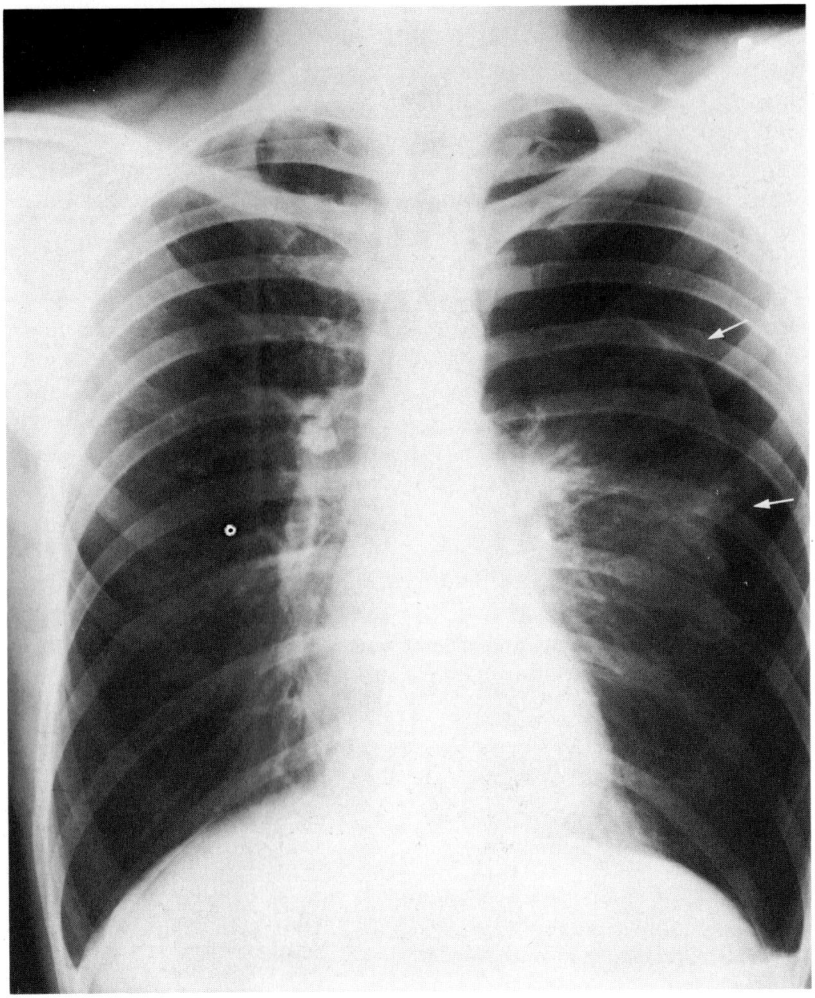

Figure 9–3. Postero-anterior chest radiograph of a 31-year-old previously healthy man who presented with sudden sharp, anterior, left chest pain and dyspnea. Note left pneumothorax and thin-walled bullae (arrows) on surface of lung.

the growth period.[61] Studies of Vawter, Matthews, and West[62] provide a theoretical basis for the occurrence of pneumothorax in young adults with long, narrow chests. They showed that as the lung height increases, volume strain near the apex rises both absolutely and relatively when compared to strain at the base of the lung. The added strain on the apical parenchyma of the lung could provide an explanation for bleb development in these otherwise healthy young adults.

While primary spontaneous pneumothorax occurs in apparently healthy young males, most patients who undergo surgery for a pneumothorax have subpleural blebs (Fig. 9–3), sometimes scattered throughout the lung.[63,64] DeTroyer et al.[65] studied 21 healthy subjects aged 16 to 38 years who had recovered from a spontaneous pneumothorax. Four of the patients had physiologic evidence of generalized emphysema, including a decrease in diffusing capacity, a high compliance, and a decreased elastic recoil. Despite normal lung mechanics, most of the remaining 17 patients showed increased residual volume and a decreased diffusing capacity; the authors suggested that these findings reflected the presence of widely disseminated blebs, occurring with a high ventilation/perfusion ratio. Only long-term studies will answer the question of whether such persons are more likely to develop diffuse emphysema than the general population.

Alveolar rupture with the formation of subpleural blebs may be related to small airway obstruction by mucus or inflammatory processes. It has been shown that young men with spontaneous pneumothorax smoke more cigarettes than do those without this condition.[66]

The relation between cigarette smoking, mucus gland hyperplasia, small airway obstruction, and the development of spontaneous pneumothorax is interesting. The work of the Macklins in the 1930s and 1940s provided useful information on the mechanism of air accumulation outside the alveoli.[67,68] With regard to this, it can be logically postulated that since approximately 10 percent of newborns develop mediastinal emphysema, air may traverse the lung parenchyma peripherally as well as centrally, with the formation of subpleural blebs.[69] These blebs would, therefore, be formed in the neonatal period and would rupture at a later time for a variety of reasons.

Cooley and Gillespie[70] have suggested that there are both marginal alveoli (which are in proximity to the perivascular sheaths and have no intercommunicating pores) and partitional alveoli (which represent all other alveoli and have intercommunicating pores). It is the marginal alveoli, in proximity to the blood vessels and without communicating pores, which rupture when the intra-alveolar pressure exceeds the interstitial pressure, with a resulting flow of air into the perivascular sheaths and the creation of blebs.

Why preformed subpleural blebs rupture is not clear. Their rupture does not appear to be related to effort, since most primary spontaneous pneumothoraces occur with the patient at rest. Some pneumothoraces have occurred with an ascent to high altitudes, but this mechanism cannot be invoked in the majority of cases.[71]

Interest in the physiologic consequences of pneumothorax was stimulated by the therapeutic use of pneumothoraces in the era before tuberculosis chemotherapy was available. The studies of Christie in the 1930s provided much of the early information about the physiologic consequences of pneumothorax.[72] His early findings were that only about 30 percent of the air introduced into the pleural space in a pneumothorax leads to collapse of the ipsilateral lung, the remainder causing enlargement of the thoracic cage. In Christie's studies, some of the air in a pneumothorax also caused expansion of the contralateral lung. Beyond this, it was noted that in otherwise normal individuals, pneumothorax did not have a profound effect on cardiac and respiratory function.

Two problems with some of the earlier human experiments on the physiologic effects of pneumothorax were that the patients who were studied often had underlying parenchymal lung disease from tuberculosis and that sophisticated measurement techniques were not available and could not be used in many situations. Recent work by Moran et al. in awake dogs has shown that a moderate-sized unilateral pneumothorax causes an immediate increase in respiratory rate and tidal volume; however, alveolar ventilation remains unchanged.[73] The same work showed a decrease in the arterial oxygen tension and an increase in shunt fraction, while the cardiac output and systemic vascular resistance were unaffected by the unilateral pneumothorax. The pulmonary vascular resistance and heart rate both rose sharply following the induction of a pneumothorax. Following the creation of a unilateral pneumothorax, there was a decrease in ventilation to the ipsilateral lung and a compensatory increase in ventilation to the contralateral lung. Regional perfusion was not significantly altered from control valves during a unilateral pneumothorax. Thus, during a unilateral pneumothorax there is a relative underventilation of the collapsed lung with a reduction in the ventilation/perfusion ratio and an overventilation of the contralateral lung with an increase in the ventilation/perfusion ratio. The carbon dioxide tension and arterial pH remained constant.

Following the expansion of unilateral pneumothoraces in dogs, the respiratory rate and tidal volume decreased to control levels within several minutes, the arterial oxygen tension and shunt fraction returned quickly to control values, and the pulmonary vascular resistance fell immediately to near control levels and decreased further by 2 hours after resolution of the pneumothorax.[73]

The changes in respiratory rate, tidal volume, arterial oxygen tension, and shunt fraction during unilateral pneumothorax in dogs agree with the findings of Rutherford et al.[74] in the experimental production of stepwise progressive tension pneumothorax in goats and monkeys. Other studies of pneumothorax in dogs[75-77] agree with findings of Moran et al.[73] that the respiratory rate and tidal volume increase immediately upon induction of a pneumothorax.

The inefficiency of ventilation following the development of a unilateral pneumothorax is caused by an increase in the respiratory rate with a decreased tidal volume in the ipsilateral lung and a constant physiologic dead space. Any decrease in physiologic dead space in the collapsed lung is compensated by an increased ventilation of the contralateral lung.[73]

While pulmonary vascular resistance increases following the development of a unilateral pneumothorax, regional blood flow distribution and perfusion appear to be unchanged. This implies a diffuse increase in the pulmonary vascular resistance in both lungs, rather than a regional increase in the pulmonary vascular resistance in the partially collapsed, underventilated lung. The increased pulmonary vascular resistance probably results from a combination of several factors known to lead to pulmonary vasoconstriction, including: (1) systemic hypoxemia mediated through chemoreceptors; (2) increased sympathetic stimulation; and (3) local hypoxia in the ipsilateral, underventilated lung.[78-80]

The mechanism of hypoxemia during pneumothorax involves the ventilation/

perfusion imbalance that is created by the pneumothorax, with a lowering of the ventilation/perfusion ratio in the ipsilateral lung. A unilateral pneumothorax decreases the tidal volume and alveolar ventilation of the ipsilateral lung, while the perfusion of this lung remains unchanged. The unchanged perfusion in the affected lung causes the decrease in the ventilation/perfusion ratio, increasing the shunt fraction and decreasing the arterial oxygen tension. Local reflexes do not appear to be operative in a unilateral pneumothorax, as they are in pulmonary artery occlusion and regional atelectasis.

Fabel et al.[81] showed in rabbits that a pneumothorax of 50 ml of air takes approximately 92 hours to be reabsorbed. The reabsorption period is decreased to about 4 hours if air is replaced by oxygen, and to about ½ hour if air is replaced by carbon dioxide. The more rapid reabsorption of oxygen and CO_2 from the pleural space is due to a greater diffusion gradient for oxygen and a more advantageous diffusion coefficient for CO_2. The consumption of oxygen by pleural tissues appears to be of minimal importance in the more rapid reabsorption of oxygen. The purpose of oxygen therapy in the conservative treatment of spontaneous pneumothorax would therefore be to displace nitrogen.

An important physiologic role of transpleural permeability is to maintain the pleural space free of gas and to remove any gas that has entered it. It has been well established that gas pockets in the body are absorbed because the sum of the partial pressures of all gases in the venous blood and in the tissues is lower than the partial pressures of alveolar gas or ambient air.[82] Therefore, a cavity filled with air, such as the pleural space following a pneumothorax, eventually reaches a state of equilibrium in which the oxygen and carbon dioxide tensions in the cavity are close to their values in the surrounding tissues and venous blood, and the tension of nitrogen is higher by a value which approximates the difference between the sum of the partial pressures in the gas cavity and the sum of the partial pressures in the surrounding tissues. The absorption rate of a pneumothorax is therefore essentially limited by nitrogen. The major part of the gas absorbed from a pneumothorax is transported by diffusion through the pleura into the alveoli.

Rist and Strohl[83] found the following approximate gas composition of a pneumothorax: $FO_2 = 0.061$, $FCO_2 = 0.060$, $FN_2 = 0.879$. Thus, the corresponding PN_2 is 0.879×713 mmHg = 626 mmHg, assuming a barometric pressure of 760 mmHg. Since the PN_2 in alveolar gas and in the arterial blood is approximately 573 mmHg (assuming a PO_2 of 100 mmHg and PCO_2 of 40 mmHg), the PN_2 difference between pneumothorax gas and alveolar gas results in a driving pressure of 53 mmHg. Using these estimates, Magnussen et al.[84] calculated that the absorption rate of 175 ml of nitrogen in excised dog-lung lobes would be approximately 50 hours. However, the absorption should in reality be slower, because the surface of a partially collapsed lung is reduced, and the entire pleura does not have access to the pneumothorax gas.

Pulmonary function following recovery from a primary spontaneous pneumothorax is generally normal, with no residua from the episode of air in the pleural space.[85] However, some authors have found evidence of emphysema in a small percentage of young persons with a primary spontaneous pneumothorax.[65,85] Long-term follow-up of these patients will be necessary in order to evaluate the question of whether or not primary spontaneous pneumothorax is an early signal of diffuse pulmonary emphysema.

CLINICAL PRESENTATION

The clinical syndrome in pneumothorax is usually sufficiently typical for the clinician to suspect this diagnosis. Only rarely is the development of pneumothorax associated with minimal or no symptoms. Of the 1674 episodes of pneumothorax compiled by Killen and Gobbel,[86] 1642 (98 percent) were symptomatic episodes. It is probable that the "asymptomatic" patients did have minimal symptoms which were transient, and that when the pneumothorax was discovered on a routine chest radiograph, they could not remember these minor symptoms of several days to weeks previously.

Chest pain and dyspnea are the most common presenting symptoms of pneumothorax. The chest pain, which occurred in 92 percent of the 1316 cases compiled by Killen and Gobbel,[87] is generally constant from its inception, but may have a pleuritic component. Dyspnea is the second most common symptom of pneumothorax; it occurred in 79 percent of the 1316 cases compiled by Killen and Gobbel.[87] The degree of dyspnea will depend on the extent of the pneumothorax and the underlying pulmonary function of the patient. A complete pneumothorax in a previously healthy young male may not produce the degree of dyspnea as a small pneumothorax in someone with severe chronic obstructive pulmonary disease. Cough has been reported in about 10 percent of cases of spontaneous pneumothorax, and is usually nonproductive.[87]

Symptoms other than chest pain, dyspnea, and cough are rare in spontaneous pneumothorax. Hemoptysis is distinctly unusual, as is wheezing, unless the patient has underlying obstructive airways disease. Epigastric pain has been described in a small number of patients; this probably occurs only in the unusual case of a localized pneumothorax in the medial diaphragmatic area.

The onset of pneumothorax is sudden in 65 to 70 percent of cases; therefore, approximately one-third of patients will give a history of insidious symptoms.[88,89] The symptoms of pneumothorax may only be of a transient nature but may progress if the air leak continues.

Pneumothorax has been noted to occur with sedentary activity approximately 75 percent of the time; with strenuous activity such as running, jumping, lifting, and competitive sports 20 percent of the time; and with coughing, sneezing, or wheezing in 4 percent of cases.[90] One would surmise that any activity that would increase intra-alveolar pressure would make the individual more prone to the development of spontaneous pneumothorax. It is possible that in many instances the individual who develops a pneumothorax is not aware of subtle coughing, a modified Valsalva maneuver, and other phenomena that would increase the intra-alveolar pressure.

The physical findings in spontaneous pneumothorax are often subtle, especially when the pneumothorax is small. When the pneumothorax is large, the patient may present with marked respiratory distress and be cyanotic. Palpation will rarely reveal any evidence of subcutaneous emphysema. The percussion note shows hyperresonance, and fremitus is diminished on the side of the pneumothorax. On auscultation there are diminished or absent breath sounds. Cardiac examination will, rarely, reveal a crackling sound with each cardiac cycle. This physical finding, known as Hamman's sign, can best be heard with the patient in the left lateral decubitus position, and is due to the presence of mediastinal air. In one series, Hamman's sign was noted in only 2 percent of 298 cases of pneumothorax.[91,92]

In 1961 Lawson[93] described the "scratch sign" as a specific physical finding in pneumothorax. In order to detect this, the stethoscope is placed over either the sternum or vertebrae, and the surface of symmetrical areas of each hemithorax is scratched. The sound is detected more easily when the side of the pneumothorax is scratched.

The clinical findings in tension pneumothorax may be more dramatic, with marked air hunger and evidence of cardiovascular collapse. The incidence of tension pneumothorax in primary spontaneous pneumothorax is small (about 5 percent),[94] but this incidence is higher in patients who develop pneumothorax on mechanical ventilation. With tension pneumothorax there may be asymmetric enlargement of the chest, a complete absence of breath sounds, and a contralateral shift of cardiac sounds (Figs. 9–2A and 9–4A).

The diagnosis of pneumothorax in the absence of tension can only be confirmed by identifying the visceral pleural line on a chest radiograph (Figs. 9–2A, 9–3, and 9–5); one cannot depend on the change in density of the collapsed normal lung for a diagnosis of pneumothorax. Dornhorst and Pierce[95] observed that blood flow decreases through the progressively collapsed lung and, therefore, does not substantially alter the density of that lung.

The radiographic changes with pneumothorax may vary, depending upon the presence of other conditions, the degree of lung collapse, and the presence of tension. A small pneumothorax may be difficult to detect, since the underlying lung maintains its normal density and since only about one-third of the pneumothorax gas is compensated by lung collapse[72]; most of the pneumothorax gas is accommodated by chest-wall expansion, which may not be obvious with a small pneumothorax. When a pneumothorax is suspected but the visceral pleural line cannot be visualized absolutely—possibly because of an overlying rib—two procedures can facilitate its recognition: (1) an erect expiration radiograph, which causes a reduction in lung volume while maintaining a constant gas volume in the pleural space (Figs. 9–6A and B); and (2) a lateral decubitus radiograph allowing the pneumothorax gas to rise to the highest point in the hemithorax, where it is more clearly visible over the lateral chest wall than over the apex.

Clinically it is important to differentiate a small pneumothorax from cavitary and bullous lung disease, a chest wall abnormality, a skin fold, clothing, or tubing artifacts. A diagnosis of "pneumothorax" in any of the foregoing settings will result in the unnecessary insertion of a chest tube, while a missed diagnosis may lead to

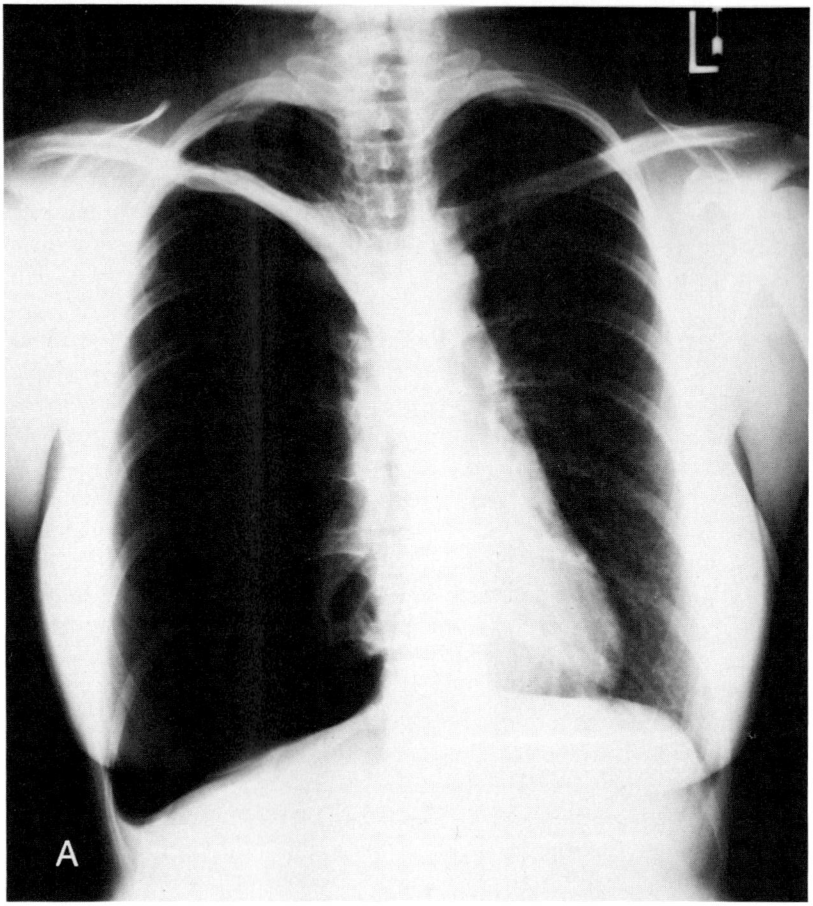

Figure 9–4. (A) Antero-posterior chest radiograph of a 28-year-old female from Texas with a 3-month history of progressive dyspnea. Upon arrival at the Denver airport she had a sudden increase in dyspnea without chest pain. Note large right radiolucency which either represents a loculated pneumothorax or a hyperinflated bulla. There is evidence of tension with a contralateral mediastinal shift, ipsilateral diaphragmatic depression, and rib-cage expansion.

marked respiratory distress and even death. In the absence of underlying lung disease, the visceral pleural line in a case of pneumothorax tends to parallel the shape of the chest wall. Artifactual lines may simulate the visceral pleural curve but do not, in general, parallel the course of the chest wall over its entire length. When the line can be shown to extend beyond the thorax, it represents an artifact. Skin-fold artifacts, particularly with critically ill patients in intensive care units who have had a supine portable radiograph, can be difficult to differentiate from pneumothorax. However, the density of the skin-fold is different from that of the visceral pleural line. The density of a skin-fold line tends to increase until it reaches its tangent, after which it becomes more lucent. With a pneumothorax,

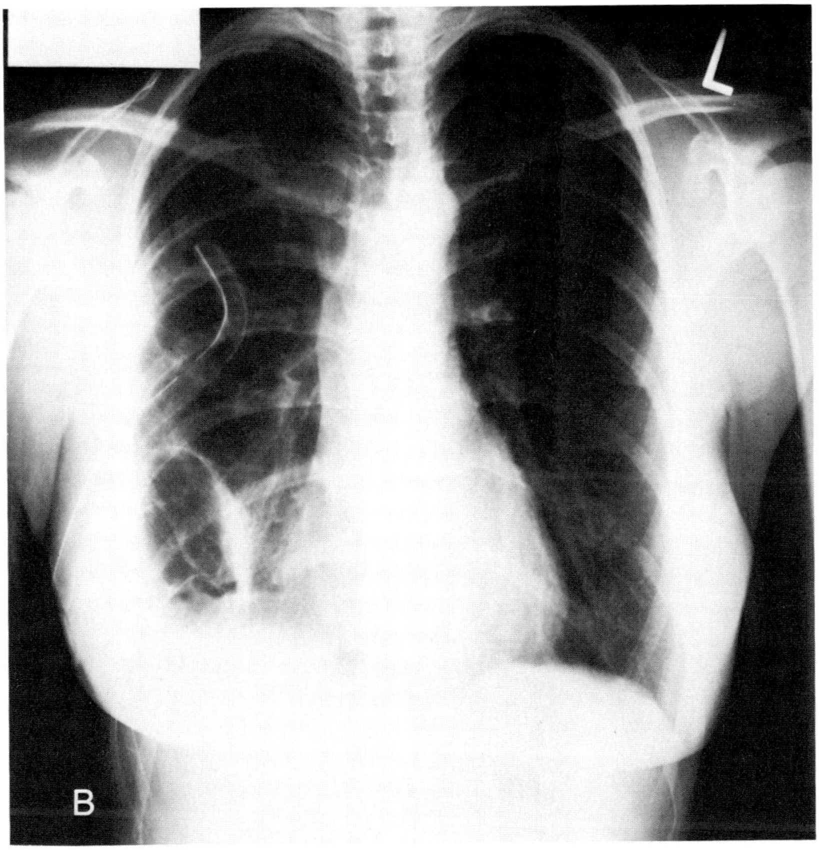

Figure 9–4 (continued). (B) Follow-up radiograph shows re-expansion of the lung and a right lower-lobe bulla. This case represented an example of a loculated tension pneumothorax from lung disease with bullae.

the uniform lucency of the lung and pleural space is interrupted by the thin visceral pleural line.[96] Other artifacts that can simulate a pneumothorax are usually easily discernible with the use of a bright light to demonstrate the presence of pulmonary vasculature distal to the artifact. Avascular cysts or blebs may be more difficult to differentiate from a pneumothorax (Fig. 9–4A). Bullae have concave rather than convex inner margins and do not tend to conform to the normal shape of the costophrenic sulcus when they occur at the lung base.[97]

Killen and Gobbel[98] found that 53 percent of nearly 2000 episodes of either primary or secondary spontaneous pneumothorax in adults occurred on the right side. This presumably is due to the fact that the volume and surface area of the right lung are slightly greater than those of the left lung. Bilateral simultaneous pneumothorax occurred in 1.6 percent of cases in the same series.

In a compilation of slightly over 1500 adult cases of primary or secondary spontaneous pneumothorax, 326 (21 percent) had evidence of a pleural effusion[99]

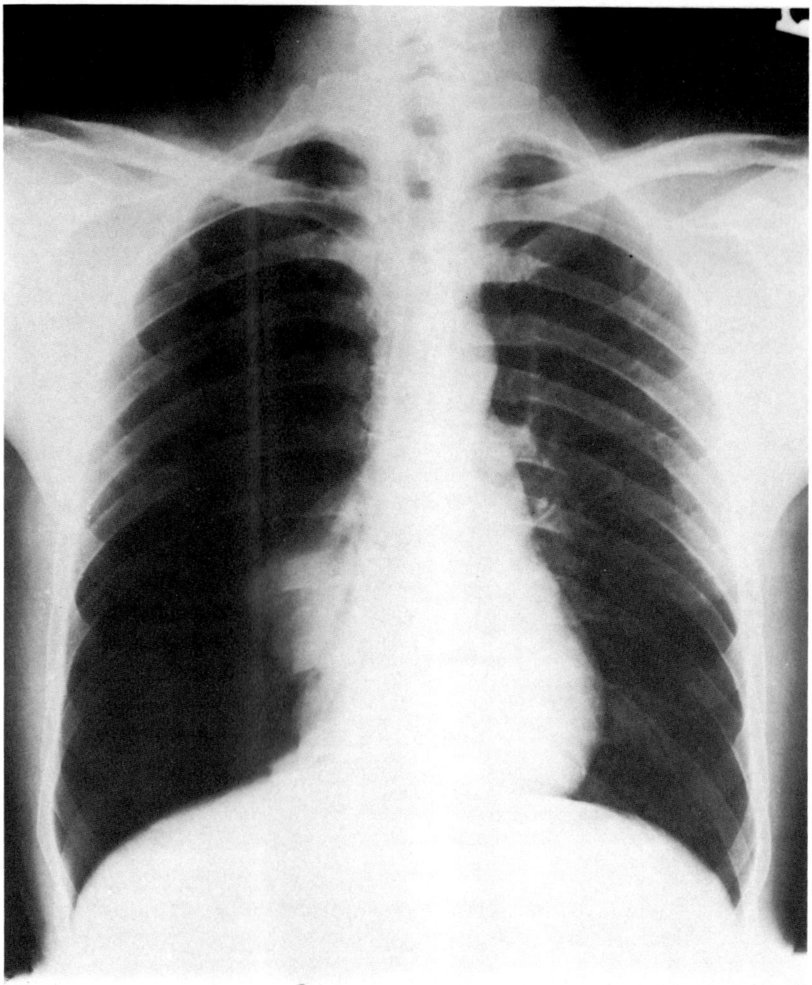

Figure 9–5. Postero-anterior chest radiograph of a 44-year-old man seen for an upper respiratory infection. Two weeks prior to this visit, he had transient right anterior chest pain and persistent dyspnea. A total right pneumothorax was found, with the lung hanging limply from the hilum. Note that the margins of the lobes can be identified and there is contralateral mediastinal shift.

Figs. 9–1, 9–2B). Pleural effusions are found more commonly with secondary spontaneous pneumothorax from active tuberculosis, pneumonia, or lung abscess than from primary spontaneous pneumothorax. If one examines the hydrostatic and oncotic pressures that act on the pleural space, the increased intrapleural pressure resulting from a pneumothorax would be considered as tending to prevent the development of pleural fluid collections. The development of a pleural fluid collection from a primary spontaneous pneumothorax would, therefore, be the result either of irritation by intrapleural air causing an increased capillary permeability or the tearing of a vessel causing a hemopneumothorax.

Pneumomediastinum is a common accompaniment of spontaneous pneumothorax in the neonate and can be found in episodes of secondary pneumothorax associated with increased airway pressure. However, it has only rarely been detected radiographically in adults with spontaneous pneumothorax. Killen and Gobbel[100] reviewed several series of approximately 650 cases of either primary or secondary spontaneous pneumothorax in adults and found that only 10 patients, or 1.5 percent, had pneumomediastinum.

Frequently, pneumomediastinum is undetectable by chest radiography, while in some instances only the lateral chest radiograph will reveal the presence of mediastinal air. Since interstitial pulmonary emphysema represents an air-on-air interface, it rarely can be demonstrated radiographically.

Since the symptoms of spontaneous pneumothorax are nonspecific, other entities are usually considered in the differential diagnosis. Besides such other lung diseases as pneumonia with pleurisy, diseases of other organ systems are often considered. Some of these include pericarditis, perforated peptic ulcer, esophageal rupture, hiatus hernia, intercostal neuralgia, acute cholecystitis, herpes zoster, and dissecting aortic aneurysm. It is important to remember that spontaneous pneumothorax should be considered when patients with underlying pulmonary disease develop a worsening of symptoms. When spontaneous pneumothorax is considered in the differential diagnosis, a chest radiograph should be obtained to evaluate the possibility of its existence.

MANAGEMENT

Immediate management of the patient with spontaneous pneumothorax can range from observation to tube thoracostomy (Table 9–2). The initial management decision made by the clinician will depend on the degree of the pneumothorax, the patient's symptoms, any underlying lung pathology, and whether or not the pneumothorax is progressing.

Nonoperative management or observation, including bed rest and the inhalation of oxygen, probably can be recommended in previously healthy patients with small pneumothoraces who are asymptomatic and show no indication that the pneumothorax is progressing, and for whom the facilities for close follow-up are available. Of the 778 cases compiled by Killen and Gobbel,[101] only 19, or 7.9 percent, were nonoperative treatment failures. However, this low failure rate is undoubtedly due to a lack of uniformity in data reporting.

While nonoperative management will be successful in certain selected cases of pneumothorax, the condition will require on the average of 3 to 4 weeks for resolution in such instances. Kircher and Swartzel[102] calculated that intrapleural air is absorbed at a rate of approximately 1.25 percent of the hemithorax volume per day. Thus, a 10 percent pneumothorax would require approximately 8 days for complete resolution. Leach[103] reported a mean of 19.4 days for the complete re-

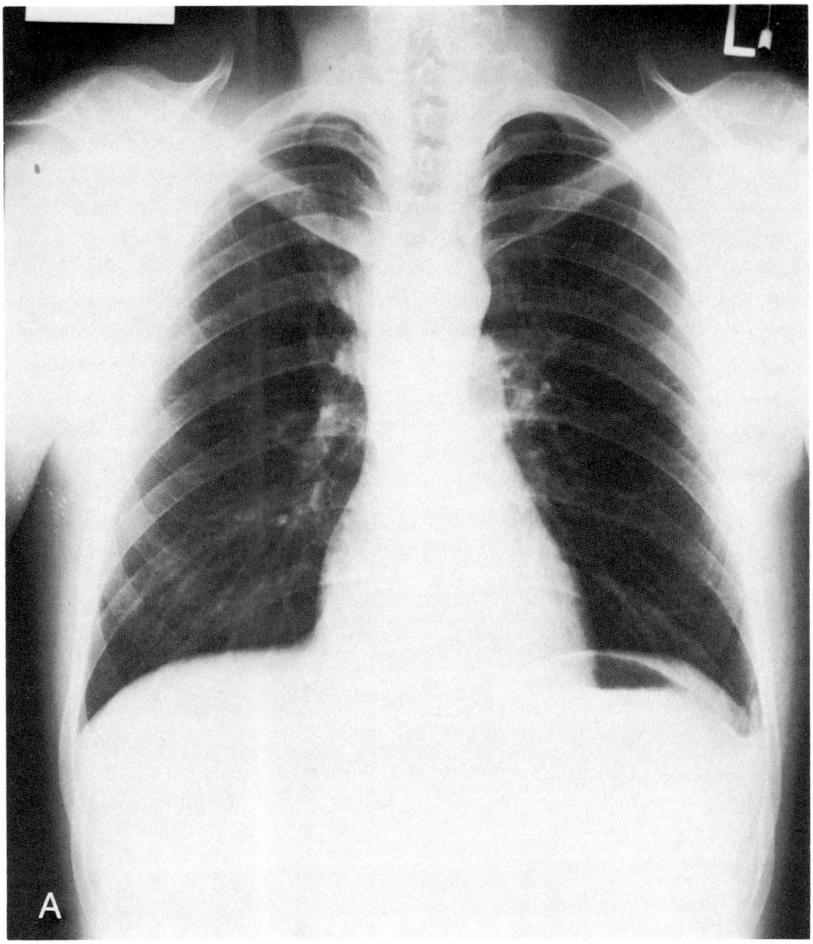

Figure 9–6. (A) Postero-anterior inspiratory chest radiograph of a 22-year-old male involved in a motorcycle accident. He presented with left chest wall and shoulder pain. There is a small left apical pneumothorax; the visceral pleural line cannot be visualized well.

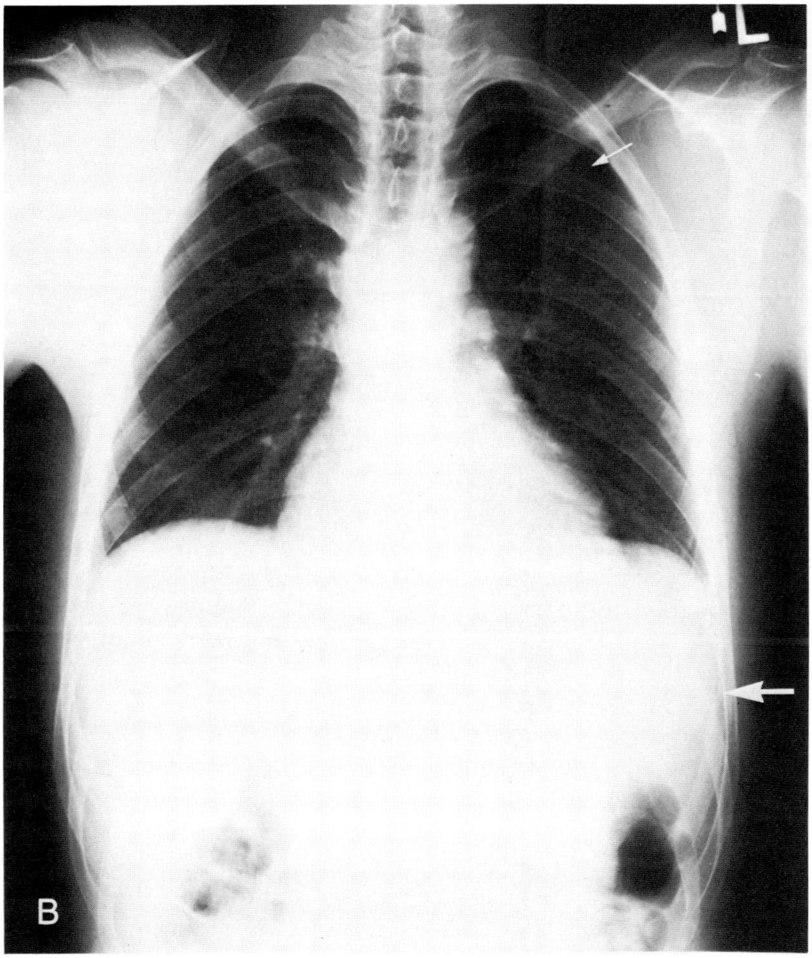

Figure 9–6 (continued). (B) Postero-anterior expiratory chest radiograph demonstrating apical pneumothorax more readily (small arrow). The large arrow denotes the left rib fracture.

Table 9–2. Management of Spontaneous Pneumothorax

Immediate Treatment	Comment
1. Observation	Small pneumothorax with minimal symptoms
2. Needle aspiration	Effective only if air leak has ceased
3. Tube thoracostomy with valve drainage system	May be used in outpatient setting
4. Tube thoracostomy to underwater seal drainage	Most common therapy, effective in 90% of cases
Prevention of Recurrence	
5. Tube thoracostomy with sclerosing agent	May be useful in the poor surgical risk with short expected survival (cystic fibrosis)
6. Thoracoscopy with talc insufflation	May be associated with fibrothorax and tumor
7. Thoracotomy	
a. Talc poudrage	As above
b. Pleural abrasion	Very effective, possibly with less morbidity than pleurectomy
c. Parietal pleurectomy	Virtually 100% effective without loss of pulmonary function

expansion of lungs with pneumothoraces of up to 50 percent of the lung volume, and 48.4 days for cases with greater than 50 percent pneumothoraces. The administration of a high inspired oxygen fraction to the patient will enhance the reabsorption of pleural gas because of the greater diffusion gradient for oxygen.

Needle aspiration of the pleural space would allow the more rapid removal of intrapleural gas than conservative, nonoperative therapy, but would only be effective when the air leak from the lung has ceased. When the air leak has stopped, needle aspiration can convert a large into a small pneumothorax which may then be suitable for nonoperative management.

Needle aspiration of the pleural space has been reported to be less successful than nonoperative management, having a failure rate of 39 percent in 146 patients.[104] This is most likely due to the use of needle aspiration for larger pneumothoraces and a lack of uniformity in reporting. In those patients satisfactorily treated with this method, the resolution time was approximately 20 days. Complications of needle aspiration are reopening of an air leak by an increasingly negative intrapleural pressure, puncture of the lung, and, rarely, empyema.

Needle aspiration probably has little value in the treatment of pneumothorax. If the pneumothorax is large enough to warrant aspiration, it is likely to require the insertion of a chest tube for management. A small pneumothorax can probably be treated best with observation; additionally, needle aspiration carries the risk of complications.

With the recent emphasis on more cost-effective medical care and the appropriate utilization of existing hospital facilities, there has been increasing interest in the treatment of spontaneous pneumothorax on an outpatient basis. The use of a valve drainage system has been advocated. The concept is not new, however, since Fuld[105] described an emergency procedure for use in pneumothorax in the battlefield, employing an inverted air inlet valve from a transfusion set. A recognized emergency treatment for tension pneumothorax is the insertion of an intrapleural needle and the tying of a punctured rubber glove finger over the needle end.[106] Heimlich, in 1965,[107] described the valve which bears his name in a drainage procedure that avoided the need for intrapleural suction following thoracotomy. The main disadvantage with this valve is in situations in which a pneumothorax is associated with a pleural effusion. In this setting the valve leaves tend to adhere, leading to blocking of the outward flow of air.

Bernstein et al.[108] reported on the use of the Heimlich valve in 18 pneumothoraces. Complete lung expansion occurred in 17 of these cases by 5 days, while 12 (66 percent) cases showed full expansion within 1 hour. Valve blockage occurred in 1 patient whose pneumothorax was associated with a pleural effusion. One patient failed to respond to both the Heimlich valve and underwater seal drainage; in this case a large apical bulla was found at thoracotomy. Mercier et al.,[109] in a series of 226 patients with spontaneous pneumothorax, reported on 167 (74 percent) who were managed successfully on an outpatient basis by observation (20 percent), or by intercostal tube drainage and a flutter valve (54 percent). In the latter situation, an intercostal catheter was put into the pleural space, and underwater drainage was used temporarily. After an observation period of 1 to 12 hours and a chest radiograph demonstrating that the lung was re-expanded adequately, the underwater drainage was removed and a disposable flutter valve—of either the Heimlich or Vycon, type—was connected to the chest tube and the patient was discharged. These patients were seen in the outpatient clinic 3 or 4 days later, and when lung expansion was complete and no air leak persisted the tube was removed. Of the 169 patients who were treated with a chest tube and flutter valve, 121 had complete resolution of their pneumothoraces without the need for further treatment. Complete recovery was achieved in less than 1 week in most cases. The length of drainage varied from 1 to 18 days, with an average of 5.1 days. No complications resulted from this ambulatory treatment, with the exception of a superficial wound infection in 1 patient.

In properly selected patients, the avoidance of hospitalization—with both its economic and psychologic burden—and the more rapid return to normal activity (as compared to non-operative management) is certainly important. However, 48 of the 169 patients reported by Mercier et al.[109] required further treatment. There were no data reported concerning these patients' ages, any underlying lung disease, any further treatment rendered, or the time to resolution following failure of the flutter valve. Thus, the consequences of flutter valve failure in this group of patients are unknown.

Tube thoracostomy has been advocated as the prime method of management in the patient with spontaneous pneumothorax. The insertion of a chest tube leads to rapid re-expansion of the lung even if there is a continued air leak. Chest tubes may be inserted in different locations depending upon the area and extent of the pneumothorax and the preference of the surgeon. The anterior second interspace and infra-axillary area are the two most common areas of insertion. The loculated pneumothorax requires careful insertion of the chest tube on the basis of radiographic localization.

A moderate-sized chest tube (18 to 28 French) should be used for evacuating a pneumothorax. Small catheters should be avoided since they can become clotted with fibrin. The chest tube should be inserted to a limited extent, with the tip of the tube in the most upright aspect of the hemithorax, the area to which air will gravitate following its escape from the lung. A tube that drops into the most dependent part of the pleural space may not allow the complete evacuation of air. In most instances, connection of the thoracostomy tube to an underwater-seal drainage system is effective for resolution of the pneumothorax. In certain instances, application of negative pressure to the thoracostomy tube is necessary to assure complete lung expansion.

Following the institution of thoracostomy tube drainage, the tube must be checked frequently for patency and continued communication with the pleural space. The thoracostomy tube should be left in place until there is no evidence of continued air leakage from the lung, as can be checked from the bedside, and the lung is fully re-expanded in a chest radiograph. As a margin of safety, most clinicians will leave the thoracostomy tube in place for an additional 24 to 48 hours following the last evidence of an air leak.

Of 605 cases of spontaneous pneumothorax compiled by Killen and Gobbel,[110] only 31, or 8.7 percent, were not treated successfully by tube thoracostomy. The average hospital stay in this series of patients was 10 days. Tube thoracostomy is the most effective means of immediate lung expansion and maintenance of this expansion in spontaneous pneumothorax. It definitely is indicated in the presence of a large pneumothorax, when there is evidence of a continued air leak, and if there are severe, persistent respiratory symptoms. In most patients with secondary spontaneous pneumothorax, tube thoracostomy is necessary.

It rarely is necessary to insert more than one chest tube in the treatment of a pneumothorax. The most common cause of failure of the initial thoracostomy tube is occlusion of the tube by fibrin or blood. Loculation of air in the pleural space may be another reason for insertion of a second chest tube. Rarely, when the pleural air leak is extremely large, a second chest tube is necessary to completely evacuate air from the pleural space. In four series reported in the early to mid-1960s, 227 (85 percent) of 266 episodes of pneumothorax were treated effectively with one chest tube.[111]

Complications with tube thoracostomy include massive subcutaneous emphysema, empyema (especially when the chest tube has been in place for a long period of time), erosion into the lung, communication of the lumen of the thoracostomy tube or its collecting system with ambient air, and re-expansion pulmonary edema.[112] Re-expansion pulmonary edema is rare, but seems to occur when there is a large pneumothorax that has been present for several days.

The intrapleural instillation of sclerosing agents is well-accepted therapy for patients with intractable malignant pleural effusions.[113] The use of sclerosing agents has also been reported for the treatment of spontaneous pneumothorax in certain high-risk groups of patients, including those with cystic fibrosis and chronic obstructive pulmonary disease. Boat et al.[114] were among the first to report the successful treatment of spontaneous pneumothorax in patients with cystic fibrosis with intrapleural quinacrine. Kattwinkel and associates[115] reported the use of intrapleural quinacrine in 1 patient with cystic fibrosis with bilateral pneumothoraces; there was no recurrence at 23 months and 11 months following intrapleural instillation of the drug. Goldszer et al.[116] reported the successful use of intrapleural tetracycline for spontaneous pneumothorax in chronic obstructive pulmonary disease.

Larrieu et al.[117] compared the use of intrapleural quinacrine for the treatment of recurrent spontaneous pneumothorax to the treatment of this condition with thoracotomy with either scarification or pleurectomy, and with tube thoracostomy alone. Twenty patients were treated with the instillation of quinacrine; of these 20, 1 had a pneumothorax immediately following tube removal which necessitated repeat tube thoracostomy, and 1 had late ipsilateral recurrence 2 years after treatment. The follow-up in this group of patients ranged from 6 months to more than 4 years, with only one late recurrence. In the thoracotomy group, 8 of 19 patients had postoperative complications, while in the tube thoracostomy group the recurrence rate was 23 percent during the first year.

Complications with sclerosing agents include all of the complications associated with tube thoracostomy, since the lung must be completely expanded with the use of chest tube drainage prior to instillation of the sclerosing agent. In addition, sclerosing agents cause chest pain and systemic reactions such as fever, chills, and malaise. Rarely, chest wall tumors have been reported following the use of iodized talc.[118]

Quinacrine hydrochloride in a powdered form for use as a sclerosing agent is no longer manufactured by Winthrop Laboratories. Tetracycline, one of the most common agents now used in this country for the treatment of malignant effusions, has been shown to be effective in that setting,[113,119,120] and has been shown to cause pleural symphysis in a dose-dependent manner.[121]

The use of such sclerosing agents as tetracycline hydrochloride would probably be effective in the treatment of recurrent spontaneous pneumothorax in the high-risk patient, especially the patient who is not expected to have a prolonged survival. The concern about this modality is its use in the young patient with primary spontaneous pneumothorax who has a normal expected survival. Careful follow-up data must be obtained concerning the possible development of fibrothorax in these patients before tetracycline hydrochloride is an accepted form of therapy.

Talc poudrage has been used successfully in the treatment of recurrent spontaneous pneumothorax. Talc can be insufflated into the pleural space either through a thorascope or with a technique that utilizes the Venturi principle. Nandi[122] reported on 24 patients with limited pulmonary function who had this form of therapy. Effective pleurodesis was obtained in all of the patients, with 22 being followed from 2 to 24 months after the procedure without evidence of recurrence or symptoms.

Patients who have a persistent air leak for many days despite tube thoracostomy, or those with recurrent pneumothoraces, should be taken to thoracotomy. At thoracotomy, several procedures can be done to promote pleural symphysis. These include talc insufflation, pleural abrasion, and parietal pleurectomy. These procedures are done following correction of the pulmonary lesion; the bleb can either be excised or oversewn at thoracotomy.

Only by thoracotomy can the lung lesion in a pneumothorax be managed effectively. In a total of 611 thoracotomies, blebs, bullae, or cysts were found in 428, or 70 percent.[123] In addition, there are patients in whom a focal area of fibrosis or a tear at the base of a pleural adhesion has been found to be the cause of a pneumothorax.[124] In 1956, Gaensler[18] introduced the technique of parietal pleurectomy in spontaneous pneumothorax. Anterior thoracotomy and posterolateral thoracotomy have been the incisions used most frequently in this procedure. The parietal pleura is mobilized from the chest wall superiorly to the apex, posteriorly to the costovertebral angle, anteriorly to the parasternal region, and inferiorly as far as can be reached conveniently through the thoracotomy incision. No attempt is made to remove the mediastinal or diaphragmatic pleura. Complete pleurectomy is more critical in the superior aspect of the chest, since this is the region in which subpleural blebs are prone to occur.

Parietal pleurectomy is virtually 100 percent effective for the treatment of recurrent pneumothorax. Of 364 patients treated with parietal pleurectomy for recurrent spontaneous pneumothorax, only 1 developed a recurrence.[125] Complications of parietal pleurectomy occur in about 10 percent of patients, the most common being intrapleural hemorrhage, contralateral pneumothorax, and bronchopleural fistula. The mortality from this procedure in a compilation of 308 parietal pleurectomies was 2.3 percent (7 patients).[126]

Thoracotomy for spontaneous pneumothorax has the risks inherent in the performance of any major surgical procedure. The mortality in elective thoracotomy is probably in the range of 1 percent.[127] The resection of blebs and the addition of procedures to promote pleural symphysis adds to the morbidity and probably to the mortality in thoracotomy.

Pulmonary function studies following recovery from parietal pleurectomy were evaluated in a series of patients by Gaensler.[18] He found there was no loss of pulmonary function as a result of parietal pleurectomy. Experimental studies have shown that while parietal pleurectomy does create effective pleural symphysis, there is not much fibrous tissue and, therefore, not as much ventilatory restriction as follows the application of certain sclerosing agents.[128] The post-parietal-pleurectomy chest radiograph is essentially normal in most patients.

Two recent series in which parietal pleurectomy was used for recurrent pneumothorax in 150 patients found 1 recurrence and no deaths.[129,130] Six patients required additional surgery for further complications. The average hospital stay was 10 days.

There is no study available comparing parietal pleurectomy with pleural abrasion in the treatment of spontaneous pneumothorax. However, Hampton-Rich et al.[131] reported using this procedure in cystic fibrosis patients with pneumothorax 31 times, with only 1 recurrence (3 percent). In their opinion, the low incidence of recurrence after an abrasion procedure makes pleurectomy unnecessary. The small added benefit that pleurectomy might offer probably is not worth the risk of increased postoperative bleeding and a pulmonary complication arising from the added anesthetic time.

Thoracotomy with either parietal pleurectomy or a pleural abrasion procedure should be regarded as the treatment of choice for patients with recurrent spontaneous pneumothorax who are able to undergo major surgery.

Tension pneumothorax is a condition that requires immediate action. The degree of symptomatology and the rapidity with which cardiovascular collapse occur depend on the amount of tension and the underlying cardiovascular status of the patient. Obviously, patients with severe chronic obstructive pulmonary disease or interstitial fibrosis are those who are most devastated by a tension pneumothorax.

The treatment of tension pneumothorax is immediate decompression of the pleural space. This can be done simply and quickly by inserting a large-bore needle into the second anterior intercostal space. In the patient with severe cardiopulmonary distress, the clinician should insert the needle into the hemithorax where his clinical examination dictates that a tension pneumothorax has occurred. If the clinical decision is correct, a rush of air will be heard through the needle, or the barrel of a glass syringe will be raised by air exiting under pressure. There will be an immediate response by the patient, with a decrease in tachycardia, an increase in blood pressure, improvement in oxygen saturation, and a decrease in the respiratory rate. If tension pneumothorax is suspected but the patient is tolerating this complication adequately, a chest radiograph should be obtained immediately to substantiate the diagnosis. When the patient has been stabilized with needle decompression, insertion of a thoracostomy tube is effective in gaining control of the pneumothorax. In most cases tube thoracostomy through an underwater seal will be effective definitive treatment of a tension pneumothorax.

Some have suggested a one-way valve attached to the thoracostomy tube for the treatment of tension pneumothorax.[105,106,132] This may be advantageous in the patient treated in the field who has severe chronic obstructive pulmonary disease. However, the key factor is relief of the tension with simple needle insertion, since most patients, except the severe pulmonary cripple, can tolerate a pneumothorax as long as it is not under tension.

Pneumomediastinum is common in neonatal spontaneous pneumothorax and secondary spontaneous pneumothorax associated with bronchial obstruction. Its incidence appears to be rather low, at less than 2 percent, in adult spontaneous pneumothorax.[133] Therapy for the condition consists of observation. Even when pneumomediastinum and subcutaneous emphysema are massive, they usually cause no cardiorespiratory compromise to the patient. Breathing of high concentrations of oxygen will facilitate the movement of nitrogen from the mediastinal air into the plasma and may decrease the time that air is in the interstitial tissues.[53] Rarely, tension mediastinum can occur with cardiopulmonary compromise. In this situation decompression of the mediastinum must be done immediately as in tension pneumothorax. Needle aspiration of the mediastinum, an incision in the suprasternal notch, or tracheostomy in less urgent cases will be effective in relieving the increased mediastinal pressure.

Patients who develop pneumomediastinum or subcutaneous emphysema on mechanical ventilation must be observed carefully, with chest tubes at the bedside, for the development of pneumothorax. These patients should be ventilated with the lowest peak cycling pressures and given adequate time for the expiratory phase of the cycle to be completed.

REFERENCES

1. Paré A: Les ocuvres d'Ambroise Paré. 8th ed., Ch. 7, 1628.
2. Emerson CP: Pneumothorax: A historical, clinical and experimental study. Johns Hopkins Rep 11:1, 1903.
3. Meckel: Sur de l'air répandu remassé dans la cavité du thorax qui arrêtait la respiration et qui a causé la mort. Mem Acad Roy Sci Berlin 1759.
4. Itaad JMG: Dissertation sur le Pneumo-thorax ou les Congestions Gazeuses qui Deforment dans la Poitrine. Thesis, Paris, 1803.
5. Laennec, R: De l'Auscultation Médiate. 1819.
6. Davy J: Observations on air found in the pleura in pneumothorax, with experiments on the absorption of various kinds of air introduced into the pleura. Philos Trans 1823.
7. Devilliers: Du Pneumothorax Déterminé par la Rupture de la Plèver et d'une Vésicule Aérienne Emphysémateuse. Thesis, Paris, 1826.
8. Noble D: Some particulars of treatment in a case of pneumothorax. Br Med J 2:425, 1873.
9. Biach A: Zur aetiologie des pneumothorax. Wien Med Wochenschr 30:1880.
10. Martin EW: A case of pneumothorax shown by the roentgen rays. Lancet 2:846, 1901.
11. Fussell MD, Riesman D: Spontaneous non-tuberculous pneumothorax. Am J Med Sci 124:218, 1902.
12. Spengler L: Zur chirurgie des pneumothorax, mitteslung über 10 eigene falle von geheilten tuberculosen pneumothorax; verbunden in 6 fallen mit gleichzeitiger heilung der lungentuberculose. Beitr Z Klin Chir 49:80, 1906.
13. Kjaergaard H: Spontaneous pneumothorax in the apparently healthy. Act Med Scand (Suppl) 43:1, 1932.
14. Bethune N: Pleural poudrage: A new technic for the deliberate production of pleural adhesions as a preliminary to lobectomy. J Thorac Surg 4:251, 1935.
15. Bigger IA: Operative Surgery. St. Louis, C.V. Mosby, 1937, p 605.
16. Hamman L: Spontaneous mediastinal emphysema. Bull Johns Hopkins Hosp 64:1, 1939.
17. Ellis FH Jr, Carr DT: The problem of spontaneous pneumothorax. Med Clin North Am 38:1065, 1954.
18. Gaensler EA: Parietal pleurectomy for recurrent spontaneous pneumothorax. Surg Gynecol Obstet 102:293, 1956.
19. Killen DA, Gobbel WG Jr: Spontaneous Pneumothorax. Boston, Little, Brown, 1968, pp 38–39.
20. Ludwig J, Kienzle GD: Pneumothorax in a large autopsy population. A study of 77 cases. Am J Clin Pathol, 70:24, 1978.

21. Watt AG: Spontaneous pneumothorax. A review of 210 consecutive admissions to Royal Perth Hospital. Med J Aust 1:186, 1978.
22. Baum GL: Textbook of Pulmonary Diseases. Boston, Little, Brown, 1965, p 689.
23. Dines DE, Clagett OT, Payne WS: Spontaneous pneumothorax in emphysema. Mayo Clin Proc 45:481, 1970.
24. Holsclaw DS: Common pulmonary complications of cystic fibrosis. Clin Pediatr (Phila) 9:346, 1970.
25. Turiaf J, Marland P, Mathieu H: Spontaneous pneumothorax, mediastinal and subcutaneous emphysema associated with asthma. Poumon Coeur 11:999, 1955.
26. Jorgensen JR, Falliers CJ, Bukantz SC: Pneumothorax in mediastinal and subcutaneous emphysema in children with bronchial asthma. Pediatrics 31:824, 1963.
27. Wilder RJ, Beacham EG, Ravitch MM: Spontaneous pneumothorax complicating cavitary tuberculosis. J Thorac Cardiovasc Surg 43:561, 1962.
28. Sokoloff MJ, Farrell JT Jr: Spontaneous pneumothorax in anthracosilicosis. JAMA 112:1564, 1939.
29. Segarra FO, Sherman DS: Spontaneous pneumothorax during steroid therapy in pulmonary tuberculosis. Dis Chest 41:354, 1962.
30. Sabiston DC Jr, Hopkins EH, Cooke RE, et al: The surgical management of complications of staphylococcal pneumonia in infancy and childhood. J Thorac Cardiovasc Surg 38:421, 1959.
31. Killen DA, Gobbel WG Jr: Spontaneous Pneumothorax. Boston, Little, Brown, 1968, p 101.
32. Hausmann W, Karlish AJ: Staphylococcal pneumonia in adults. Br Med J 2:845, 1956.
33 Janetos GP, Ochsner SF: Bilateral pneumothorax in mediastatic osteogenic sarcoma. Am Rev Resp Dis 88:73, 1963.
34. Zavala DC, Schoell JE: Ultrathin needle aspiration of the lung in infections and malignant disease. Am Rev Resp Dis 123:125, 1981.
35. George RB, Herbert SJ, Shames JM, et al: Pneumothorax complicating pulmonary emphysema. JAMA 234:389, 1975.
36. Finucane KE, Colbatch HJH: Elastic behavior of lungs in patients with airway obstruction. J Appl Physiol 26:330, 1969.
37. Bernhard WF, Malcolm JA, Berry RW, et al: A study of the pathogenesis and management of spontaneous pneumothorax. Dis Chest 42:403, 1962.
38. Killen DA, Gobbell WG Jr: Spontaneous Pneumothorax. Boston, Little, Brown, 1968, p 87.
39. Scoggin CH, Sahn SA, Petty TL: Status asthmaticus: A nine-year experience with 811 patients with 19 requiring mechanical ventilation. JAMA 238:1158, 1977.
40. Hardy HL: Clinical and epidemiologic aspects of the beryllium problem. In Pneumoconiosis, ed. Vorwald, AJ, New York, Paul B Hoeber, 1950, p 133.
41. Shaver CG, Riddell AR: Lung changes associated with the manufacture of alumina abrasives. J Ind Hyg Toxicol 29:145, 1947.
42. Aho A, Heinivarra O, Mahonen H: Boeck's sarcoid as a cause of spontaneous pneumothorax. Ann Med Int Fenn 47:163, 1958.
43. Roland AS, Merdinger WF, Froeb HF: Recurrent spontaneous pneumothorax. A clue to the diagnosis of histiocytosis X. N Engl J Med 270:73, 1964.
44. Carlson RA, Hattery RR, O'Connell EJ, et al: Pulmonary involvement by histiocytosis X in the pediatric age group. Mayo Clin Proc 51:542, 1976.

45. Lundgren R, Stjernberg N: Spontaneous pneumothorax as first symptom in bronchial carcinoma. Acta Med Scand 207:329, 1980.
46. Nelson SW: Large pneumothorax and associated massive collapse of the homolateral lung due to intrabronchial obstruction: A case report. Radiology 68:411, 1957.
47. Schulman P, Cheng E, Cvitkovie E, et al: Spontaneous pneumothorax as a result of intensive cytotoxic chemotherapy. Chest 75:194, 1979.
48. Laws HL, Fox LS, Younger B: Bilateral catamenial pneumothorax. Arch Surg 112:627, 1977.
49. Kovarik JL, Tall GD: Thoracic endometriosis with recurrent spontaneous pneumothorax. JAMA 196:221, 1966.
50. Lillington GA, Mitchell SP, Wood GA: Catamenial pneumothorax. JAMA 219: 1328, 1972.
51. Rossi NP, Goplerud CP: Recurrent catamenial pneumothorax. Arch Surg 109:173, 1974.
52. Burgener L, Solmes JG: Spontaneous pneumothorax and pregnancy. Can Med Assoc J 120:19, 1979.
53. Chernick V, Avery ME: Spontaneous alveolar rupture at birth. Pediatrics 32:816, 1963.
54. Ebner H: Spontaneous pneumothorax of the newborn. Anesth Analg 38: 64, 1959.
55. Avery ME: The Lung and Its Disorders in the Newborn Infant. Philadelphia, WB Saunders, 1964, p 144.
56. Kirschner PA, Strauss L: Pulmonary interstitial emphysema in the newborn infant. Precursors and sequelae. Dis Chest 46:417, 1964.
57. Oztalay AG, Beard AG: Possible relationship of high intratracheal pressure and tension pneumothorax. South Med J 55:1322, 1962.
58. Grimes OF, Farber SM: Air cysts of the lung. Surg Gynecol Obstet 113:720, 1961.
59. Feraru F, Morrow CS: Surgery of subpleural blebs: Indications and contraindications. Am Rev Resp Dis 79:577, 1959.
60. Lichter I, Gwynne JF: Spontaneous pneumothorax in young subjects. A clinical and pathological study. Thorax 26:409, 1971.
61. Withers JN, Fishback ME, Kiehl PV, et al: Spontaneous pneumothorax. Suggested etiology and comparison of treatment methods. Am J Surg 108:772, 1964.
62. Vawter DL, Matthews FL, West JB: Effect of shape and size of lung and chest wall on stresses in the lung. J Appl Physiol 39:7, 1975.
63. Baronofsky ID, Warden HG, Kaufman JL, et al: Bilateral therapy for unilateral spontaneous pneumothorax. J Thorac Surg 34:310, 1957.
64. Driscoll PJ, Aronstam EM: Experiences in the management of recurrent spontaneous pneumothorax, J Thorac Cardiovasc Surg 42:174, 1961.
65. DeTroyer A, Yernault JC, Rodenstein D, et al: Pulmonary function in patients with primary spontaneous pneumothorax. Bull Eur Physiopathol Respir 14:31, 1978.
66. Jansveld CAF, Dijkman JH: Primary spontaneous pneumothorax and smoking. Br Med J 4:559, 1975.
67. Macklin CC: Pneumothorax with massive collapse from experimental local overinflation of the lung substance. Can Med Assoc J 36:414, 1937.
68. Macklin MT, Macklin CC: Malignant interstitial emphysema of the lungs and mediastinum as an important occult complication in many respiratory diseases and other conditions. An interpretation of the clinical literature in the light of laboratory experiment. Medicine 23:281, 1944.

69. Holt LE Jr, McIntosh R: Pediatrics, 12th ed. New York, Appleton-Century-Crofts, 1953.
70. Cooley JC, Gillespie JB: Mediastinal emphysema: Pathogenesis and management. Report of a case. Dis Chest 49:104, 1966.
71. Dernaksian G, Lamb LE: Spontaneous pneumothorax in apparently healthy flying personnel. Ann Intern Med 51:39, 1959.
72. Christie RV, McIntosh CA: The lung volume and respiratory exchange after pneumothorax. Q J Med 5:445, 1936.
73. Moran JF, Jones RH, Wolfe WG: Regional pulmonary function during experimental unilateral pneumothorax in the awake state. J Thorac Cardiovasc Surg 74:396, 1977.
74. Rutherford RB, Hurt HH Jr, Brickman RD, et al: The pathophysiology of progressive tension pneumothorax. J Trauma 8:212, 1968.
75. Kilburn H: Cardiorespiratory effects of large pneumothorax in conscious and anesthetized dogs. J Appl Physiol 18:279, 1963.
76. Simmons DH, Hemingway A: Acute respiratory effects of pneumothorax in normal and vagotomized dogs. Am Rev Tuberc 76:195, 1957.
77. Simmons H, Hemingway A: The pulmonary circulation following pneumothorax and vagotomy in dogs. Circ Res 7:93, 1959.
78. Fishman AP: Respiratory gases in the regulation of the pulmonary circulation. Physiol Rev 41:214, 1961.
79. Comroe JH Jr: Physiology of Respiration, 2nd ed. Chicago, Year Book Medical Publishers, 1974, p 155.
80. West JB: Respiratory Physiology. Baltimore, Williams and Wilkins, 1974, pp 40–46.
81. Fabel H, Wettengel, Tollner D: Reabsorption of nitrogen, oxygen and carbon dioxide in pleural tissue. Respiration 29:229, 1972.
82. Piiper J: Physiological equilibria of gas cavities in the body. In Handbook of Physiology, vol 2, Section 3: Respiration. eds. Fenn WO, Rahn H. Washington, DC, American Physiological Society.
83. Rist E, Strohl A: Etudes expérimentales et critiques sur le pneumothorax. Ann Med 8:223, 1920.
84. Magnussen H, Perry SF, Willmer H, et al: Transpleural diffusion of inert gases in excised lung lobes of the dog. Respir Physiol 20:1, 1974.
85. Williams MH Jr, Kane C: Pulmonary function in patients who have recovered from spontaneous pneumothorax. Dis Chest 47:153, 1965.
86. Killen DA, Gobbel WG Jr: Spontaneous Pneumothorax. Boston, Little, Brown, 1968, p 160.
87. Killen DA, Gobbel WG Jr: Spontaneous Pneumothorax. Boston, Little, Brown, 1968, p 161.
88. Crowther JS: Spontaneous pneumothorax. Tubercle 36:265, 1955.
89. Lenox-Smith I: Spontaneous pneumothorax: A study of ninety-four cases. Br J Dis Chest 56:1, 1962.
90. Killen DA, Gobbel WG Jr: Spontaneous Pneumothorax. Boston, Little, Brown, 1968, p 163.
91. Shefts LM, Gilpatrick C, Swindell H, et al: Management of spontaneous pneumothorax. Dis Chest 26:273, 1954.
92. Thomas PA: Spontaneous pneumothorax: Modern concepts in etiology and treatment of an important syndrome in military practice. Mil Med 124:116, 1959.

93. Lawson JD: The scratch sign: A valuable aid in the diagnosis of pneumothorax. N Engl J Med 264:88, 1961.
94. Killen DA, Gobbel WG Jr: Spontaneous Pneumothorax. Boston, Little, Brown, 1968, p 220.
95. Dornhorst AC, Pierce JW: Pulmonary collapse and consolidation: the role of collapse in the production of lung field shadows and the significance of segments in inflammatory lung disease. J Fac Radiol 5:276, 1954.
96. Greene R, McLoud TC, Stark P: Pneumothorax. Sem Roentgenol 12:313, 1977.
97. Berg RA: Giant congenital bronchogenic cyst, "Pseudopneumothorax." Postgrad Med 48:121, 1970.
98. Killen DA, Gobbel WG Jr: Spontaneous Pneumothorax. Boston, Little, Brown, 1968, p 171.
99. Killen DA, Gobbel WG Jr: Spontaneous Pneumothorax. Boston, Little, Brown, 1968, p 173.
100. Killen DA, Gobbel WG Jr: Spontaneous Pneumothorax. Boston, Little, Brown, 1968, p 230.
101. Killen DA, Gobbel WG Jr: Spontaneous Pneumothorax. Boston, Little, Brown, 1968, p 190.
102. Kircher LT Jr, Swartzel RL: Spontaneous pneumothorax and its treatment. JAMA 155:24, 1954.
103. Leach JE: Pneumothorax in young adult males: Descriptive characteristics in 126 cases. Arch Intern Med 76:264, 1945.
104. Killen DA, Gobbel WG Jr: Spontaneous Pneumothorax. Boston, Little, Brown, 1968, p 194.
105. Fuld H: Simple device for control of tension pneumothorax. Br Med J 2:503, 1944.
106. Birch CA: Emergencies in Medical Practice, 8th ed. London and Edinburgh, Livingstone, 1967, p 164.
107. Heimlich JH: Heimlich flutter valve: Effective replacement for drainage bottle. Hosp Top 43:122, 1965.
108. Bernstein A, Waqaruddin M, Shah M: Management of spontaneous pneumothorax using a Heimlich flutter valve. Thorax 28:386, 1973.
109. Mercier C, Page A, Verdant A, et al: Outpatient management of intercostal tube drainage in spontaneous pneumothorax. Ann Thorac Surg 22:163, 1976.
110. Killen DA, Gobbel WG Jr: Spontaneous Pneumothorax. Boston, Little, Brown, 1968, p 199.
111. Killen DA, Gobbel WG Jr: Spontaneous Pneumothorax. Boston, Little, Brown, 1968, pp 203–204.
112. Waquaruddin M, Bernstein A: Re-expansion pulmonary edema. Thorax 30:54, 1975.
113. Sahn SA, Good JT Jr, Potts DE: The pH of sclerosing agents: A determinant of pleural symphysis. Chest 76:198, 1979.
114. Boat TF, di Sant Agnese PA, Warwick WJ, et al: Pneumothorax in cystic fibrosis. JAMA 209:1498, 1969.
115. Kattwinkel J, Taussig LM, McIntosh CL, et al: Intrapleural instillation of quinacrine for recurrent pneumothorax. JAMA 226:557, 1973.
116. Goldszer RC, Bennett J, Van Campen J, et al: Intrapleural tetracycline for spontaneous pneumothorax. JAMA 241:724, 1979.
117. Larrieu AJ, Tyers GFO, Williams EH, et al: Intrapleural instillation of quinacrine for treatment or recurrent spontaneous pneumothorax. Ann Thorac Surg 28:146, 1979.
118. Jackson JW, Bennett MH: Chest wall tumour following iodized talc pleurodesis. Thorax 28:788, 1969.

119. Wallach HW: Intrapleural tetracycline for malignant pleural effusions. Chest 68:510, 1975.
120. Rubinson R, Bolooki H: Intrapleural tetracycline for control of malignant pleural effusions. South Med J 65:847, 1972.
121. Sahn SA, Potts DE: The effect of tetracycline on the pleural membrane of rabbits. Am Rev Resp Dis 117:493, 1978.
122. Nandi P: Recurrent spontaneous pneumothorax; an effective method of talc poudrage. Chest 77:493, 1980.
123. Killen DA, Gobbel WG Jr: Spontaneous Pneumothorax. Boston, Little, Brown, 1968, p 269.
124. Brewer LA III, Dolley FS, Evans BH: The surgical management of chronic "spontaneous" pneumothorax. J Thorac Surg 19:167, 1950.
125. Killen DA, Gobbel WG Jr: Spontaneous Pneumothorax. Boston, Little, Brown, 1968, pp 274–275.
126. Killen DA, Gobbel WG Jr: Spontaneous Pneumothorax. Boston, Little, Brown, 1968, pp 276–281.
127. Killen DA, Gobbel WG Jr: Spontaneous Pneumothorax. Boston, Little, Brown, 1968, p 272.
128. Frankel A, Krasna I, Baronofsky ID: An experimental study of pleural symphysis. J Thorac Cardiovasc Surg 42:43, 1961.
129. Askew AR: Parietal pleurectomy for recurrent pneumothorax. Br J Surg 63:203, 1976.
130. Singh SV: Current status of parietal pleurectomy in recurrent pneumothorax. Scand J Thorac Cardiovasc Surg 13:93, 1979.
131. Hampton Rich R, Warwick WJ, Leonard AS: Open thoracotomy and pleural abrasion in the treatment of spontaneous pneumothorax in cystic fibrosis. J Pediatr Surg 13:237, 1978.
132. Wayne MA, McSwain NE: Clinical evaluation of a new device for the treatment of tension pneumothorax. Ann Surg 191:760, 1980.
133. Killen DA, Gobbel WG Jr: Spontaneous Pneumothorax. Boston, Little, Brown, 1968, p 230.

10

Pulmonary Infection in the Immunosuppressed Patient

Richard A. Matthay, M.D.
William H. Greene, M.D.
Ernest D. Moritz, M.D.

INTRODUCTION

Advances in the fields of chemotherapy and transplantation have greatly improved the prognosis for patients with many malignant and chronic disorders. An unfortunate corollary of this has been the growth of a population with modified host defense mechanisms in whom infection is a common cause of death.[1,2] Such patients are a hallmark of latter twentieth century medicine, and further progress in their management must include methods of preventing, diagnosing, and effectively treating the infectious complications of immunosuppression.[1–5]

The lungs represent the single most commonly documented site of infectious disease among adults[6] and children[3] with cancer, and pneumonia accounts for as much as 25 to 50 percent[3,7] of all infectious-disease mortality among patients with hematologic malignant disease. For renal-transplant patients, the lungs rank second only to the operative site and urinary tract as a source of septicemia and infectious mortality.[8,9] In earlier series, the mortality within the first year after transplantation of cadaver kidneys was 28 percent,[10] and much of this was secondary to infection, with infectious morbidity from all causes being as high as 83 percent.[9] Some recent changes in the prophylaxis and management of renal-transplant patients appear responsible for a decline in infectious morbidity and mortality, especially from extrapulmonary sources, in this group.[10] Nevertheless, in most centers, pulmonary infection remains a substantial problem in patients who have received a transplant.[1]

The spectrum of organisms that infect the immunosuppressed patient is wide, including bacteria, mycobacteria, viruses, fungi, and protozoa.[1,2] The relative incidence of the different types of infection varies in different parts of the world and at different periods in the natural history of the underlying primary diseases.

The clinical presentation includes one or more of the following: cough, dyspnea, fever, and infiltrates on radiographs of the chest.[1] This clinical picture is nonspecific, and is common not only to the pulmonary infections caused by many different organisms, but also to several noninfective pulmonary complications[2,11–13]; these are listed below under "General Considerations."

The diagnosis and successful management of pulmonary complications in the immunocompromised patient is an enormous clinical challenge, which can be met most effectively by a team with collective knowledge of the probable types of complication in different clinical settings. The team members should be able to obtain pulmonary tissue transbronchially, percutaneously, or by open-lung biopsy when indicated, and should have bacteriologic and histopathologic expertise. In addition, intensive care facilities should be available to care for critically ill patients.[2]

This chapter has five major purposes: (1) to outline the general considerations in immunosuppressed patients with pulmonary complications; (2) to detail the defenses that are impaired in immunosuppressed hosts; (3) to critically evaluate diagnostic methods for establishing the etiology of pulmonary infiltrates in immunosuppressed patients; (4) to underscore the variety of infectious agents causing pulmonary disease in these patients; and (5) to outline the appropriate treatment of opportunistic pulmonary infections.

GENERAL CONSIDERATIONS

There are several important general considerations regarding pulmonary abnormalities in the immunocompromised patient.[1,2]

1. Although infection is the most common pulmonary complication of a compromised immune defense, several noninfective problems may produce a similar clinical picture.[2,11–13] These include malignant disease, pulmonary infarction, intrapulmonary hemorrhage, drug-induced pulmonary disease, radiation pneumonitis, pulmonary edema (cardiogenic and noncardiogenic), and nonspecific interstitial pneumonitis.
2. Although almost any organism can be responsible for a fatal infection in the immunocompromised patient, bacterial infection is the most frequent cause of this, and *Pseudomonas, Klebsiella, Escherichia coli,* and *Staphylococcus aureus* are the most commonly responsible agents.
3. Even though the lung may appear to be the primary site of infection, this may not be the case; the patient must be examined carefully for alternative sites of primary infection from which dissemination may have occurred.
4. Infection is often already disseminated at the time of presentation; therefore, blood cultures, examination of the cerebrospinal fluid, and a careful search for skin lesions for biopsy may provide the etiologic diagnosis.
5. Because infection in the immunocompromised patient may be rapidly fatal, treatment must be instituted early, often on an empirical basis. Subsequent

Table 10–1. Conditions Impairing Host-Defense Mechanisms

Depression of leukocyte bactericidal function
Myelocytic leukemias
Chronic granulomatous disease
Drug-induced granulocytopenia
Corticosteroid therapy
Acidosis
Burns
Depression of humoral immune response
Lymphocytic leukemias and lymphomas
Multiple myeloma
Paraneoplastic syndrome
Congenital hypogammaglobulinemias
Antimetabolite or cytoxic drug therapy
Childhood splenectomy
Depression of cellular immune response
Hodgkin's disease
Corticosteroid therapy
Uremia
Sarcoidosis
Terminal cancer
Antimetabolite or cytotoxic drug therapy
Severe malnutrition
Depression of mucocutaneous boundary function
Patients that are intubated
Patients with catheters (intravenous or urethral)
Patients with mucositis, decubiti, mucosal ulceration
Patients with alterations of normal flora (the debilitated, those receiving antibiotics)
Patients with secretory IgA deficiency

(Adapted from Matthay RA, Greene WH: Pulmonary infections in the immunocompromised patient. Med Clin North Am 64:529, 1980.)

identification of the infecting organisms allows the appropriate modification of therapy.

6. Outbreaks of particular infections may occur in localized geographic areas, and a knowledge of these may help in making the diagnosis in individual cases.
7. Infection with more than one organism is common.
8. The outcome of any infective complication in the immunocompromised patient depends upon many factors, the most important of which (in the presence of appropriate treatment for the infection) are the extent of underlying primary disease, its response to therapy, and the degree and duration of neutropenia.[1,2]

CONCEPTS OF IMMUNOSUPPRESSION AND INFECTION

The major mechanisms protecting the body from infection are the mucocutaneous boundaries, polymorphonuclear leukocytes, circulating immunoglobulins, and cellular immune mechanisms.[1,14] Some of the conditions adversely affecting these sources of defense against infection are listed in Table 10–1.[1] For example, patients with acute granulocytic leukemia tend to have both a severe reduction in number and severe impairment in the functional capability of polymorphonuclear leukocytes. In patients with chronic lymphatic leukemia, lymphocytic lymphoma, or multiple myeloma, the basic defect in host defense mechanisms resides primarily in the effect these diseases have on circulating immunoglobulins. Such patients have a tendency to hypogammaglobulinemia and depressed or absent antibody responses to test antigens. Hodgkin's disease exemplifies the third major variety of deficits in host defense, in which there appears to be a depression or absence of cell-mediated immune mechanisms, with the absence of delayed hypersensitivity to common skin-test antigens. All patients with the foregoing conditions are subjected additionally to transgressions of the mucocutaneous boundaries and to functional alterations of these boundaries, such as changes in the normal flora.[1]

Pulmonary defense mechanisms are incompletely understood, but the alveolar macrophage, the major initial line of defense against particles deposited on the respiratory membrane, and both humoral and cell-mediated immunity appear important in protecting against pathogens.[1,5] Alterations in any of these sources of defense may lead to pulmonary infection.

DIAGNOSIS OF PULMONARY INFECTIONS IN IMMUNOSUPPRESSED HOSTS

Since therapy is now available for almost all of the pathogens causing infection in immunosuppressed hosts, and since infection in these individuals may be rapidly fatal, appropriate diagnostic procedures for the specific cause of a pulmonary infection in such an individual is vital.[15] A suspected infection in the immunocompromised host should be pursued far beyond the routine evaluation of fever.[5] The routine evaluation in such a case primarily includes obtaining material for appropriate stain tests and culture from multiple, easily accessible sources, such as the sputum, blood, throat, nares, stool, urine, and skin. Properly collected and processed sputum specimens are valuable and simple diagnostic tools in the majority of patients with uncomplicated pneumonia; however, because expectorated sputum is contaminated by oropharyngeal flora, it is not always a reliable indicator of the microorganisms present in the lower respiratory tract.[15-18]

In patients with pulmonary infiltrates, skin testing for tuberculosis, the measurement of cold agglutinins for *Mycoplasma pneumoniae*, serologic tests for *M. pneumoniae*, *Toxoplasma gondii*, candida, and cryptococcus, and, depending on exposure, *Histoplasma capsulatum* and *Coccidioides immitis* are indicated.[5,15] In some cases, serial serologic studies for viruses (*Herpes simplex*, varicella-zoster and cytomegalovirus), or indirect fluorescent antibody studies of material from viral skin lesions may be helpful.[5,15] After this workup, antibacterial chemotherapy is administered to the severely compromised patient with apparent infection. If the initial workup does not establish a specific infectious diagnosis, repeated physical examinations, chest radiographs, and further cultures during empiric antibiotic therapy are indicated. The etiologic agent may be discovered after antimicrobial drug therapy has been started, and repeated cultures may detect multiple infections or superinfections.[5] Failure to reach a diagnosis during a routine workup mandates a step-by-step utilization of invasive methods,[1,5,15] particularly if a course of empiric antibiotic therapy has been given without an adequate response. Four invasive procedures will be reviewed extensively: transtracheal aspiration, aspiration lung biopsy, fiberoptic bronchoscopy, and open-lung biopsy.

Transtracheal Aspiration

Transtracheal aspiration is the next logical procedure when a sputum examination is unrewarding or when no sputum is produced,[5] perhaps because of an inadequate inflammatory response.[4] Transtracheal aspiration was proposed by Pecora et al.[18,19] as a method for obtaining a representative specimen of lower-respiratory-tract secretions without contamination by the flora of the oropharynx. Modifying the transtracheal anesthesia technique, he introduced the concept of direct percutaneous endotracheal aspiration, a method simple enough to be used at the bedside.[15] Kalinske et al.[20] described tracheal aspiration using a percutaneous approach through the cricothyroid membrane, the technique now utilized widely (Fig. 10–1).[21-23] This minor refinement was intended to avoid complications resulting from blind needle puncture of the more richly vascularized region anterior to the trachea. Current technique involves the intratracheal instillation of 2 to 3 cc of sterile saline when this is needed to aspirate a specimen.[22] A vacuum suction apparatus also may be used, to facilitate the return of material from the airway.[21]

Diagnostic Yield

When done properly, transtracheal aspiration is a safe technique for sampling lower-respiratory-tract secretions,[20-24] and the bacteriologic data obtained have been more reliable than those obtained from the evaluation of routine sputum samples. Comparative studies of paired cultures of tracheal aspirates and expectorated specimens have repeatedly demonstrated that transtracheal aspiration yields more pulmonary pathogens and fewer varieties of bacterial contaminants in patients with clinical and radiographic evidence of pneumonitis.[22,23] As an alternative to the use of expectorated sputum for identifying pathogenic organisms, transtracheal aspiration appears to be superior as a sampling technique; however, an appraisal of the sensitivity and specificity of transtracheal aspiration as a diagnostic technique must extend beyond comparing its results with the results of sputum sampling.[15]

Bartlett et al.[21] examined the diagnostic accuracy of tracheal aspirates in 488 patients, 23 of whom had bacteremic pneumonia. In all patients with bacteremia, the blood-borne pathogen was also recovered from the transtracheal specimen. Potential pathogens in addition to those isolated from blood cultures were found in seven tracheal aspirates in this group. Similar indications of the sensitivity of transtracheal aspiration are found in reports favorably comparing the culture

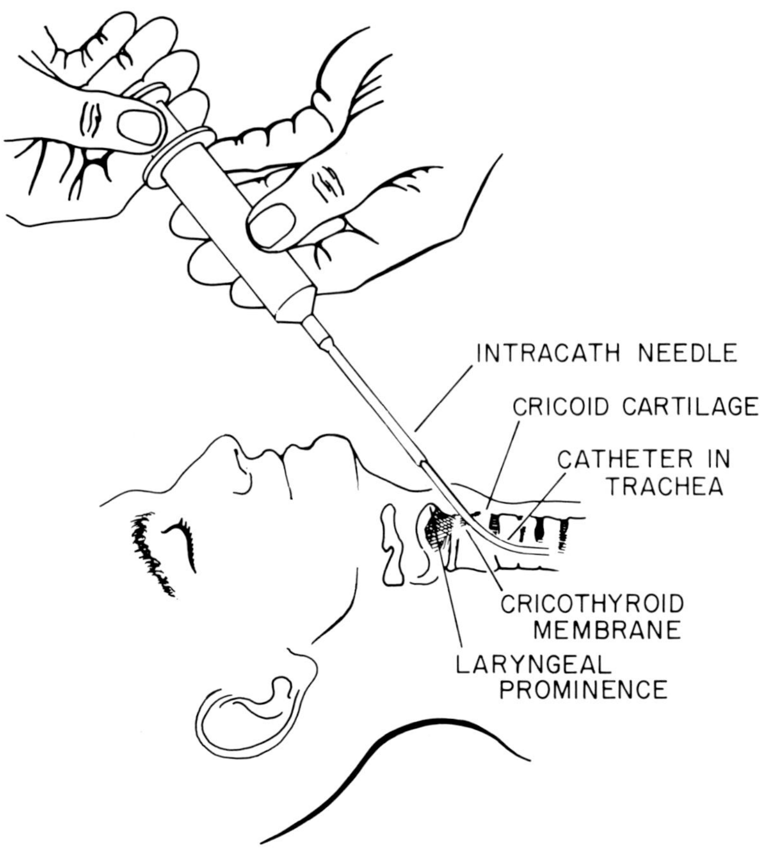

Figure 10–1. Illustration of technique for transtracheal aspiration. (Matthay RA, Moritz ED: Invasive procedures for diagnosing pulmonary infection: A critical review. Clin Chest Med 2:3, 1981).

results from tracheal aspirates with culture material obtained at autopsy in patients who died within 24 hours of the procedure.[20]

Transtracheal aspiration may yield negative results in certain patients with clinically and radiographically apparent pulmonary infection. This may be explained by previous antimicrobial therapy, which can cause misleading culture information,[21] or by a nonbacterial lower-respiratory-tract process. In one study, a small number of patients who had received no antibiotics had tracheal aspirates that were sterile despite a diagnosis of bacterial infection of the pulmonary parenchyma confirmed by alternative methods.[21] Such false-negatives can be anticipated in approximately 1 percent of patients from whom tracheal aspirates are taken for culture, and are probably related to the location of the infectious lesion and the patency of the airways between the trachea and the nidus of the bacterial process.[15]

The incidence of false-positive tracheal aspirate cultures is incompletely under-

Table 10–2. Complications of Transtracheal Aspiration

Series	No. of Procedures	Moderate to Severe Subcutaneous Emphysema[a]		Significant[b] Hemorrhage		Paratracheal Infection	
		No.	(%)	No.	(%)	No.	(%)
Pecora[19]	300	0		0		2	(0.7)
Kalinske[20]	102	2	(2)	0		0	
Hahn[22]	61	1	(1.6)	0		0	
Schreiner[23]	103	0		0		0	
Bartlett[21]	544	0		1	(0.2)	0	
Pratter[24]	100	3	(3)	1	(1)	0	
Totals	1210	6	(0.5)	2	(0.2)	2	(0.2)

[a]Other than confined to the anterior neck; includes pneumomediastinum.
[b]Other than blood-streaking of sputum.
(Matthay RA, Moritz ED: Invasive procedures for diagnosing pulmonary infection: A critical review. Clin Chest Med 2:3, 1981.)

stood.[21,25] In classifying patients according to the presence or absence of acute bacterial lung infection, the latter category represents an extremely heterogenous population. The "normal" lower respiratory tract of any patient is subject to a multitude of acute and chronic effects, many of which will influence whether a recoverable microbial flora will be present or not. As a general rule, in the setting of acute infection of the lower respiratory tract, we regard the presence of pathogenic microorganisms as diagnostic of parenchymal lung infection, and therefore as an indication for specific therapy.[15] This may not be true in all cases, since certain patients may have bacterial or fungal colonization of a major airway without lung parenchyma invasion.[5]

Statistics on the diagnostic accuracy of transtracheal aspiration presuppose familiarity with the principles and practice of the technique, prompt transfer of the specimen to the laboratory, and optimal methods of aerobic and anaerobic bacteriologic processing.[15,21] No single aspect of this sequence should be assumed to be adequate in itself, since the value of transtracheal aspiration depends on maximal care in both sampling and processing.

Complications

The safety of transtracheal aspiration has been documented by several large series in which experienced or closely supervised physicians have achieved acceptably low morbidity and mortality with the technique.[20–24] As with any invasive procedure, complications have been encountered, and the physician must carefully judge patient benefit against potential hazards.

Reported complications of transtracheal aspiration are listed in Table 10–2. Blood-streaking of the sputum occurs with such frequency that patients should be advised to anticipate mild hemoptysis during and after the procedure. This hemoptysis, however, is self-limited and usually remits within minutes. Isolated instances of life-threatening bleeding have been described,[26] and deaths from endotracheal hemorrhage and hematoma of the posterior wall of the trachea have been reported.[27,28] However, in a recent retrospective study of 100 consecutive patients who underwent transtracheal aspiration, gross but self-limited hemoptysis occurred in only one individual among subjects who were screened for clotting abnormalities prior to tracheal puncture.[24]

Localized subcutaneous emphysema has been reported in 5 to 10 percent of patients undergoing transtracheal aspiration.[20,22] The occurrence and severity of this complication are related to the amount of coughing during and after the procedure. Extensive subcutaneous emphysema of the neck, face, and chest wall, and pneumomediastinum have been described.[20] One case report documents bilateral pneumothorax occurring in a patient who underwent bronchoscopy and positive pressure (IPPB) respiratory therapy after a transtracheal aspiration-induced pneumomediastinum and pneumopericardium.[29]

While most infections with transtracheal aspiration have been localized to the region of the cricothyroid membrane, infection of the paratracheal puncture site has been reported,[19,30,31] although with far less frequency than might be anticipated with the withdrawal of a contaminated catheter through the pretracheal soft tissues; damage to the posterior tracheal wall may also predispose patients to infection.[31] A wide range of pathogens has been recovered from the soft tissues in such instances, including aerobic and anaerobic bacteria, *Mycobacterium tuberculosis*, and fungal microorganisms. While it would seem that the etiologic agent of the infectious complication would be among the organisms recovered from the transtracheal aspiration, this has not always been the case.[31]

Unusual episodes of acute respiratory failure and, in some instances, sudden death without substantial hemorrhage have been reported.[26,32] A specific event related to the procedure itself, such as the aspiration of gastric contents, may have been responsible for acute decompensation in these cases. However, these life-threatening complications have more often occurred in patients prone to arrhythmias or respiratory arrest as a result of severe hypoxemia or acidosis. In the more than 1200 procedures referred to in Table 10–2, no deaths occurred.

Recommendations

The decision to perform transtracheal aspiration in a patient with suspected infection of the lower respiratory tract is ultimately made by weighing the likelihood of obtaining information which will alter patient management against the risk of carrying out the procedure. Experience has shown that the greatest benefit from transtracheal aspiration is derived in the patient who is unable to raise sputum.[22] In the obtunded patient, transtracheal aspiration offers a simple, high-yield opportunity to obtain an uncontaminated sample of lower-respiratory-tract secretions.[15] The procedure also should be considered in patients with community-acquired infection who are unable to produce satisfactory sputum specimens despite adequate hydration or sputum induction. Particularly in cases noteworthy for atypical clinical or chest radiographic features, direct tracheal sampling usually allows some conclusion regarding the presence of a bacterial or nonbacterial process, and directs early therapy.[20,21]

Transtracheal aspiration has been useful in patients with suspected pneumonia and sputum production in whom routine sputum examination gives no indication of a likely pathogen, or in whom multiple microorganisms (particularly staphylococci or Gram-negative rods) are identifiable, but with no clearly predominant form.[20] Early transtracheal sampling may confirm the presence of bacterial infection and permit early, specific therapy based on Gram-stain findings. Patients for whom we presently favor such an aggressive early diagnostic approach include immunocompromised hosts. However, no data regarding outcome are available to substantiate this position. Regardless of the state of the particular host, transtracheal aspiration in this setting may minimize the need for nonspecific and potentially toxic broad-spectrum antibiotic coverage.[15]

We have discussed the limitations of transtracheal aspiration in patients who have received antibiotics, and have noted that the prior use of antibiotics may account for sterilization of the tracheobronchial tree. In one study, 44 of 48 patients with probable bacterial infection of the pulmonary parenchyma but with negative tracheal-aspirate cultures had received antimicrobial agents before the procedure.[21] However, Schreiner et al.[23] recovered bacteria from tracheal aspirates in 9 of 25 patients who had undergone antimicrobial therapy. Nevertheless, the difficulty in separating pathogens from nonpathogens in the setting of prior antimicrobial therapy is obvious, and current opinion would discourage transtracheal aspiration in such patients.[21,25]

On the basis of reported complications and experience with the successful use of protocols in performing the procedure,[21,24] certain recommendations can be made for increasing the safety of transtracheal aspiration.[15] The procedure should only be undertaken by experienced or well-supervised physicians on cooperative patients in whom the cricothyroid membrane and landmarks of the anterior neck are easily identified (Fig. 10–1). Before the procedure, abnormalities of clotting function, platelet count, and arterial oxygen tension should be measured and corrected. If such abnormalities persist, the potentially increased risk which they represent must be considered. During and for several minutes following the procedure, pressure should be maintained over the cricothyroid puncture site to minimize subcutaneous emphysema and soft-tissue bleeding. While severe or intractable cough represents a relative contraindication to transtracheal aspiration, the use of pressure over the cricothyroid membrane, cough suppressants, and the avoidance of any cough-inducing procedures will often be sufficient for preventing major complications.[22] Similarly, while marked hemoptysis is considered a contraindication to transtracheal aspiration, mild blood-streaking in the sputum of patients with normal clotting function and a normal platelet count may be handled with bed-rest and cough suppression following the aspiration.[28]

Aspiration Lung Biopsy

Diagnostic lung puncture was first described nearly 100 years ago,[33] but only during the last decade has it enjoyed a high level of acceptance. The use of image-intensified fluoroscopic guidance has increased the diagnostic capability of percutaneous puncture, while allowing the procedure to be practiced widely with an acceptable morbidity and low mortality.[34] Several large series have reported the use of percutaneous aspiration biopsy,[35] needle biopsy,[36] and trephine biopsy of the lung,[37,38] primarily as methods for diagnosing suspected neoplastic disease. Although the diagnostic yield of closed lung biopsy in inflammatory states has not been documented extensively, current opinion favors the use of fluoroscopically-guided needle aspiration in the taking of percutaneous biopsies for the diagnosis of localized pulmonary disease.

Although pneumocentesis was originally practiced in the setting of pulmonary infection, it has never become a popular method for the diagnosis of pneumonia. In 1936, Sappington and Favorite[40] showed it to be a simple and safe method, providing useful diagnostic and prognostic information in lobar pneumonia. However, enthusiasm for lung puncture declined with the advent of the antibiotic era and the de-emphasis of type-specific therapy for the pneumococcus. With the recognition of the need for specificity in antimicrobial treatment and the failure of routine culture specimens to direct therapy adequately, interest in the study of "lung juice" was rekindled.[41] This was particularly true in the pediatric literature, which includes a number of reports on the utility and safety of lung aspiration, often without the benefit of fluoroscopic guidance.[42–44]

The need for specificity in the therapy for infectious diseases has never been greater than today, when the immunocompromised population is confronted with an ever-increasing list of potential pathogens.[5] It is in this setting that aspiration lung biopsy has re-emerged as a promising modality, primarily in the immunosuppressed host.[15] For a discussion of lung aspiration techniques, the reader is referred to two quality reviews.[34,35]

Diagnostic Yield

The ability to directly sample an abnormal area of the lung is the greatest attribute of any form of lung puncture.[15] In the presence of suspected pulmonary infection, aspiration lung biopsy allows sampling of the parenchymal focus without the risk of contamination by upper-airway material.[15,36] Early experience indicated that positive lung cultures occurred in approximately 50 percent of cases of lobar pneumonia. However, Sappington and Favorite[40] described positive cultures in 90 percent of 60 patients with this entity, isolating essentially pure cultures of the pneumococcus in 51 cases, and a hemolytic streptococcus in 3.

Aspiration lung biopsy in the immunologically compromised host with focal pulmonary infiltrates has been described with encouraging results. Of 21 such biopsies described by Bandt et al.,[45] 16 (76 percent) demonstrated an infectious agent despite multiple inconclusive examinations of sputum, blood, and, in most cases, transtracheal aspirates. Infectious agents were later demonstrated in 3 of the 5 patients in whom aspiration lung biopsy was nondiagnostic.

In 1979, Castellino and Blank[46] published an update of the experience with aspiration lung biopsy in immunocompromised patients at the same institution at which Bandt and co-workers had done their study, describing 108 additional, presumed infectious episodes, with pulmonary infiltrates in 82 patients. As in the earlier study, patients were considered for aspiration lung biopsy when a prior diagnostic workup, including transtracheal aspiration, was negative or inconclusive. Aspiration yielded one or more infectious agents in 79 instances (73 percent), in 61 of which there was a single agent. In the remaining 29 negative aspirates, infection was established later in 15 and was presumed to be present in 9.

As part of their extensive experience with aspiration lung biopsy in 1211 patients, Sagel et al.[35] reported 31 immunosuppressed patients in whom a localized pneumonic infiltrate was aspirated. Cultures from 24 of these 31 aspirates showed an infectious agent; in all of these, the organism was demonstrable on a stained smear immediately following the aspiration procedure. The diagnostic rate of 77 percent is not detailed further, except for a note that some patients were receiving antibiotics at the time of aspiration lung biopsy. Recent reports describe the rapid diagnosis of Legionnaire's disease by direct immunofluoroscent staining of lung aspirates.[47,48]

Zavala and Schoell[47] have described their experience with "ultrathin (24- or 25-gauge) needle" aspiration biopsies in 50 patients, 25 of whom were thought to have pulmonary infection. Aspiration lung biopsy revealed pathogenic organisms in 15 of the 18 patients (83 percent) in whom an infectious process was actually present. This diagnostic sensitivity compares very favorably with that cited in earlier studies in which larger bore needles of 18 to 20 gauge were employed.

While we would conclude from these data that aspiration lung biopsy yields an impressive percentage of positive cultures in patients with suspected pulmonary infection, we are troubled by the apparent lack of sensitivity of this technique in patients shown subsequently to have infectious agents present in the pulmonary areas under study. To a certain extent, sampling techniques and the prior use of antibiotics will influence the rate of false-negative results. However, we wonder if the timing of the procedure (typically after a less invasive workup is not productive) may in some way affect the recovery of an organism from the area of radiographic abnormality. In this regard, a helpful study has been reported in which pediatric and adolescent immunocompromised patients suspected of having *Pneumocystis carinii* pneumonia were studied prospectively to determine the efficacy of aspiration lung biopsy.[49] Of the 202 patients examined, *P. carinii* was identified by lung aspiration in 121 (60 percent). Among this group, 13 patients died within 2 weeks of the onset of antimicrobial therapy, and *P. carinii* pneumonitis was found at autopsy in each. Of the 81 patients in whom *P. carinii* was not identified in the aspirate, 18 died and 63 recovered without trimethoprim-sulfamethoxazole or pentamidine therapy. Among the 18 who died, there were 6 cases of *P. carinii* pneumonitis recognized in 13 autopsies. Therefore, of 127 patients found to have *P. carinii* pneumonitis, 121 (95 percent) were diagnosed correctly by aspiration lung biopsy. Of particular interest was that all 6 of the patients in whom *P. carinii* was recognized at autopsy, but in whom lung aspirates did not yield this organism, had their aspirates taken before the use of fluoroscopically directed aspiration biopsy became routine.

Complications

We regard the low rate of reported complications with percutaneous aspiration biopsy, relative to that with other forms of lung puncture, as being of great importance.[15,37,50–54] The most common complication of aspiration lung biopsy in any series is pneumothorax, which occurs in approximately 25 percent of all cases.[51] A smaller percentage of pneumothorax cases will actually require some form of chest-tube drainage. Castellino and Blank,[46] who used an 18-gauge spinal needle for aspiration biopsy, reported pneumothorax in 28 (26 percent) of the 108 aspirations they performed in immunosuppressed hosts, with 14 patients (13 percent of the total group) requiring thoracostomy for relief of the complication.

In their experience with ultrathin-needle aspiration in 50 patients, Zavala and Schoell[47] report an 8 percent overall incidence of pneumothorax, with 2 patients (4 percent) requiring chest tube drainage. If the low rate of pneumothorax cited in this study is maintained as experience with fine needle aspirations increases, the overall complication rate of aspiration lung biopsy will decrease substantially.

Accumulated experience with 5300 needle aspirations for a variety of indications in 2726 patients resulted in moderate but self-limited hemoptysis in 5 percent of aspirations of central lesions and in 2 percent of aspirations of peripheral lesions.[51] In none of the smaller series describing aspiration lung biopsy in the compromised host does the incidence of hemoptysis exceed this. Greenman et al.[52] describe a significantly increased risk of bleeding complications of aspiration in patients with thrombocytopenia (platelet count less than 110,000/μl) or a prothrombin time of less than 60 percent of control values. Chaudhary et al.[49] report a fatal bleeding complication in a patient who had received platelets before lung aspiration. In contrast to this low rate of hemoptysis are the results, collected from two studies,[45,52] in a group of 16 patients at similar risk who underwent cutting-needle biopsy; 4 developed bleeding, which required transfusion in 3 cases, and 1 patient died.

Minor local bleeding in the vicinity of the aspirated lesion may occur in 11 percent of all patients undergoing aspiration lung biopsy.[51] There is no indication of a higher incidence of this complication among immunocompromised subjects. Nonetheless, we re-emphasize the aforementioned precautions regarding platelet count and clotting activity.

Because the needle used in aspiration lung biopsy is small, extension of disease from the lung parenchyma to the pleural space via the needle tract is an exceedingly rare complication of the procedure.[51] Implantation metastasis following the aspiration of malignant lesions has been reported,[51] and emphysema has been noted after lung aspiration for pneumonitis[40]; however, both are apparently very rare events.

An additional unusual complication of aspiration lung biopsy is air embolism.[53] This uncommon occurrence deserves mention not just because it is life-threatening, but also because the risk is decreased greatly by careful management of the needle hub and carefully instructed breathing on the part of the patient. Although deaths have been attributed to aspiration lung biopsy,[54] the mortality is acceptably low, especially when compared to that in other techniques of lung puncture which provide a larger specimen, such as cutting-needle biopsy or Trephine-drill biopsy.

Recommendations

Fluoroscopically directed aspiration lung biopsy results in an accurate diagnosis in approximately 90 percent of all patients.[35,39] Available data indicate that a specific etiologic diagnosis in suspected instances of pulmonary infection can be made in 75 to 80 percent of cases. Higher levels of accuracy may be obtained with certain pathogens.

In the immunocompromised patient with localized pulmonary infiltrates, aspiration lung biopsy should be considered early, as part of an orderly but prompt diagnostic evaluation. Future reports describing the respective yield, morbidity, and mortality of aspiration lung biopsy, bronchoscopy, and open-lung biopsy under such circumstances will be welcomed. At present, we would advise aspiration lung biopsy under conditions in which prompt and accurate processing of the aspirated sample would allow alternative diagnostic methods to proceed without unreasonable delay, should the results of lung aspiration be inconclusive.

As with any invasive procedure, patient selection for aspiration lung biopsy is very important, and screening for abnormalities of platelet count, clotting function, and arterial oxygen tension is essential. Patient cooperation is also essential, since respiration must be controlled according to the stage of the procedure.[34] Preexisting lung disease, particularly bullous emphysema, represents a relative contraindication to lung puncture,[35] and, because of the relatively high incidence of pneumothorax, the ability of the patient to withstand additional pulmonary embarrassment as opposed to the need for the procedure must be considered.[15]

Fiberoptic Bronchoscopy

Since its introduction by Ikeda and co-workers approximately 10 years ago,[55,56] the flexible fiberoptic bronchoscope has been employed widely to diagnose a variety of pulmonary disorders.[15,57–62] The procedure is performed easily,[56,60] is associated with few complications,[63,64] and affords greater visualization of the endobronchial tree than does rigid bronchoscopy.[54,55] Furthermore, patients can undergo fiberoptic bronchoscopy with minimal discomfort, and biopsy of previously inaccessible areas of the lung may be accomplished through the use of biopsy forceps with the fiberscope.[15,57,58,61,62]

Details of techniques for passing the fiberoptic bronchoscope, and methods for obtaining specimens with this instrument have been published.[57,60–62,65–69] The transnasal approach is employed most often,[57,59,66,67,70–72] but some investigators[37,58,61,73–75] prefer to pass the fiberscope through either a rigid bronchoscope or endotracheal tube. This method permits removal and reinsertion of the instrument atraumatically, and guarantees adequate control of the airway if a cardiorespiratory complication occurs during the procedure. In general, experience at centers that utilize the transnasal approach to routine flexible fiberoptic bronchoscopy almost exclusively does not support the need for intubation or rigid bronchoscopy prior to this procedure.[57,59,66,70] Removal and reinsertion of the instrument are unnecessary except under unusual circumstances, and life-threatening emergencies are rare if the procedure is performed properly.[59] When fiberoptic bronchoscopy is done on the critically ill patient with obtundation and severe hypoxemia, passage of the fiberscope through an endotracheal tube is advisable.

Several types of specimens can be obtained through the fiberscope for culture or histologic diagnosis of lower respiratory tract disease, or for both purposes. These include washings from the bronchi and alveolar spaces,[66,69,76–79] brush specimens,[37,57,66,67,80,81] and transbronchial forceps biopsies.[37,57,58,61,67–70,74,81]

Contamination of washings and brush specimens obtained during fiberoptic bronchoscopy by bacteria from the upper airways has raised the question whether cultures from these specimens reflect the microflora of the lower respiratory tract.[65,82] Bartlett et al.[65] report that contamination of fiberoptic bronchoscopy specimens by oropharyngeal flora is a frequent occurrence, even when the bronchoscopy is done through an endotracheal tube. In their study, 80 strains of bacteria were isolated from 17 patients who had no evidence of pulmonary infection at the time the bronchoscopy specimens were obtained.[65] However, a recently developed, telescoping double catheter with a plugged tip, passed through the fiberoptic bronchoscope, may achieve more reliable culture results.[83] Moreover, transbronchial forceps biopsies obtained during fiberoptic bronchoscopy can provide an accurate diagnosis of fungal and protozoal lung infections in immunocompromised hosts.[37,66–71,81]

Diagnostic Yield

The broadest experience with fiberoptic bronchoscopy in diagnosing lung infections has been with immunocompromised patients. The results of eight studies utilizing transbronchoscopic forceps and brush biopsies in immunocompromised patients are summarized in Table 10–3. A specific etiologic diagnosis, usually infection or pulmonary involvement by the underlying disease, was made after 121 of 234 procedures (52 percent). Forceps biopsies provided a specific diagnosis in an average of 41 percent of the cases (range 26 to 68 percent), while brushing was diagnostic in 27 percent (range 8 to 63 percent). The studies showing forceps-biopsy diagnostic yields at the two extremes of 26 percent and 68 percent[66,80] are balanced by the results in five other studies in which the yield was 38 to 46 percent (average 42 percent) (Table 10–3).[37,66,68,70,71] The less favorable forceps biopsy diagnostic results reported by Nishio and Lynch[81] are due in part to failure to obtain lung parenchyma in 7 of 47 cases. The higher-than-average yield (68 percent) achieved by Matthay et al.[67] may have been due to a bacterial diagnosis in 9 of 25 cases. This 36 percent incidence of bacterial lung infection is higher than

Table 10–3. Specific Etiologic Diagnosis by Fiberoptic Bronchoscopy Procedures in Immunocompromised Patients

	Transbronchial Biopsy			Bronchial Brushing			Combined Biopsy and Brushing		
		Specific Diagnosis			Specific Diagnosis			Specific Diagnosis	
Author	No.	No.	(%)	No.	No.	(%)	No.	No.	(%)
Nishio[81]	47	12	(26)	56	8	(14)	47	14	(30)
Pennington[68]	14	6	(43)	14	0	(0)	14	6	(43)
Feldman[70]	38	16	(42)	38	3	(8)	38	17	(45)
Poe[71]	35	16	(46)	ND	ND	(ND)	ND	ND	(ND)
Cunningham[37]	31	13	(42)	31	9	(28)	31	15	(48)
Lauver[66]	24	9	(38)	36	18	(50)	37	22	(59)[a]
Phillips[69]	ND	ND	(ND)	ND	ND	(ND)	42	26	(62)[a]
Matthay[67]	25	17	(68)	25	16	(63)	25	21	(84)
Totals	214	87	(41)	200	54	(27)	234	121	(52)[b]

ND = no data.
[a]Combined yield from transbronchial biopsy, bronchial brushing, and bronchoalveolar washing.
[b]Combined yield excluding Lauver and Phillips is 47 percent (73/155).
(Matthay RA, Moritz ED: Invasive procedures for diagnosing pulmonary infection: A critical review. Clin Chest Med 2:3, 1981.)

that reported by the other seven groups of investigators in their immunosuppressed hosts undergoing bronchoscopy (Table 10–3).[37,66,68–78,81]

Lung infections diagnosed by forceps or brush biopsies of lung parenchyma in the eight studies summarized in Table 10–3 and in other studies[57,80,82–87] included those caused by *Pneumocystis carinii* (Fig. 10–6), fungi (aspergillus [Figs. 10–4B, C and 10–5], candida, cryptococcus, histoplasma, blastomyces), viruses (*Herpes simplex*, cytomegalovirus), *Mycobacterium tuberculosis* (Fig. 10–3), nocardia (Fig. 10–4A), and a variety of Gram-positive and Gram-negative bacteria. In many cases, bacterial diagnoses made by bronchoscopy were subsequently confirmed by positive blood cultures or at autopsy, or both. Forceps and brush biopsies were particularly successful in diagnosing *Pneumocystis carinii* infections.[57,67,80,86]

Although forceps biopsies gave a higher diagnostic yield than brush specimens, the latter added to the diagnostic yield of forceps biopsies in at least four studies[37,67,70,81] (Table 10–3). These data suggest that brush specimens in addition to forceps biopsies should be obtained at bronchoscopy. Moreover, although adequate data are not yet available for critical analysis, two groups of investigators[66,69] have indicated that bronchoalveolar washings add to the yield of both forceps and brush biopsies. In other studies, lung lavage alone has provided a diagnosis of lung infection, including that caused by *Pneumocystis carinii.*[76–79] The true diagnostic yield of bronchoalveolar lavage relative to forceps and brush biopsies in the immunocompromised patient requires further study.

Forceps biopsies reveal nonspecific inflammation in as many as 30 to 50 percent of bronchoscopy procedures in immunocompromised patients with diffuse pulmonary infiltrates.[68,71,81] Nishio et al.[81] have questioned the adequacy of nonspecific diagnoses obtained with transbronchial biopsies in immunocompromised hosts. The investigators reported nonspecific inflammatory or fibrotic changes in 16 of 47 procedures (34 percent). In 7 of these 16, a specific diagnosis was obtained subsequently at open lung biopsy or by other techniques. Among the diagnoses missed by transbronchial biopsy were Hodgkin's disease, squamous cell carcinoma, cryptococcosis, and *H. influenza* and *Pneumocystis carinii* infection.[81] In contrast, Poe et al.[71] reported that 12 of 15 immunosuppressed patients having nonspecific transbronchial biopsy results responded clinically and radiographically to specific therapy or were shown to have untreatable disease. The data from three other studies,[57,67,70] involving a total of 108 patients, corroborate the findings of Poe and co-workers. In these studies, the overall sensitivity (true-positive ratio) was 83 percent, and the specificity (true-negative ratio) was 100 percent, figures nearly identical to those of Poe et al.[71] Moreover, of the 13 "false negative" biopsies (a negative or misleading biopsy result), in the three studies just mentioned only 4 cases were of an infectious etiology.[57,67,70]

Unfortunately, even with the accurate diagnosis of lung infiltrates in the immunocompromised host with hematologic malignancy, there is little evidence that subsequent application of specific therapy has improved the outcome for the affected patients. In fact, Pennington et al.[68] showed no improvement in mortality after fiberoptic bronchoscopy was introduced and utilized to diagnose a variety of lung infections and other entities in patients with hematologic malignancy. Thus, although a specific diagnosis can be made with bronchoscopic techniques in approximately 50 percent of immunosuppressed patients with pulmonary infiltrates (Table 10–3), the prognosis for these patients remains poor.

Plugged Telescoping Brush-In Catheter System

Previous studies[65,82] have established that in most cases, brush and wash material cultured from the lower respiratory tract during bronchoscopy is likely to be contaminated with oropharyngeal microorganisms. Moreover, anesthetic agents introduced into the airways during bronchoscopy inhibit the growth of potential bacterial isolates.[11] The new, plugged telescoping brush-in catheter system[83] is under investigation as an alternative method for obtaining lower-respiratory-tract secretions without contamination from the channel of the fiberscope. Wimberly and co-workers,[83] who developed this catheter, suggest that it may provide more specific bacteriologic information.

Data on 10 patients from a recent study by Hayes et al.[88] suggest that the plugged telescoping catheter successfully delivers a sterile brush via a bronchofiberscope into the lower respiratory tract for specimen collection without contamination by upper airway flora. When these investigators passed the plugged catheter brush through a fiberoptic bronchoscope into the trachea, cultures from the brush demonstrated no growth. This is in contrast to a nonplugged, sterile bronchial brush-in-catheter system, which gave positive cultures in 5 of 9 patients.

Fletcher et al.[89] using the plug-protected specimen brush in patients with pneumonia, failed to diagnose postmortem-confirmed Gram-negative pneumonias in 75 percent of the cases. Moreover, upper respiratory contaminants were isolated from the brush specimen. In 13 patients with presumed pulmonary infection, LeGrand et al.[90] reported discrepancies between aerobic and anaerobic organisms isolated by transtracheal aspiration and those isolated by the telescoping catheter. These two studies[89,90] suggest that further, careful evaluation of the plugged brush-in-catheter system is required before it is accepted as a standard clinical tool for the diagnosis of lung infection.[15]

Complications

Bronchoscopy is generally considered a safe procedure. Two large-scale retrospective studies of 24,000 and 48,000 procedures, respectively, revealed few serious complications and a total of only 11 deaths.[63,64] Periera et al.[91] reported 16 cases of transient postbronchoscopy fever and 6 of increasing pulmonary infiltrates among 100 patients on whom the procedure was done. Aelony et al.[92] and Webb et al.[93] each reported 3 cases of new postbronchoscopy pneumonia. In 1975, Flick and coworkers[94] reported a case of fatal hemorrhage following forceps biopsy of the middle lobe. Zavala[62,74] subsequently emphasized the importance of wedging the fiberscope into the biopsied subsegment for several minutes in order to reduce bleeding and the escape of blood into the other airways. This method is now practiced widely and, although prospective controlled studies documenting this conclusion are unavailable, the wedging technique, as practiced at our institution, seems to reduce the bleeding complications of bronchoscopy.

The complications noted by seven groups of investigators who performed 231 bronchoscopies in immunocompromised patients are listed in Table 10–4. Moderate hemorrhage ($\geq$ 25 ml) occurred in 17 cases and pneumothorax in 17, an incidence of 7 percent for each complication. These data suggest that even in the severely compromised host, bronchoscopy is safe provided that proper precautions are taken. In patients with thrombocytopenia (platelet count $<$ 100,000/μl), platelet transfusions are indicated to obtain a count of 100,000/μl or greater before bronchoscopy is done.[66,91] A markedly abnormal prothrombin time or partial thromboplastin time may increase the bleeding tendency, and uremia has been demonstrated to cause bleeding after bronchoscopic lung biopsies.[37] The occurrence of bleeding in 8 of 31 patients (26 percent) in a study by Cunningham et al.[37] represents a higher incidence than in most other series, primarily due to the large number of uremic patients who underwent biopsy (Table 10–4).

Arterial hypoxemia with a 10 to 20 mmHg decrease in oxygen tension is common during bronchoscopy.[95,96] Albertini et al.[95,96] and others[68,74] have emphasized the need for oxygen supplementation during bronchoscopy, especially in patients who have an arterial oxygen tension of less than 50 to 60 mmHg while breathing room air.

Table 10–4. Complications of Fiberoptic Bronchoscopy Procedures in Immunocompromised Patients

Author	No. of Procedures	Hemorrhage[a]		Pneumothorax	
		No.	(%)	No.	(%)
Nishio[81]	47	2	(4)	2	(4)
Pennington[68]	14	0	(0)	0	(0)
Feldman[70]	38	0	(0)	4	(11)
Cunningham[37]	31	8	(26)	6	(19)
Lauver[66]	34	2	(6)	0	(0)
Phillips[69]	42	3	(7)	3	(7)
Matthay[67]	25	2	(8)	2	(8)
Totals	231	17	(7)	17	(7)

[a]Hemorrhage ≥ 25 ml.

(Matthay RA, Moritz ED: Invasive procedures for diagnosing pulmonary infection: A critical review. Clin Chest Med 2:3, 1981.)

Recommendations

In immunocompromised hosts with fever and focal or diffuse pulmonary infiltrates, it is reasonable to examine the sputum, a transtracheal aspirate, or both, and to start antibiotic therapy on the basis of the microorganisms identified. However, if no diagnosis is evident after such specimens have been obtained, or if the patient fails to respond to directed antibiotic therapy, fiberoptic bronchoscopy should be done to obtain forceps and brush biopsies, as well as wash specimens. Oxygen supplementation should be used during the procedure, and a platelet transfusion administered to achieve a platelet count of at least 100,000/μl before the procedure is begun.

Open-Lung Biopsy

In 1949, Klassen et al.[97] reported the first large series of open-lung biopsies. At that time, they introduced the small thoracotomy incision, entering the pleural space through the anterior fourth interspace without rib resection. Subsequently, Klassen and Andrews[98] reported the results of 270 open-lung biopsies done with the foregoing technique in patients with diffuse pulmonary lesions. A number of other investigators have used this or similar techniques to diagnose diffuse lesions in both immunocompromised and nonimmunocompromised hosts.[52,98–105]

Patients undergoing open-lung biopsies usually receive general anesthesia and endotracheal intubation.[98,101] Generally, two techniques are employed for the biopsy: a conventional posterolateral thoracotomy with or without rib resection, and a small anterior intercostal incision.[97,98,101,102] The posterolateral thoracotomy permits detailed evaluation of the intrathoracic structures and biopsy not only of the lung and pleura, but also of the peribronchial, hilar, and mediastinal lymph nodes.[98] Frequently, however, patients undergoing open-lung biopsy have extensive bilateral lesions, a low respiratory reserve with a low arterial oxygen tension and, occasionally, a low blood volume. The lateral position can interfere with pulmonary ventilation, and the posterolateral thoracotomy incision is associated with an average blood loss of 500 cc.[98] Therefore, this procedure is generally

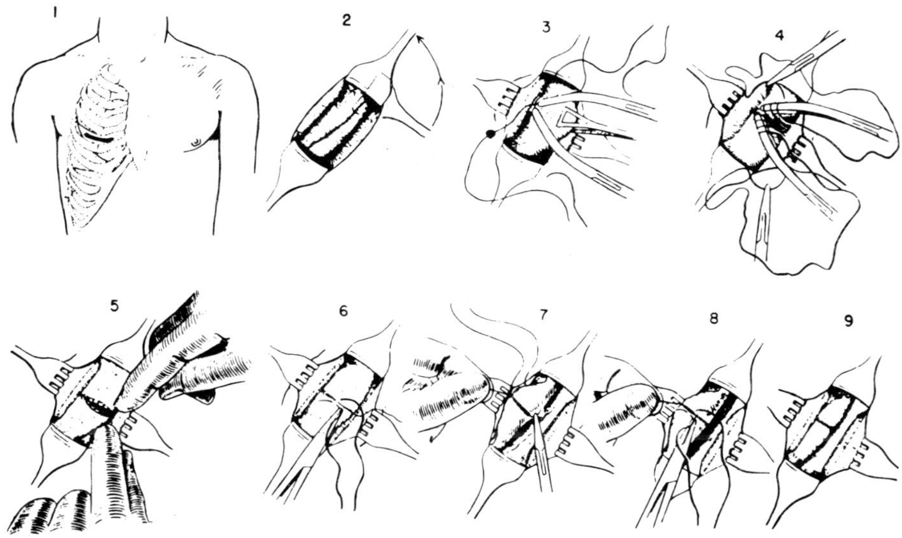

Figure 10–2. Illustration of technique for anterior thoracotomy. (Adapted from Klassen KP, Anlyan AJ, Curtis GM: Biopsy of diffuse pulmonary lesions. Arch Surg 59:694, 1949. Copyright 1949, American Medical Association.)

reserved for patients in good clinical condition in whom lymph node biopsy as well as lung biopsy is required.[98,101]

In most cases, a small anterior thoracotomy (4 to 10 cm) is performed, usually through the fourth intercostal interspace, utilizing a submammary incision (Fig. 10–2).[97,98,102] In patients with more extensive involvement of the posterior and apical portions of the lung, an axillary approach can be used. This exposes the fourth rib between the posterior border of the pectoralis major and the anterior border of the latissimus dorsi muscles. The entire thoracic cavity is inspected and palpated. Excision of several wedges of pulmonary tissue from representative areas is advisable. To perform the biopsy, the margin of the lobe is grasped with a noncrushing forceps and brought into the field, and a wedge-shaped specimen is resected. A thoracostomy tube is left in the pleural space for controlled suction for approximately 24 hours, and removed after a chest radiograph shows complete expansion of the lung.[98]

The biopsy specimens taken from the lung can be sent for routine, fungal, and acid-fast cultures, and a complete pathologic evaluation. Touch preparations can be made immediately and processed rapidly for special stains designed to reveal organisms, including fungi and *Pneumocystis carinii.* Care must be taken to handle the surgical specimen in a sterile manner if cultures are to be done.

Diagnostic Yield

Examination of the tissue from 288 open-lung biopsies performed on immunocompromised patients in six studies revealed a specific, potentially treatable entity, usually infection or pulmonary involvement by the underlying disease, in 198 (69

Table 10–5. Specific Etiologic Diagnosis Obtained by Open-Lung Biopsy in Immunocompromised Patients

Author	No. of Procedures	Specific Diagnosis	
		No.	(%)
Rossiter[106]	83[a]	46	(55)
Singer[105]	44	27	(61)
Greenman[52]	48	31	(65)
Leight[102]	42	30	(71)
Wolff[107]	24	21	(88)
Rosen[103]	47	43	(91)
Totals	288	198	(69)

[a]Thirteen of 83 patients were not immunocompromised.
(Matthay RA, Moritz ED: Invasive procedures for diagnosing pulmonary infection: A critical review. Clin Chest Med 2:3, 1981.)

percent) (Table 10–5). The specific yield in these six studies ranged from 55 to 91 percent.[52,102,103,105–107] As in bronchoscopy, a wide range of organisms was isolated, including *Pneumocystis carinii*, aspergillus, candida, nocardia, *Mycobacterium tuberculosis*, viruses (adenovirus and cytomegalovirus), and Gram-negative and Gram-positive bacteria.

Four studies[52,102,105,106] demonstrate the incidence of a nonspecific diagnosis, inflammation, fibrosis, or both, obtained at open-lung biopsy. Nonspecific diagnoses were noted in 13 percent,[52] 29 percent,[102] 39 percent,[105] and 45 percent,[106] of cases, respectively, in the four studies. Thus, about 32 percent of open-lung biopsy procedures in the immunosuppressed host result in nonspecific diagnoses (range: 13 to 45 percent).

Rossiter and co-workers[106] reported that 46 of their patients in whom open-lung biopsies yielded a specific diagnosis fared no better than those without diagnoses (a hospital mortality of 26 percent [12 of 46 patients] versus 24 percent [9 of 37 patients], p = N.S.). These figures are similar to those in bronchoscopy studies done by Pennington et al.[68] However, Singer et al.[105] reported a 28 percent survival in immunosuppressed patients who did not undergo lung biopsy versus 48 percent in those who had an open-lung biopsy.

Complications

The relative safety of open-lung biopsy has been documented in the literature in both nonimmunocompromised [97,98,101,104] and immunocompromised patients. [52,102,103,105–107] The complications observed in 288 open-lung biopsies are listed in Table 10-6. Pneumothorax was the most common complication, occuring in 8 percent of cases. Bleeding complications (hemothorax, wound hematoma, and hemoptysis) were rare. In six series [52,102,103,105–107] the overall complication rate was 11 percent (Table 10-6)—a rate similar to that for fiberoptic bronchoscopy (Table 10-4). Thus, with the open-lung biopsy techniques now utilized widely, this procedure can be performed safely. Of 288 consecutive procedures there have been only two definite biopsy-related deaths reported (0.6 percent).

Table 10–6. Complications of 288 Open-Lung Biopsy Procedures in Immunocompromised Patients[a]

Complication	No. of Occurrences	(%)
Pneumothorax	22	(8)
Hemothorax	2	(0.6)
Wound hematoma	1	(0.3)
Hemoptysis	1	(0.3)
Wound dehiscence	1	(0.3)
Incisional neuritis	1	(0.3)
Tumor recurrence at chest-tube site	1	(0.3)
Death	2	(0.6)
Totals	31/288	(11)

[a]Adapted from references 52,102–107.
(Matthay RA, Moritz ED: Invasive procedures for diagnosing pulmonary infection: A critical review. Clin Chest Med 2:3, 1981.)

Recommendations

In most centers, open-lung biopsy is indicated in immunocompromised patients with diffuse or focal pulmonary infiltrates and suspected lung infection if no specific diagnosis is obtained after bronchoscopy with transbronchial forceps and brush biopsies, after percutaneous needle aspiration, or after all of these procedures. The results of at least one study of immunocompromised hosts [71] suggest that open-lung biopsy is not required if nonspecifc inflammation, fibrosis, or both are found on bronchoscopic forceps biopsies of involved lung parenchyma. However, the study by Nishio and Lynch [81] revealed treatable entities at open-lung biopsy that were missed by transbronchial forceps biopsies at bronchoscopy. These results may be closer to the overall experience. Until more definitive data are available, we must in most cases recommend proceeding to open-lung biopsy after obtaining negative or nonspecific fiberoptic bronchoscopy biopsies. Each center attempting to determine the etiology of pulmonary infiltrates in immunosuppressed hosts should evaluate its own yield, and the complications from percutaneous needle aspiration, bronchoscopy biopsies, and open-lung biopsy. If percutaneous lung aspiration, bronchoscopy biopsies, or both are nonspecific in an immunosuppressed patient, the chances of identifying a treatable entity by open-lung biopsy at the investigating institution must be determined.

PULMONARY INFECTIONS ENCOUNTERED IN IMMUNOCOMPROMISED PATIENTS

Although some pathogens, such as *S. aureus*, in immunosuppressed patients also can cause disease in normals, most of the organisms that cause infections in immunocompromised patients are opportunistic pathogens. The term opportunistic infection implies infection by an organism that is not normally pathogenic, and which the normal host encounters without evidence of disease. Normally harmless

Table 10–7. Opportunistic Pathogens Causing Pulmonary Infection in Immunocompromised Hosts

Bacteria	Fungi	Protozoa and Parasites	Viruses
Escherichia coli	*Aspergillus*	*Pneumocystis*	Cytomegalovirus
Pseudomonas	*Candida*	*Toxoplasma*	*Herpes simplex*
Klebsiella	*Coccidioides*	*Strongyloides*	Varicella-Zoster
Serratia	*Cryptococcus*		Measles
Nocardia	*Phycomycetes*		Adenoviruses
Tubercle bacillus	*Torulopsis*		Epstein-Barr virus
Listeria			
Legionella pneumophila			
Atypical mycobacteria			

(Adapted from Matthay RA, Greene WH: Pulmonary infections in the immunocompromised patient. Med Clin North Am 64:529, 1980.)

organisms invade the host when there is an alteration in host defense because of disease or cytotoxic drugs. Examples of such organisms are listed in Table 10-7[108]

Common pathogens isolated in immunosuppressed patients, and the associated immunologic deficit in these patients, are shown in Table 10-8.[108] In general, patients whose underlying defect involves polymorphonuclear leukocyte production and function seem to become infected primarily by S. *aureus* , and especially by the aerobic, Gram-negative enteric bacilli that account for the majority of nosocomial infections.[4,5] Primary nonbacterial infection, pulmonary or otherwise, is uncommon in the purely leukopenic or leukocyte-dysfunctional states. Such infection occurs mainly among patients who also have received corticosteroids or broad-spectrum antibiotics or both which depress cell-mediated defense mechanisms and promote nonbacterial growth. Among patients whose major defect involves the synthesis of normal immunoglobulin, or who have decreased reticuloendothelial function (such as postsplenectomy patients, particularly children), the clearance of bacteria that have antiphagocytic capsules is impaired. Thus, prior to the era of myelosuppressive chemotherapy, *Streptococcus pneumoniae* (pneumococcus) and *Hemophilus influenzae* were particularly common among patients with multiple myeloma,[109] and remain so for those with congenital or acquired hypogammaglobulinemia or hyposplenism.[110] Individuals whose underlying deficit relates to cell-mediated immune mechanisms are uniquely susceptible to tuberculosis, candidiasis, cryptococcosis, listeriosis, and other infections (Table 10-8). In these diseases, adaptation to an intracellular residence has allowed such pathogens to escape extinction by neutrophil and antibody-complement-mediated attack.[108] Defense against these invaders depends upon an intact T cell–macrophage alliance that results in macrophage activation and in the generation of cytotoxic effector cells. Depression of these defenses is particularly common among patients with Hodgkin's disease or transplants, or those receiving steroids. Finally, the most common abnormality in host defense is some mucocutaneous boundary alteration that results in a change of normal flora or a break in the physical intactness of the mucosa or skin (Table 10-8). Common mucocutaneous portals of entry for infecting organisms include: (1) the respiratory tract, via tracheostomies or aspirated oro-

Table 10–8. Association of Pathogens in Immunocompromised Patients with Underlying Immunologic Deficit

Depression of Leukocyte Bacterial Functions	Depression of Humoral Immune Response	Depression of Cellular Immune Response	Depression of Mucocutaneous Boundary Functions
Pseudomonas	Pneumococci	Tubercle bacillus	Staphylococci
Serratia	*Hemophilus*	*Candida*	*Escherichia coli*
Staphylococci	*Pseudomonas*	*Listeria*	*Klebsiella*
Nocardia	*Pneumocystis*	Herpes simplex	*Pseudomonas*
Candida		*Toxoplasma*	Anaerobes, esp. *Bacteroides*
Aspergillus		*Pneumocystis*	*Candida*
		Cytomegalovirus	

(Adapted from Matthay RA, Greene WH: Pulmonary infections in the immunocompromised patient. Med Clin North Am 64:529, 1980.)

pharyngeal flora; (2) the skin, via indwelling intravenous catheters or decubitus ulcerations; and (3) the urinary tract via indwelling Foley catheters.[108]

Thus, a broad variety of common as well as uncommon and opportunistic pathogens (Tables 10-7 and 10-8) cause infection in immunosuppressed patients. The following discussion focuses upon those organisms typically encountered in compromised hosts with pulmonary infection.

Bacteria

Although there is variation in the epidemiology and frequency of bacterial pneumonia among different classes of compromised hosts, all have shared the general upward trend in the frequency of Gram-negative pneumonia. This has been particularly true among patients with cancer. In several recent studies of cancer patients, 90 percent of all bacterial pneumonias were caused by Gram-negative organisms.[4,6,7,111] Similarly, in transplant patients, more than 70 percent of bacterial pneumonias are due to Gram-negative organisms. In contrast, only about 50 percent of all nosocomial pneumonias and no more than 10 to 20 percent of community-acquired pneumonias are due to Gram-negative bacilli.[112] Because Gram-negative bacilli are opportunistic pathogens, elements that compromise the host enhance the development of pneumonia with these organisms. In the general hospital population, such elements may include gross aspiration of pharyngeal contents, the bypassing of upper airway defenses via intubation or tracheostomy, or interference with the cough reflex by drugs or surgery. The classic compromised hosts are individuals with malignant disease or transplants, or those requiring immunosuppressive therapy. Additional predisposing factors to Gram-negative bacterial pneumonia include: (1) interference with the granulocytic response to infection (by virtue of granulocytopenia or corticosteroid administration); (2) impairment of pulmonary alveolar macrophage function (by steroids or cytotoxic agents)[113]; and (3) improper pulmonary drainage (caused by an obstructing tumor or decreased cough).

The epidemiology of these pneumonias is of interest. Among patients with adult acute leukemia, substantial myelosuppression is induced at the very onset of the disease. At this stage, infection, especially pneumonia, may mitigate effective chemotherapy or, if fatal, may abrogate an anticipated prolonged survival. In contrast, bacterial pneumonia as a complication of the treatment of lymphoma or most solid tumors usually occurs near the end of useful therapy and less commonly compromises survival statistics.[114] It can be anticipated, however, that as myelosuppressive chemotherapy achieves greater responses (as, for example, in testicular cancer), the risks of toxicity will be balanced by the potential gains, and opportunistic pneumonia will become even more common. The pattern among patients with renal transplants is different, reflecting the differing periods of maximal immunosuppression. In general, bacterial disease is especially evident during the first posttransplant month and at 4 months or more after transplantation.[115,116] The intervening period (from 1 to 4 months) appears to be a time of particular susceptibility to nonbacterial infections, particularly by cytomegalovirus. Of note, however, is the high mortality in this population when bacterial infection presents not as a primary infection but as a superinfection imposed upon preceding viral or other pulmonary processes.

The organisms most commonly causing pneumonia in the immunodeficient host are the aerobic Gram-negative enteric bacilli. *Escherichia coli, Klebsiella* species, *Pseudomonas aeruginosa*, and mixed bacterial infections predominate. Other organisms such as *Enterobacter* species, *Proteus* species, and *Serratia marcescens* usually are less predominant. Among the less frequently seen Gram-positive pathogens, *Staphylococcus aureus* continues to be important.[117] However, there is considerable interinstitutional variation, not only in the major bacterial species causing pneumonia in immunocompromised patients, but also in their antibiotic susceptibilities.[118] Thus, each institution has a responsibility to determine its own offending pathogens and their susceptibilities in order to design rational empiric antibacterial therapy. A confounding aspect of choosing such therapy is the recent recognition of *Legionella pneumophila* as a part of the differential diagnosis of pneumonia in compromised hosts, especially those with renal disease requiring dialysis or transplants, those with cancer, and those who are taking immunosuppressive drugs.[119]

Few features of Legionnaires' disease distinguish it from the more common Gram-negative enteric bacillary pneumonias; patients receiving corticosteroids and those with renal transplants seem particularly predisposed to the disease.[120,121] Because of difficulties in establishing the diagnosis, many empirical regimens for pneumonia now include erythromycin. Among immunosuppressed hosts, recommendations have been made for parenteral use of this drug in doses of 2 to 4 gm per day for 3 weeks. If Legionnaires' disease is established, or seems very likely, and the patient is not responding to erythromycin, some have suggested the addition of rifampin[120,121] based on in vitro susceptibilities.

Another bacterium, distinct from *Legionella pneumophila* but now classified as a species of *Legionella*, has been described as an opportunistic pulmonary pathogen. This Gram-negative, weakly acid-fast organism has been visualized or recovered and grown from lung tissue in several institutions.[17,122,123] Initially called the "Pittsburgh pneumonia agent," it has infected with particular frequency renal transplant patients and those taking corticosteroids, and appears to be susceptible to erythromycin, rifampin, and trimethoprim-sulfamethoxazole.

In patients with severe neutropenia, the classic clinical presentation of pneumonia may be obscured.[46,124] Sputum may be produced in only 50 percent of these patients,[4,6] and whatever sputum is produced may be difficult to identify as such because of a lack of purulence. Similarly, on physical examination, rales may be absent in 25 percent of neutropenic patients with pneumonia, and signs of consolidation may be absent in more than 50 percent. Clinically, the most reliable finding in both cancer and transplant patients is the presence of fever. In the severely compromised host, fever should prompt an immediate chest radiograph. Even if initially negative, the chest radiograph should be repeated frequently, since a pulmonary infiltrate will be found in from 83 percent[6] to 96 percent[4] of such infections. Radiographically, bacterial pneumonias in these patients tend to be multifocal, involving the lower lobes especially; lobar consolidation and abscess formation are infrequent. With rare exception, it is impossible to implicate a specific organism from the chest radiograph. A specific diagnosis is obtained from cultures of blood, pleural fluid (if present), and appropriately obtained pulmonary specimens, as outlined previously.

Nocardia

Although nocardia is a bacterium, it is considered separately, since it occurs primarily in immunosuppressed hosts. Nocardiosis is being diagnosed with increasing frequency.[1] Prior to 1957, only 50 cases were reported, but an additional 180 cases were reported during the next 4 years.[125] Patients with serious underlying disease are especially susceptible to this infection, and the rapid increase in its incidence has been largely in these patients. Typical antecedent illnesses include lymphoma, carcinoma, sarcoidosis, and alveolar proteinosis. In addition, nocardia infections occur in patients who have had organ transplants.[125-128] Approximately 80 percent of nocardiosis occurring in cancer patients occurs in those with hematologic malignant diseases, especially lymphomas,[128] and most of these patients are receiving antitumor agents and adrenal corticosteroids when the infection develops. About 20 percent of nocardia infections occur in patients receiving corticosteroids.[129] Neutropenia is not an important predisposing factor, and only about 25 percent of affected patients are neutropenic.[125]

Although there are several species of nocardia, only *N. asteroides* is a frequent pulmonary pathogen.[1] This organism is a Gram-positive, partially acid-fast bacillus; it forms delicate branching filaments, but may appear as fragmented bacillary coccoid forms. It grows aerobically but may require several weeks incubation, and often is not isolated from culture specimens.

The infection may be chronic or fulminant. The respiratory tract is the site of entry in 70 percent of cases of nocardiosis, the skin in 27 percent, and the gastrointestinal tract in 3 percent.[125] About 30 percent of patients have disseminated infection.[125] The organs most commonly involved include the lungs, skin, brain, spleen, kidney, heart, liver, bone, and lymph nodes. Nocardial pulmonary infection may present as lobar pneumonia, a single nodule (Fig. 10-4 A) or multiple nodules, miliary abscesses, or thick-walled cavitary lesions.[125,130] The pulmonary infection also may be associated with pleural effusion, empyema, and occasionally with sinus tracts. The usual clinical symptoms are fever, night sweats, and a productive cough.[125]

Tubercle Bacillus

Among the many patients being treated with long-term immunosuppressive drug therapy are those, particularly the elderly, who have been exposed to tuberculosis in the past and have old, healed primary or postprimary tuberculous lesions which may harbor viable *Mycobacterium tuberculosis.* Long-term immunosuppressive therapy, especially with corticosteroids, may allow these previously dormant organisms to multiply and cause life-threatening, progressive pulmonary or disseminated tuberculosis (Fig. 10-3 A and B). In one series of patients with neoplastic disease,[131] there was a 17 percent mortality as a direct result of tuberculous infection. The records of patients who died as a result of tuberculosis indicated that in most cases this diagnosis was not considered antemortem. Had the diagnosis been made earlier, the mortality from tuberculosis could certainly have been reduced.[1]

There appears to be a correlation between high doses of immunosuppressive drugs and the severity of tuberculosis at the time of its diagnosis.[132] Tuberculosis is also a common complication of lymphoma, particularly Hodgkin's disease and chronic lymphocytic leukemia. Before effective therapy was available for either malignant disease, tuberculosis developed in 20 percent of patients with Hodgkin's disease.[125,133] However, during the past two decades, tuberculosis has developed in less than 1 percent of patients with any form of cancer. Tuberculosis is most prevalent in patients with bronchogenic carcinoma, lymphoma, gastric carcinoma, and multiple myeloma.[125] The infection is most likely to be disseminated in patients with lymphoma and in those receiving radiotherapy, corticosteroids, and chemotherapy. While the overall mortality among immunosuppressed patients with tuberculosis is 17 percent, it is nearly 50 percent in individuals with lymphoma.[125]

Cancer patients appear to have an unusually high incidence of atypical mycobacterial infections. During a 5-year period at one cancer hospital, 50 percent of mycobacterial infections were caused by an atypical strain of the organism,[125] either *M. kansasii* or *M. fortuitum.* These infections can be difficult to treat because the organisms are resistant to many antituberculous agents.[1]

Careful assessment of the risk of tuberculosis should be made in any patient for whom long-term immunosuppressive therapy is contemplated.[132] As mentioned above, the risk seems to be highest in patients receiving prednisone (above 10 mg per day), particularly in association with additional immunosuppressive agents. All patients should have a tuberculin skin test as well as chest and abdominal radio-

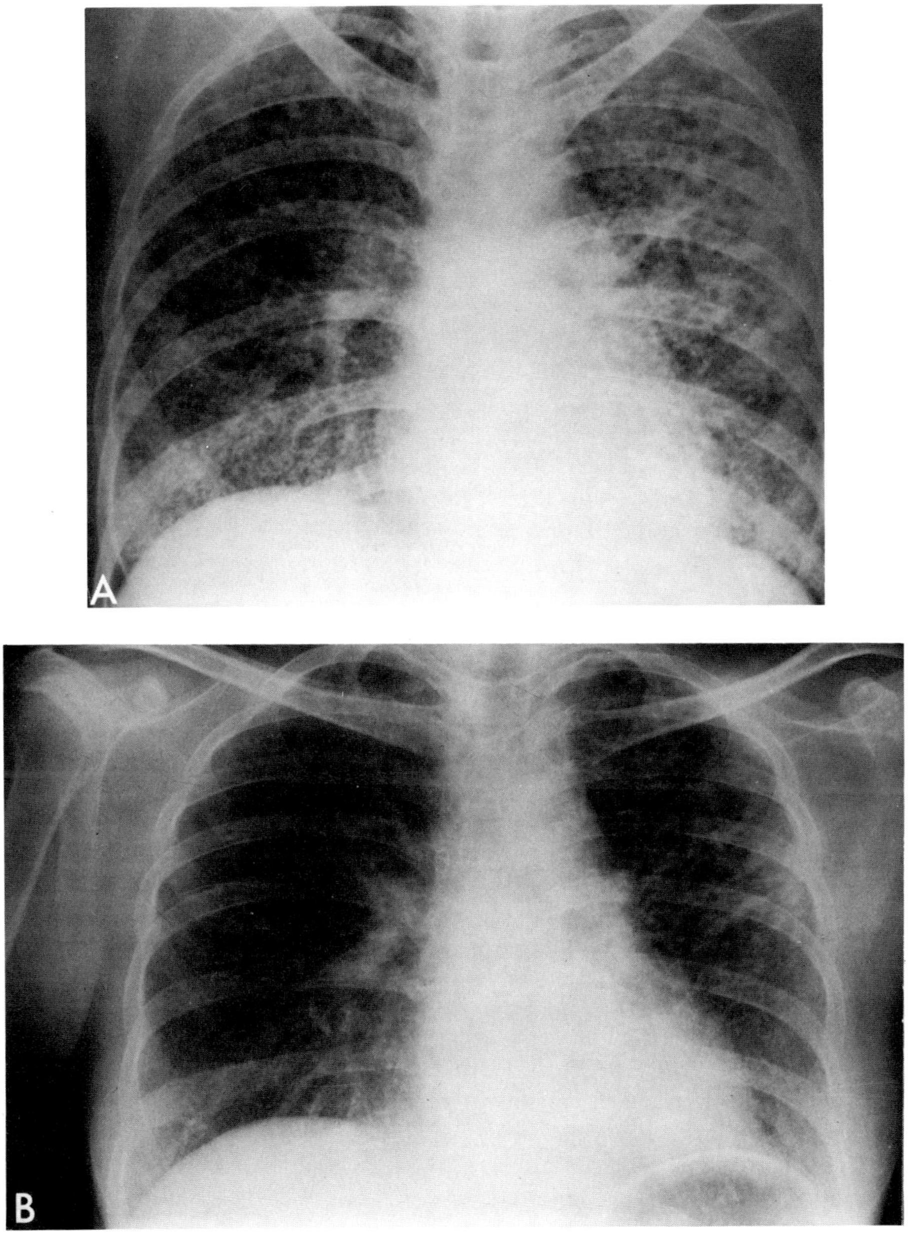

Figure 10–3. Pulmonary tuberculosis. (A) Posteroanterior chest radiograph shows new-onset diffuse, bilateral small nodules in a 31-year-old Korean woman receiving 60 mg of prednisone per day for systemic lupus erythematosus. Sputum cultures revealed tubercle bacilli. (B) Posteroanterior chest radiograph after 3 months of treatment with isoniazid, ethambutol, and streptomycin reveals dramatic clearing. (Matthay RA, Greene WH: Pulmonary infections in the immunocompromised patient. Med Clin North Am 64:529, 1980.)

graphs before long-term immunosuppressive therapy is started. Isoniazid chemoprophylaxis (300 mg per day) for as long as the immunosuppressive therapy is prescribed has been recommended in patients with a positive tuberculin skin test, in those with old, healed calcified lesions on a chest radiograph, or in those with calcified abdominal nodes on radiographs.[132]

Any abnormality of the chest radiograph should be assessed carefully to exclude tuberculosis. Radiographically, the chest infiltrates of tuberculosis in immunosuppressed hosts are variable. Among the many patterns that occur are upper lobe cavitary lesions, lobar consolidation, and a miliary infiltrate (Fig. 10-3 A and B).

In all immunosuppressed patients, regular clinical, bacteriologic, and radiologic review is essential; and in view of the suppression of symptoms by corticosteroids, the development of a cough, of sputum production, or of dyspnea should be viewed with suspicion.[1] The sputum in such patients should be routinely evaluated for tubercle bacilli by smear and culture. Any patient in whom lesions highly suggestive of tuberculosis develop should be treated with at least two antituberculous drugs while awaiting the results of smear and culture. The foregoing and other precautions should reduce further the incidence of severe tuberculosis associated morbidity and perhaps mortality in the immunosuppressed patient.

Fungal Infection

Among patients with acute leukemia and lymphoma, fungi cause 30 percent of fatal infections[7,134,135] and 15 to 20 percent of fatal pneumonias.[7,134] In renal transplant patients the incidence of fungal infections is lower, but seems clearly related to the vigor and frequency of therapy for rejection episodes.[136] Some factors responsible for this phenomenon are prolonged granulocytopenia, corticosteroid administration, the prolonged administration of broad-spectrum antibiotic agents, and conditions or drugs which suppress cell-mediated host defenses (Table 10–8).[5] A limited number of different genera of fungi are being isolated with increasing frequency in the compromised host.[4,7] These primarily include aspergillus (Figs. 10–4B and C; 10–5A and B), candida, mucorales, and, perhaps, torulopsis. In addition, cryptococcus and histoplasma may be found with greater frequency and with greater likelihood of dissemination among patients with leukemia, lymphoma, and transplants, but there is little evidence of any increasing incidence of these infections among such patients. Finally, there are a large number of fungi, among them sporothrix, coccidioides, and blastomyces, which cause sporadic disease in both normal and compromised hosts but which are much more likely to disseminate in the latter.

Candida and *aspergillus* species (Figs. 10–4B and C; 10–5A and B) account for more than 90 percent of all fungal infections in patients with malignant disease,[3,4,7,137] and are the predominant fungal pathogens following organ transplantation.[9,138] The host-defense abnormalities that occur in the general hospital setting are primarily alterations in mucocutaneous boundaries, such as those among patients undergoing abdominal surgery and receiving broad-spectrum antibiotics. Fungal infection in such cases is usually caused by one of the *candida* species (Table 10–8).

Two recent studies[139,140] have established that the extension of candidal infection to the lungs occurs via two routes with similar frequency: (1) hematogenous dissemination, as part of multiple organ involvement; and (2) aspiration of pharyngeal contents. In the former case, candidal overgrowth in another organ, usually the gastrointestinal tract,[139] results in invasion of the blood with miliary extension to other organs, particularly the kidneys and lungs. In the latter case, tracheal, laryngeal, pharyngeal, esophageal, or gastric candidasis associated with aspiration leads to candidal bronchitis and bronchopneumonia.[139,140]

Although pathologically one may see solid nodules, abscesses, consolidation, or bronchopneumonia,[4,139,140] the clinical and radiologic picture in candidal infection is so variable and so often obscured by associated infectious and noninfectious pulmonary involvement that no "typical" presentation can be described. Rather, the appropriate setting, evidence of widespread colonization or local invasion or both on mucosal surfaces of the gastrointestinal and genitourinary tracts, and the presence of a pulmonary infiltrate, either unexplained or unresponsive to other therapeutic measures, should suggest the possibility of candidiasis. Substantiating the diagnosis may be difficult because sputum cultures, even transtracheal samples or those obtained at endoscopy, may reflect upper airway contamination. Unfortunately, even biopsies rarely document invasive pulmonary candidiasis[140]; positive blood cultures are present in no more than 25 to 33 percent of these cases. However, in the setting of immunosuppressive therapy, leukopenia, and multiple positive cultures at four or more other sites, and in the absence of a contaminated intravenous catheter, the isolation of candida from the blood should suggest clinically important dissemination.[141] Diagnosis by serologic means may be helpful, particularly if a fourfold increase in the candida precipitin titer is documented[5]; however, a negative test does not rule out invasive disease. Diagnosis by the detection of antigenemia[142] and by gas-liquid chromatography of blood specimens[143] are promising newer procedures not yet widely tested or available. Evidence of dissemination to the retina by fundoscopic examination, or to the skin by biopsy, also may aid the diagnosis in some patients with invasive candidiasis.

Invasive aspergillosis is the other major fungal infection accounting for mortality among severely immunocompromised patients. Unlike candidiasis, aspergillosis almost always (90 percent of cases) involves the lungs, from which dissemination to other organs may occur.[144,145] Occasionally, primary infection may begin in the sinuses or even the skin. One of the singular characteristics of aspergillus, and the phycomycetes (mucor) as well, is its tendency to grow across blood vessels, inducing thrombosis, infarction of tissue, and bleeding. Thus, the most common radiographic appearance of pulmonary aspergillosis is that of a multifocal necrotizing bronchopneumonia (Figs. 10–4B and 4C; 10–5A and 5B).[144] However, the infection may even appear as lobar disease, making specific radiographic diagnosis hazardous. Unfortunately, sputum is rarely helpful in making the diagnosis since the organism is not usually recovered from expectorated secretions. Until recently, only invasive measures providing biopsy material had a substantial likelihood of yielding the diagnosis. However, newer studies have suggested the utility of passive hemagglutination[146] and enzyme linked immunosorbent assays (ELISA)[147] for the detection of changes in aspergillus antibody. In one study, a

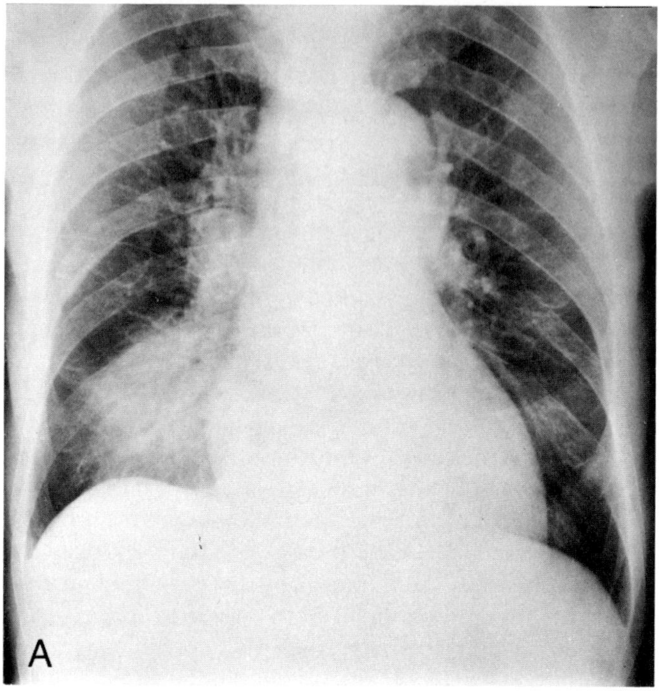

Figure 10–4. Nocardia lung infection and invasive pulmonary aspergillosis. (A) Posteroanterior chest radiograph shows a well-circumscribed, focal infiltrate in the right lower lung zone (nocardia) in a 65-year-old man receiving vincristine and prednisone for histiocytic medullary reticulosis. The patient's temperature was 101°F and the white blood cell count was 850 cells per μl.

radioimmunoassay (RIA) proved successful in detecting aspergillus antigenemia in 4 of 7 patients with systemic aspergillosis, and in the pleural fluid of a patient with aspergillus empyema.[148] The incidence of aspergillosis varies considerably from institution to institution and from time to time, and may reflect the extent of environmental contamination.[149,150]

Mucormycosis (phycomycosis) refers to infection with any of several genera of the order mucorales, predominantly ubiquitous species of absidia, mucor, and rhizopus, all of which produce similiar clinical effects and are almost solely pathogens of diabetics and severely immunocompromised hosts.[4,151–153] Disease caused by these fungi tends to present in one of three ways: (1) rhinocerebral, which occurs particularly in poorly controlled diabetics, with initial involvement of the vestibule, facial sinuses, or both, with contiguous spread to the orbit and base of the brain; (2) pulmonary, which is usually found among cancer patients, especially those with leukemia and lymphoma,[153] and among patients with transplants; and (3) gastrointestinal, which predominately involves the stomach or colon, presenting as hemorrhagic ulceration and infarction.[152] In a review of

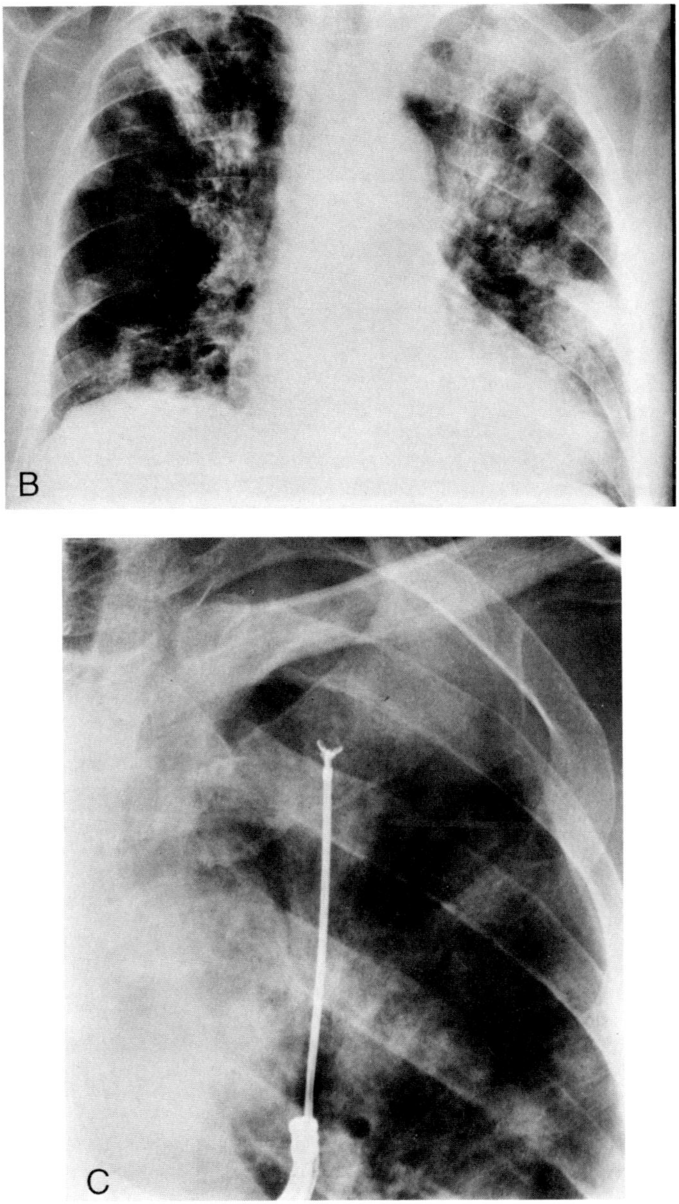

Figure 10–4 (continued). (B) Posteroanterior chest radiograph taken 3 months later shows diffuse bilateral nodular densities developing while the patient was receiving cytotoxic drugs and prednisone. (C) Chest radiograph shows biopsy forceps extending from the fiberscope into the left upper lung zone. *Aspergillus fumigatus* was isolated from brush and forceps specimens. The patient died several days later despite therapy with amphotericin B. (Matthay RA, Greene WH: Pulmonary infections in the immunocompromised patient. Med Clin North Am 64:529, 1980.)

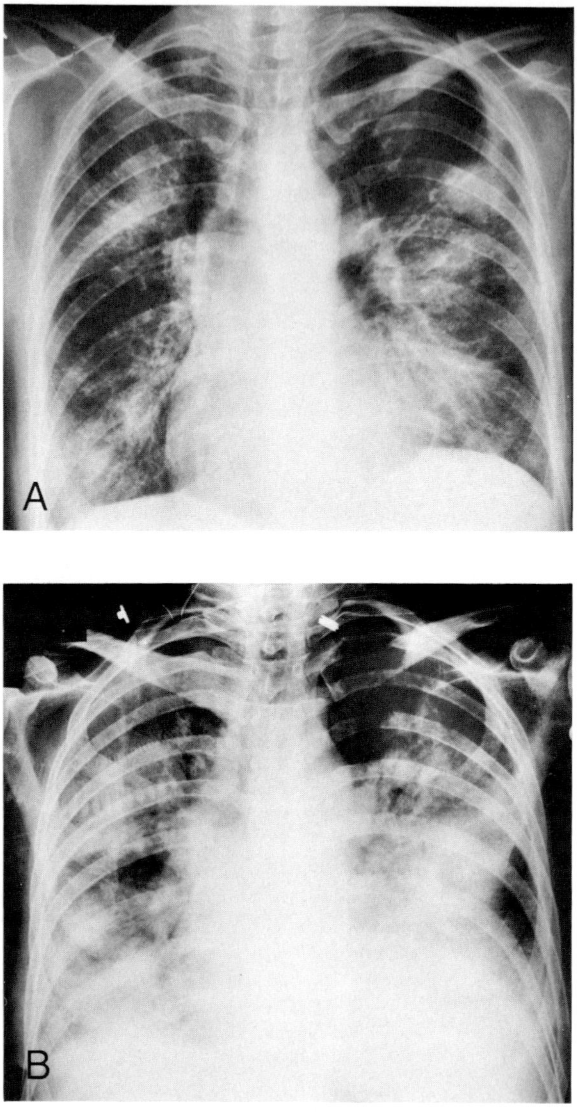

Figure 10–5. Invasive pulmonary aspergillosis. (A) Posteroanterior chest radiograph shows a bilateral patchy and nodular infiltrate in a 43-year-old woman with acute myelogenous leukemia. Brush and transbronchial forceps lung biopsies revealed *Aspergillus fumigatus*. (B) Anteroposterior chest radiograph 7 days later shows progression of the infiltrates to a more homogeneous pattern despite amphotericin B therapy. The patient never entered partial or complete remission from her leukemia, and died of overwhelming invasive pulmonary aspergillosis several days later.

mucormycosis in a cancer hospital, Meyer et al.[153] found that 21 of 26 cases had pulmonary involvement, and that 10 of these 21 also had disseminated disease. In all anatomic locations, including the lung, the clinical manifestations of mucormycosis are dominated by the tendency for these fungi, like *aspergillus sp.*, to grow across tissue lines, including organ boundaries and especially blood vessel walls. This latter tendency results in thrombosis, with organ infarction and hemorrhage. Fever is usually present and, in the pulmonary form of the infection, there is an antibiotic-resistant infiltrate on the chest radiograph. However, the latter is variable in appearance, and may range from bronchopneumonia to cavitation and fungus-ball formation.[5,153] Although the rhinocerebral presentation of mucormycosis is quite singular, the pulmonary form is not. Since serodiagnosis is essentially unavailable, the diagnosis of mucormycosis rests almost invariably on the biopsy or brushing demonstration of the wide, nonseptate hyphae in tissue specimens. Because of the infrequency of this infection (less than 3 percent of autopsied leukemia and lymphoma patients[153], and the frequent failure to diagnose it antemortem, the optimal therapy for the pulmonary form of mucormycosis is not well defined. Although some have suggested surgical resection where possible, Medoff and Kobayashi[155] reported a case of pulmonary mucormycosis, in a patient with acute lymphocytic leukemia, that was treated successfully with amphotericin B only. Thus, aggressive diagnostic procedures may allow discovery of the infection early enough to render medical therapy successful. This subject has recently been reviewed.[156]

Although the mortality for aspergillus and mucor infections remains high, there have been recent reports of the successful treatment of both diseases.[145,155] Such reports have emphasized the necessity for early diagnosis and for the prompt initiation of appropriate antifungal therapy, in some instances empirically.

Torulopsis glabrata is a yeast that has caused infection in compromised hosts under circumstances and in a manner very similar to those associated with infection by candida, to which it is taxonomically related.[157,158] *T. glabrata* is a commensal, like candida, and can be found in the normal respiratory, gastrointestinal, and vaginal flora. Thus, infection with the organism can be documented only by its isolation from a normally sterile body source, or by histologic demonstration of the yeast form in tissue, or both. The absence of pseudohyphae distinguishes *T. glabrata* infection from candida infections. Although its incidence may be increasing[157] *T. glabrata* is still a very unusual cause of pneumonitis in most hospitals. There is no defined radiographic picture of torulopsis pneumonia, and the infection is often of mixed etiology, with other fungi and bacteria.

Protozoa

Two protozoa, *Pneumocystis carinii* and *Toxoplasma gondii*, may cause severe pulmonary infection in immunocompromised hosts. *P. carinii* has been responsible for as many as 45 percent of cases of interstitial pneumonia among cancer patients.[160] Rarely, the organism disseminates to invade the liver, spleen, lymph nodes, and bone marrow.[161] Patients less than 20 years old have accounted for 35 percent of infections with this organism, and about 5 percent of children with cancer have been found to have *P. carinii* infection at autopsy.[125] In one study, a substantial number of *P. carinii* infections occurred in children with leukemia in remission and receiving maintenance therapy.[162] The attack rate per year had been estimated at 1 percent in patients with acute lymphocytic leukemia, 0.5 percent in patients with chronic lymphocytic leukemia, 0.4 percent in patients with Hodgkin's disease, and 0.2 percent in patients with acute myelogenous leukemia.[163] Infection with the organism may represent the reactivation of dormant disease or recent exposure,[1] but in recent years has markedly declined in frequency with the use of trimethoprim-sulfamethoxazole chemoprophylaxis.

The characteristic clinical features of *Pneumocystis carinii* infection are fever, a nonproductive cough, dyspnea, and cyanosis. Physical findings are usually minimal or absent.[125] The disease may develop over a 1- to 2-month period or may progress rapidly over a 4- to 5-day period. If untreated, it usually terminates in death from severe respiratory insufficiency.

The diagnosis of *Pneumocystis* pneumonia should be suspected in the patient with progressive dyspnea and cyanosis, few physical findings, and increasing pulmonary infiltrates.[1] *Pneumocystis carinii* is seldom found in smears of sputum, hypopharyngeal secretions, or tracheal aspirates. Percutaneous needle aspiration has been especially useful in diagnosing the disease in children.[164] In adults, the combination of transbronchial forceps and brush biopsies via the flexible fiberoptic bronchoscope is recommended for establishing the diagnosis.[57,67,165] Specimens obtained from the lung should be stained with Gomori's methenamine-silver nitrate impregnation technique and a polychrome stain such as that of Giemsa or Gram-Weigert, or methylene blue. The toluidine blue stain is useful for the rapid processing of specimens.[166,167]

Although the chest radiograph classically shows bilateral diffuse perihilar infiltrates extending toward the periphery, and these infiltrates have commonly been called interstitial,[125] it is clear that *P. carinii* pneumonia has atypical radiologic features.[168] In general, the infiltrate is initially a patchy reticulonodular process progressing to a diffuse alveolar consolidation (Fig. 10–6A and B). Although historically described as an "interstitial pneumonia," acute pneumocystis pneumonia is really a combination of alveolar or air-space consolidation with a variable interstitial component.[168] Early acinar involvement may be confused with interstitial disease on the chest film, but rapid progression leading to coalescence of bronchograms makes the predominantly alveolar nature of the pneumonia evident. Extensive air bronchograms were seen in 53 percent of 30 patients in a recent series.[168] Atypical radiologic features of this disease include a unilateral predominance, lobar distribution, nodular densities, abscess formation, and even a normal chest radiograph.[168]

The earliest histologic evidence of pulmonary pneumocystis infection is the presence of cysts and trophozoites within the cytoplasm of cells attached to the alveolar walls.[125] As the disease progresses, the alveoli become filled with an intense, foamy exudate, presumably derived from the organisms. The alveolar cells are markedly hypertrophied and are associated with infiltration of mononu-

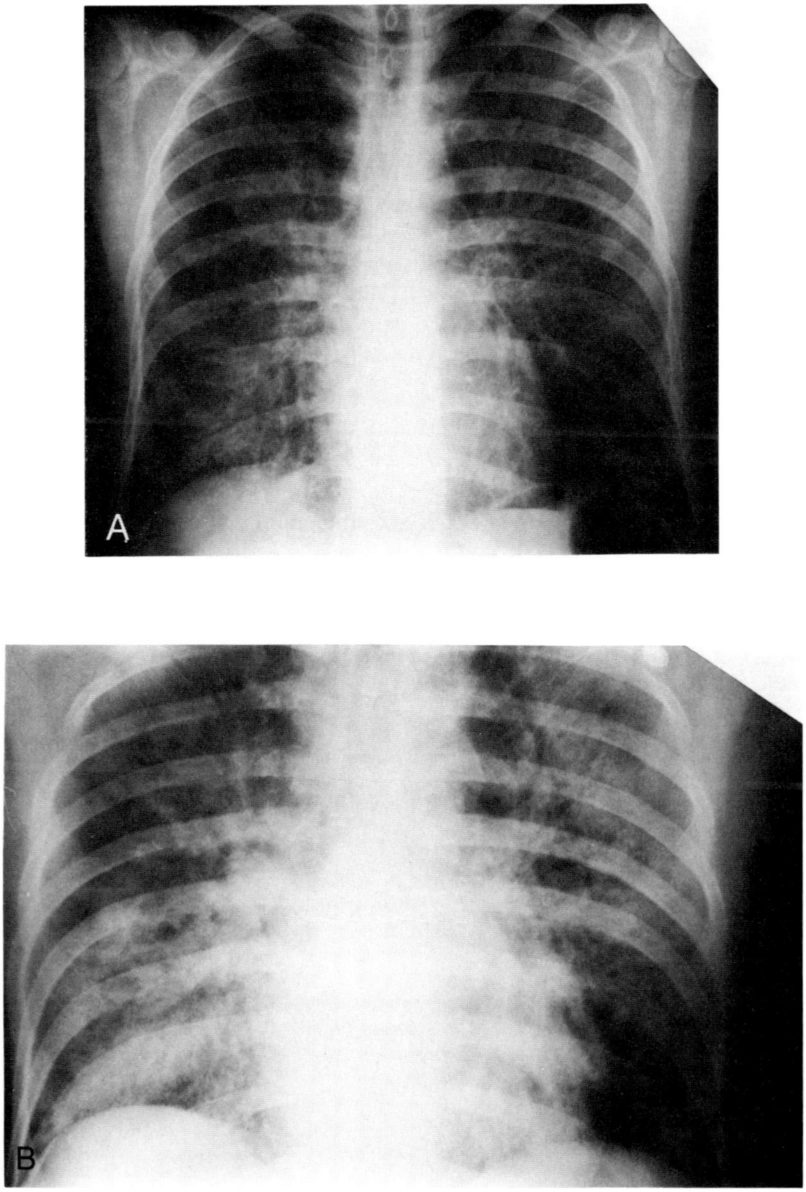

Figure 10–6. *Pneumocystis carinii* lung infection. (A) Posteroanterior chest radiograph shows diffuse, alveolar-interstitial infiltrates, most marked in the central lung zones, in a 32-year-old man with stage IV-B Hodgkin's disease. Cytotoxic chemotherapy and prednisone had been discontinued several weeks previously. Brush and forceps biopsy specimens obtained at bronchoscopy showed *Pneumocystis carinii*. (B) Anteroposterior (supine) chest radiograph taken 8 days later shows a diffuse alveolar filling process which evolved despite therapy with pentamidine and later trimethoprim-sulfamethoxazole. The patient died 6 weeks later in respiratory failure.

clear cells. Cysts of the organism can be identified in the alveoli, and consist of an outer, double-layered wall containing from two to eight internal bodies.[125]

Approximately 40 percent of pneumocystis pneumonia patients treated with pentamidine isethionate recover.[169] If the patient survives long enough to receive a week of therapy, the recovery rate is about 60 percent. Symptoms generally improve within 1 to 6 days after the institution of therapy. Nearly 50 percent of patients who receive pentamidine have adverse reactions, including azotemia (25 percent), liver function abnormalities (10 percent), hypoglycemia (6 percent), and skin rashes (2 percent). Local pain and abscess formation have been reported in 18 percent and acute hypotension in 10 percent of patients.[125]

Toxoplasma gondii is an obligate intracellular parasite that causes a variety of clinical syndromes including pneumonia, chorioretinitis, and a disease similar to infectious mononucleosis.[1,125,170] Toxoplasmosis, an infrequent but serious disease in patients with cancer, occurs most often in patients with Hodgkin's disease, but also in those with other lymphomas and leukemia.[171] This disease may represent either the reactivation of a latent infection or a newly acquired infection.[125] The organism may be transmitted by pets, by the ingestion of improperly cooked meat products, and by blood transfusion.[125]

In a collated series of 37 cases of toxoplasmosis in cancer patients, central nervous system involvement occurred in 90 percent, heart involvement in 40 percent, and lung involvement in 30 percent.[172] Other organs affected included the liver, kidney, lymph nodes, spleen, and bone marrow. In the lungs, the parasites invade alveolar cells and endothelial cells, causing intense inflammation, interstitial hemorrhage, and a homogeneous alveolar exudate.[125]

The diagnosis of toxoplasmosis is established by the identification of organisms in clinical specimens or by serologic tests. *T. gondii* can be identified microscopically in the blood, sputum, cerebrospinal fluid, and tissue of infected patients.[125] Numerous serologic tests for the organism are available, including the Sabin-Feldman dye test, the immunofluorescent antibody test, and the IgM-fluorescent antibody (IgM-IFA) test.[170,172] A single high titer ($\geq$1:80) in the IgM-IFA test or in the conventional IFA or Sabin-Feldman dye tests ($\geq$1:1000), in the setting of encephalitis in the compromised host, may be sufficient for the diagnosis of or presumptive therapy for toxoplasmosis.[173] Recently, antigenemia has been reported.[174]

Viral Infections

As indicated in Table 10–7, the major viral pathogens among compromised hosts are cytomegalovirus, *Herpes simplex*, varicella-zoster virus, and measles and adenoviruses. Vaccinia virus infections were also of concern until the abolition of routine smallpox vaccination. Unlike bacterial and fungal pneumonias, the development of pulmonary involvement with the herpes viruses occurs in relatively well-defined epidemiologic groups.

Cytomegalovirus

Although evidence of the serologic and virologic activation of cytomegalovirus infection occurs in more than 25 to 33 percent of children[175] and adults[176] with neoplasia, most infected patients are asymptomatic, and pneumonitis is an unusual accompaniment of the infection. Although cytomegalovirus is seen occasionally at autopsy and may be responsible for death, other, coexisting infectious syndromes are usually considered of greater importance. In contrast, among patients undergoing bone marrow and renal transplantation, cytomegalovirus infection is a major cause of morbidity and mortality.[154,177] Among patients receiving marrow transplants, an interstitial pneumonitis develops in 30 to 50 percent[177] within 4 months after transplantation, and is accompanied by fever, a nonproductive cough, dyspnea, and hypoxemia.[154] The mortality from respiratory failure in these patients has been from 50 to 60 percent and, at autopsy, approximately 50 percent have had histologic evidence of disseminated and pulmonary cytomegalovirus infection in the absence of other pathogens. Similarly, serologic and virologic evidence of cytomegalovirus infection was demonstrated in 73 percent of patients in a careful prospective study of renal-transplant recipients.[178] In many instances the transplanted organs themselves have been implicated as the agent of transmission of the virus. Most patients with a primary cytomegalovirus infection (those with no antibody to cytomegalovirus demonstrable prior to infection), and perhaps 25 to 30 percent of those with reactivation infection, develop clinical syndromes.[179,180] These syndromes have been characterized by one or more of the following manifestations: fever, leukopenia, atypical lymphocytosis, pneumonitis, and hepatitis. Less commonly, cytomegalovirus infection may appear as retinitis, arthritis, or gastrointestinal ulceration.[181,182] Most of these syndromes occur in the 1- to 4-month period after transplantation, and correlate with episodes of graft rejection and maximal immunosuppression.[115] Cytomegalovirus infection may appear on the chest radiograph as a diffuse, interstitial pneumonitis or, in some instances, as a diffuse small (2 to 4 mm) nodular infiltrate, with prominence in the peripheral lung zones.[5]

Diagnosis of this infection may be difficult, because fourfold serologic changes may occur without disease, and disease may occur without serologic evidence. Isolation of the virus from the urine may persist for months after a transplant and, may therefore not indicate active disease. More reliable are the isolation of cytomegalovirus from cultures of peripheral blood buffy coat[183] and the demonstration of characteristic intranuclear inclusions of the virus in lung-biopsy tissue. However, the frequent association of cytomegalovirus with other pulmonary pathogens, especially *Pneumocystis carinii* and *Toxoplasma gondii*, should alert the physician to the possibility of mixed infections, one component of which may be more treatable than the cytomegalovirus infection.

In this regard, two recent studies in renal transplant recipients have documented the frequency and severity of superinfection superimposed upon a preceding cytomegalovirus infection.[115,116] The variety of superinfecting organisms in such cases has been great, ranging from *Pseudomonas aeruginosa* and other bacteria to candida, aspergillus, and *Herpes simplex*. In many instances the superinfection seemed related to cytomegalovirus-induced or drug-induced profound granulocytopenia.

Winston and colleagues[184] recently have called attention to the role of prophylactic granulocyte transfusions in the transmission of cytomegalovirus among patients with acute leukemia or bone marrow transplants. The extent to which therapeutic blood products are also responsible for such infection is uncertain.

Varicella-Zoster Virus

Among normal children, varicella (chickenpox) is a benign illness with rare visceral manifestations and an even rarer mortality. Among immunosuppressed children, however, the frequency of visceral varicella involvement, and especially pneumonic involvement, is considerably greater and, in one series, was 14 percent (4 of 30 cases). Three of the 4 affected children died.[185] In normal adults, varicella, while rare, is more severe. Pulmonary involvement, which occurs in 15 percent of cases, is fatal in 10 percent.[186] More commonly, evidence of infection with the varicella-zoster virus among adults, as well as in some children, is the reactivation syndrome of shingles (Herpes zoster).[187] In contrast to cytomegalovirus infection, the greatest frequency of Herpes zoster is seen among lymphoma patients, particularly those with Hodgkin's disease, with estimates of its frequency of incidence ranging from 15 to 38 percent in recent series.[187,188] The frequency is lower among patients with non-Hodgkin's lymphoma, renal transplants (about 7 percent),[178] acute leukemias, and solid tumors. Indeed, the last-named group shows little increased frequency of Herpes zoster as compared to normal populations. However, this can be expected to change with the greater practice of immunosuppressive therapy for solid tumors. This increase was noted recently in two reports of an 8 to 12 percent incidence of zoster, with frequent cutaneous dissemination, among patients with small-cell carcinoma of the lung who were subjected to radiation, chemotherapy, or both.[189,190] Among immunosuppressed patients with zoster, dissemination (primarily cutaneous) occurs in from 6 to 26 percent of cases,[187] with only occasional (less than 3 percent) pulmonary involvement and mortality. However, morbidity may be considerable.

The pneumonias of varicella and zoster are similar and are characterized radiographically by a widespread, small (< 0.5 cm) nodular infiltrate in a peribronchial distribution, with greater density near the hilum and sparing of the apices.[186]

These pulmonary lesions appear clinically during the period of cutaneous dissemination of the viral infection, and are accompanied by a temperature exceeding 103°F in one-third of patients, and by cough, dyspnea, chest pain (often pleuritic), and hemoptysis. Physical examination of the chest may disclose rales, wheezing, and rhonchi, but is often unimpressive and fails to reflect the extensive radiographic involvement that is seen. Establishing the diagnosis is usually not difficult because of the constant association of the infection with the characteristic rash. However, the differentiation of varicella and zoster infections from bacterial superinfection[186] is sometimes necessary, especially in children.

It should be noted that substantial prevention or amelioration of the symptoms of varicella in immunosuppressed children can be achieved with zoster immune globulin if this is given within 72 hours of exposure to the virus.[185] Strict criteria have been devised for the use of this globulin,[187] and it should not be given to exposed adults, most of whom already have antibody to varicella-zoster virus.

Other Viruses

Herpes simplex viruses[191] have been implicated in rare cases of opportunistic pneumonias, involving patients with burns, immunosuppression, and transplants.[5,116] The chest radiographic picture in such cases may be that of an interstitial pneumonitis or bronchopneumonia, but the diagnosis has rarely been made antemortem. In the appropriate setting of host compromise and mucocutaneous herpetic disease, a search for tissue or lung specimens showing intranuclear inclusions should be undertaken. If positive specimens are found, adenine arabinoside (15 mg/kg/day) may be administered. This drug is effective in patients with *Herpes simplex* encephalitis,[192] for which it is presently licensed.

Recently, a series of 15 cases of adenovirus infection in compromised hosts was reported.[193] Generally, the illness was associated with a high fever and severe malaise (80 percent of cases), lethargy, fatigue, and night sweats. Also prominent were the gastrointestinal symptoms of anorexia, nausea or vomiting or both, and diarrhea. Eleven of the patients had pulmonary complaints, especially a cough (10 of 15 cases) and tachypnea (8 of 15 cases). Radiographic evidence of pneumonia was present in 12 cases (80 percent), being bilateral in 10 and unilateral in 2. Elevated hepatic enzymes were present in 8 of 11 patients in whom they were measured. Such alterations are therefore not helpful in distinguishing this adenovirus infection from cytomegalovirus infection. Nine of the patients died.

Epstein-Barr virus excretion, and increased titers of antibodies to this virus—the cause of infectious mononucleosis in the healthy adolescent or adult—have been documented among renal-transplant recipients. A recent report related such occurrences to cytomegalovirus-like syndromes.[194] However, only one of the patients was reported to have had fleeting pulmonary infiltrates.

Finally, patients with malignant disease and those who have been immunosuppressed, particularly if there is co-morbid cardiovascular or respiratory disease, should be immunized on a yearly basis against influenza. Although there is little evidence that influenza causes greater mortality in these patients than in normal hosts, the febrile illness associated with influenza virus infection often requires a considerable workup to exclude other causes. Furthermore, necessary chemotherapy or anti-rejection therapy in such patients may be withheld pending resolution of the fever, thus jeopardizing the efficacy of such therapy. Less commonly, respiratory syncytial virus will cause influenza-like syndromes among malignant-disease and immunosuppressed patients.[195] Equally important in these patients is the careful avoidance of immunization with live virus vaccines, including measles, polio, rubella, and, especially, vaccinia.

THERAPY OF OPPORTUNISTIC LUNG INFECTIONS

Bacteria

Once pneumonia in the neutropenic patient is suspected and appropriate cultures have been obtained, the overwhelming likelihood of a bacterial etiology, the difficulties involved in establishing the precise identity of the infecting organism(s), and the rapid mortality in the untreated patient all mandate the initiation of broad-spectrum antibiotic therapy. As previously noted, each institution must know its own organisms and use this knowledge to design a rational antibiotic combination-therapy regimen. For example, if gentamicin resistance is commonplace, tobramycin or amikacin may be better choices when therapy is initiated without knowledge of the specific susceptibilities of the infecting organisms. Despite these specific variations, certain principles underlying such empiric therapy have been established for the neutropenic cancer patient, and warrant generalization:

1. Broad-spectrum therapy should be initiated promptly and in full sepsis doses.
2. The agents used should be bactericidal rather than bacteriostatic, and should contain a broad-spectrum, cell-wall-active agent and one of the newer aminoglycosides.
3. A combination of carbenicillin (or ticarcillin) and gentamicin (or tobramycin or amikacin) has given best results.[196] The addition of oxacillin or cephalosporin as part of the initial empiric regimen appears to add little in terms of efficacy, and the latter drugs may augment aminoglycoside renal toxicity, although this may not be the case for the newer cephalosporins.[194] The role of the third-generation cephalosporins, with activity against many pseudomonas and *B. fragilis* as well as almost all other Gram-negative rods, is uncertain, but these drugs may potentially represent single-agent coverage for sepsis.
4. The antibiotic response rate among pneumonias (40 to 60 percent) is consistently less than that of nonpulmonary infections in immunocompromised hosts and aggressive diagnostic and supportive adjuncts are therefore mandatory.

Once an etiologic bacterial agent is identified and its susceptibilities determined, the antibiotics being given to an immunocompromised patient may be adjusted accordingly. If the response to therapy is not prompt, additional measures may be necessary. These include the use of a "synergistic" antibiotic combination,[197] granulocyte transfusions for the neutropenic host, and a reduction in immunosuppressive therapy in the transplant recipient.[10] Indeed, in one series, the use of lower doses of steroids for the treatment of transplant rejection was correlated with an improved survival, largely because of a decreased frequency of infectious episodes, especially sepsis and wound infections.[198]

The appearance of legionella as an opportunistic pathogen has resulted in the frequent addition of erythromycin to the empiric regimen for pneumonia of unknown origin. If this drug is added to such a regimen, the dose probably should be 2 to 4 g per day parenterally for at least 3 weeks, as noted previously.

Nocardia

Since the introduction of sulfonamide therapy, the mortality from nocardiosis has fallen from 75 to 46 percent; however, only 30 percent of patients with disseminated infection recover.[125] For maximum efficacy, the therapy should be continued for at least 3 to 6 months. Since relapse in cases of nocardia infection has occurred with the premature cessation of treatment,[199] long-term therapy of 12 months or more is recommended for serious infections.[199,200] Other drugs (tetracycline, erythromycin, ampicillin, cycloserine, gentamicin, or kanamycin) may be used in combination with a sulfonamide, especially in patients with serious infection.[125,199] The possible additional benefit from combined antimicrobial therapy has not been investigated in controlled clinical studies.

Tubercle Bacillus

Any immunocompromised patient in whom radiographic lesions highly indicative of tuberculosis develop should be treated with at least two antituberculous drugs while awaiting the results of smear and culture. The two most popular drugs are the bactericidal agents, rifampin (600 mg/day) and isoniazid (300 mg/day). These drugs may be supplemented by an injectable agent, such as streptomycin (500 to 1000 mg/day, i.m.) or ethambutol (15 mg/kg/day). It should be noted that "short-course" therapy has no role in the compromised host, and that antituberculosis medication should be given for at least the full duration of immunosuppression or for 18 to 24 months, whichever is longer.

Protozoa

Experience suggests that a combination of trimethoprim-sulfamethoxazole is useful for the treatment of *Pneumocystis carinii* infection, and this combination administered for 2 weeks is now the initial therapeutic choice in cases of such infection rather than pentamidine.[169,172] The dose suggested when oral trinethoprim-sulfamethoxazole is used has been 20 mg/kg of trimethoprim and 100 mg/kg of sulfamethoxazole per day in divided doses. The parenteral preparation of trimethoprim-sulfamethoxazole, which is still investigational, has been used at initial daily doses of 10 to 15 mg/kg of trimethoprim and 50 to 75 mg/kg of sulfamethoxazole.[201] However, with either formulation, it would appear that the response is related, at least in part, to serum levels of the drugs and that such levels are not directly predictable from the dose.[201] Therefore, levels of the drugs should be measured, with doses adjusted to yield 1½ hour serum levels of $\geq 5 \mu g/ml$ of trimethoprim or, if this test cannot be performed, of $\geq 100 \mu g/ml$ of sulfamethoxazole. Equally important is the realization that a clinical response to trimethoprim-sulfamethoxazole is not assured, and that in addition to following inadequate dosage, a worsening clinical situation may be secondary to: (1) concomitant pathogens; (2) an inadequate host immune response; and (3) organism resistance. Thus, if by day 4 of therapy the patient has not stabilized or improved, these alternatives should be considered. If alternative pathogens are unlikely, immunosuppressive therapy has been reduced to the lowest possible level, and *P. carinii* has been documented, the use of pentamidine should be seriously considered, since patients failing with trimethoprim-sulfamethoxazole have responded to this toxic agent.

The treatment for toxoplasmosis is pyrimethamine and a sulfonamide (sulfadiazine or triple sulfonamides) for a 4-week period. Since this regimen may cause myelosuppression and megaloblastic anemia, folinic acid may be administered without affecting the therapeutic results.[125] In contrast to its effect in *P. carinii* infection, trimethoprim has no activity against *T. gondii*. Hence, the fixed combination of trimethoprim-sulfamethoxazole should not be used for the treatment of toxoplasmosis.

Fungi

Although the treatment of systemic fungal infections has made only slow progress there have been some advances, which have been reviewed recently.[202] The standard of therapy for severe fungal disease remains amphotericin B, despite its many hazards and toxicities. For candidal disease of the skin and mucous membranes that is refractory to topical agents, low-dose (0.3 to 0.4 mg/kg/day) amphotericin B appears to be effective. However, in compromised hosts, pulmonary parenchymal disease with candida, and any form of aspergillus or mucor infection, warrants standard doses of amphotericin (0.6 to 1.0 mg/kg/day). Recent reports of success in the treatment of these formerly uniformly fatal illnesses probably reflects not only the benefit of their early diagnosis, but also an increased willingness to use amphotericin B empirically in the appropriate setting. Of little value when used alone, 5-fluorocytosine can spare amphotericin dosage without lowering response rates when it is used in combination with the latter drug for the treatment of cryptococcal meningitis. In vitro considerations also suggest that combinations of amphotericin B and tetracycline or rifampin may be additive or synergistic in their activity against candida and aspergillus. Although in vivo data are lacking on this point, desperate clinical situations sometimes warrant desperate attempts at therapy.

Miconazole is a marketed antifungal agent, but its present clinical value appears limited to coccidiodomycosis, paracoccidioidomycosis, and selected cases of other fungal infections in which amphotericin B cannot be administered. More exciting is the oral agent ketoconazole, recently the subject of a published symposium.[203] This drug is no longer experimental, and initial trials have shown it to have little toxicity and considerable efficacy in the treatment of histoplasmosis, coccidioidomycosis, paracoccidioidomycosis, and in some cases of invasive candidiasis (particularly chronic mucocutaneous candidiasis) and aspergillosis.

Viruses

The most exciting advances in the treatment of opportunistic infections are in the realm of viral infections, a topic recently reviewed.[204] Adenine arabinoside (ara-A) is an antiviral agent that has been proven to be effective against *Herpes simplex* encephalitis in a dose of 15 mg/kg/day for 10 days. It is also probably effective against disseminated *Herpes simplex*, a particular problem in the neonate and less commonly in the adult, and for disseminated cutaneous Herpes zoster and varicella. On the basis of these findings, and because of its relative lack of toxicity, apart from the large volumes necessary for its administration, ara-A can probably be recommended for the treatment of *H. simplex*, varicella, and zoster pneumonia, although clinical data supporting such use are lacking. Another nucleic-acid inhibitor that has a good therapeutic ratio is the investigational agent acyclovir, which has excellent in vitro activity against *H. simplex*, varicella-zoster virus, and Epstein-Barr virus. Controlled clinical trials with this agent should be published shortly. Human leukocyte interferon has been found effective in halting the cutaneous dissemination of H. zoster and in preventing the activation of *H. simplex* after trigeminal nerve division. When available, it may be useful against both of these viruses in other clinical situations.[205]

Unfortunately, none of the foregoing agents is effective against cytomegalovirus. Furthermore, a clear limitation in the treatment of any viral infection is the difficulty in establishing a diagnosis promptly. In this regard, a review of rapid viral diagnostic methods was recently published.[206] Greater potential for success lies in the prophylaxis of viral infection by isolation, by immunization, or by pharmacologic agent. The use of seronegative donors for WBC, RBC, and platelet transfusions, and possibly the use of hyperimmune cytomegalovirus globulin prophylactically may decrease the frequency of cytomegalovirus infection among patients with cancer and those undergoing bone marrow transplantation. The one published trial with a cytomegalovirus vaccine did not show a reduction in active cytomegalovirus infection in vaccinated individuals.[207] For varicella, both zoster immune globulin (for the exposed child) and transfer factor for long-term prophylaxis[208] appear to be effective in decreasing the frequency and severity of childhood infection; a live attenuated vaccine is under development.[209] Finally, influenza vaccine and amantidine are effective prophylactic agents; the latter is also of some benefit in the treatment of influenza A infections if used within the first 48 hours of illness.

REFERENCES

1. Matthay RA, Greene WH: Pulmonary infections in the immunocompromised patient. Med Clin North Am 64:529, 1980.
2. Benatar SR: Pulmonary complications in the immunocompromised patient. S Afr Med J 52:1019, 1977.
3. Hughes WT: Fatal infections in childhood leukemia. Am J Dis Child 122:283, 1971.
4. Sickles EA, Young VM, Greene WH, et al: Pneumonia in acute leukemia. Ann Intern Med 79:528, 1973.

5. Williams DN, Krick JA, Remington JS: Pulmonary infection in the compromised host. Am Rev Resp Dis 114:359, 1976.
6. Valdivieso M, Gil-Extremera B, Zornoza J, et al: Gram-negative bacillary pneumonia in the compromised host. Medicine 56:241, 1977.
7. Levine AS, Graw RG Jr, Young RC: Management of infections in patients with leukemia and lymphoma: Current concepts and experimental approaches. Semin Hematol 9:141, 1972.
8. Anderson RJ, Schafer OA, Olin DB, et al: Septicemia in renal transplant recipients. Arch Surg 106:692, 1973.
9. Murphy JF, McDonald FD, Dawson M, et al: Factors affecting the frequency of infection in renal transplant recipients. Arch Intern Med 136:670, 1976.
10. Tilney NL, Strom TB, Vineyard GC, et al: Factors contributing to the declining mortality rate in renal transplantation. N Engl J Med 299:1321, 1978.
11. Jennings FL, Arden A: Development of radiation pneumonitis: Time and dose factors. Arch Pathol 74:351, 1962.
12. Rosenow EC III: The spectrum of drug-induced pulmonary disease. Ann Intern Med 77:977, 1972.
13. Sostman HD, Matthay RA, Putnam CE: Cytotoxic drug-induced lung disease. Am J Med 62:608, 1977.
14. Eickhoff TC: Infections in immunosuppressed patients. Drug Therapy 2:19, 1972.
15. Matthay RA, Moritz ED: Invasive procedures for diagnosing pulmonary infection: A critical review. Clin Chest Med 2:3, 1981.
16. Hughes WT: Pneumocystis pneumonia: A plague of the immunosuppressed. Johns Hopkins Med J 143:184, 1978.
17. Pasculle AW, Myerowitz RL, Rinaldo CR Jr: New bacterial agent of pneumonia isolated from renal-transplant recipients. Lancet 2:58, 1979.
18. Pecora DV: A method of securing uncontaminated tracheal secretions for bacterial examination. J Thorac Surg 37:653, 1959.
19. Pecora DV, Kohl M: Transtracheal aspiration in the diagnosis of acute lower respiratory tract infection. Am Rev Resp Dis 86:755, 1962.
20. Kalinske RW, Parker RH, Brandt D, et al: Diagnostic usefulness and safety of transtracheal aspiration. N Engl J Med 276:604, 1967.
21. Bartlett JG: Diagnostic accuracy of transtracheal aspiration bacteriologic studies. Am Rev Resp Dis 115:777, 1977.
22. Hahn HH, Beaty HN: Transtracheal aspiration in the evaluation of patients with pneumonia. Ann Intern Med 72:183, 1970.
23. Schreiner A, Digranes A, Myking O: Transtracheal aspiration in the diagnosis of lower respiratory tract infections. Scand J Infect Dis 4:49, 1972.
24. Pratter MR, Irwin RS: Transtracheal aspiration. Guidelines for safety. Chest 76:518, 1979.
25. Unger KM: (Editorial) Sputum or spit? Chest 76:498, 1979.
26. Spencer CD, Beaty HN: Complications of transtracheal aspiration. N Engl J Med 286:304, 1972.
27. Pauker SG: Transtracheal aspiration (letter). Ann Intern Med 73:142, 1970.
28. Schillaci RF, Iacovoni VE, Conte RS: Transtracheal aspiration complicated by fatal endotracheal hemorrhage. N Engl J Med 295:488, 1976.
29. Parsons GH, Price JE, Auston PW: Bilateral pneumothorax complicating transtracheal aspiration. West J Med 125:73, 1976.

30. Deresinski SC, Stevens DA: Anterior cervical infections: Complications of transtracheal aspirations. Am Rev Resp Dis 110:354, 1974.
31. Yoshikawa TT, Chow AW, Montgomerie JZ, et al: Paratracheal abscess: An unusual complication of transtracheal aspiration. Chest 65:105, 1974.
32. Unger KM, Moser KM: Fatal complication of transtracheal aspiration. Arch Intern Med 132:437, 1973.
33. Leyden I: VII. Verhandlungen des vereins fur innere medicin.: Ueber infectiose Pneumonie. Dtsch Med Wochenschr 9:52, 1883.
34. Dahlgren S, Nordenstrom B: Transthoracic Needle Biopsy. Chicago, Yearbook Medical Publishers, 1966.
35. Sagel SS, Ferguson TB, Forrest JV, et al: Percutaneous transthoracic aspiration needle biopsy. Ann Thorac Surg 26:399, 1978.
36. Adamson JS, Bates JM: Percutaneous needle biopsy of the lung. Arch Intern Med 119:164, 1967.
37. Cunningham JH, Zavala DC, Corry RJ, et al: Trephine air drill, bronchial brush and fiberoptic transbronchial lung biopsies in immunosuppressed patients. Am Rev Resp Dis 115:213, 1977.
38. King EG, Bachynski JE, Mielke B: Percutaneous trephine lung biopsy. Chest 70:212, 1976.
39. Herman PG: Needle biopsy of the lung (Editorial): Ann Thorac Surg 26:395, 1978.
40. Sappington SW, Favorite GO: Lung puncture in lobar pneumonia. Am J Med Sci 91:225, 1936.
41. Finland M: Diagnostic lung puncture (Commentaries). Pediatrics 44:471, 1969.
42. Hughes JR, Sinha DP, Cooper MR, et al: Lung tap in childhood. Pediatrics 44:477, 1969.
43. Klein JO: Diagnostic lung puncture in the pneumonias of infants and children. Pediatrics 44:486, 1969.
44. Mimica I, Donosog E, Howard JE, et al: Lung puncture in the etiologic diagnosis of pneumonia. Am J Dis Child 122:278, 1971.
45. Bandt PD, Blank N, Costellino RA: Needle diagnosis of pneumonitis. Value in high risk patients. JAMA 220:1578, 1972.
46. Costellino RA, Blank N: Etiologic diagnosis of focal pulmonary infection in immunocompromised patients by fluoroscopically guided percutaneous needle aspiration. Radiology 132:563, 1979.
47. Zavala DC, Schoell JE: Ultrathin needle aspiration of the lung in infections and malignant disease. Am Rev Resp Dis 123:125, 1981.
48. Giglia AR, Morgan PN, Bates JH: Rapid definitive diagnosis of Legionnaire's disease. Chest 76:98, 1979.
49. Chaudhary S, Hughes WT, Feldman S, et al: Percutaneous transthoracic needle aspiration of the lung. Am J Dis Child 131:902, 1977.
50. Norenberg R, Claxton CP, Takaro T: Percutaneous needle biopsy of the lung: report of two fatal complications. Chest 66:216, 1974.
51. Sinner WN, Zajicek J: Implantation metastasis after percutaneous transthoracic needle aspiration biopsy. Acta Radiol (Diagn.), 17:473, 1976.
52. Greenman RL, Goodall PT, King D: Lung biopsy in immunocompromised hosts. Am J Med 59:488, 1975.
53. Westcott JL: Air embolism complicating percutaneous needle biopsy of the lung. Chest 63:108, 1973.

54. Pearce JG, Patt NL: Fatal pulmonary hemorrhage after percutaneous aspiration lung biopsy. Am Rev Resp Dis 110:346, 1974.
55. Ikeda S: Flexible bronchofiberscope. Ann Otol Rhinol Laryngol 79:916, 1970.
56. Ikeda S: Atlas of flexible bronchofiberscopy. Tokyo, Igaku Shoin, 1974.
57. Ellis JH Jr: Transbronchial lung biopsy via the fiberoptic bronchoscope: experience with 107 consecutive cases and comparison with bronchial brushing. Chest 68:524, 1975.
58. Hanson RR, Zavala DC, Rhodes ML, et al: Transbronchial biopsy via flexible fiberoptic bronchoscope: result in 164 patients. Am Rev Resp Dis 114:67, 1976.
59. Kahn MA, Whitcomb ME, Snider GL: Flexible fiberoptic bronchoscopy. (Editorial). Am J Med 61:151, 1976.
60. Sackner MA: Bronchofiberscopy. Am Rev Resp Dis 111:62, 1975.
61. Zavala DC: Diagnostic fiberoptic bronchoscopy. Techniques and results of biopsy in 600 patients. Chest 68:12, 1975.
62. Zavala DC: Pulmonary hemorrhage in fiberoptic transbronchial biopsy. Chest 70:584, 1976.
63. Credle WF, Smiddy, JF, Elliott RC: Complications of fiberoptic bronchoscopy. Am Rev Resp Dis 109:67, 1974.
64. Suratt PM, Smiddy JF, Grubert B: Deaths and complications associated with fiberoptic bronchoscopy. Chest 69:747, 1976.
65. Bartlett JG, Alexander J, Mayhew J, et al: Should fiberoptic bronchoscopy aspirates be cultured? Am Rev Resp Dis 114:73, 1976.
66. Lauver GL, Hasan FM, Morgan RB, et al: The usefulness of fiberoptic bronchoscopy in evaluating new pulmonary lesions in the compromised host. Am J Med 66:580, 1979.
67. Matthay RA, Farmer WC, Odero D: Diagnostic fiberoptic bronchoscopy in the immunosuppressed host with pulmonary infiltrates. Thorax 32:539, 1977.
68. Pennington JE, Feldman NT: Pulmonary infiltrates and fever in patients with hematologic malignancy: Assessment of transbronchial biopsy. Am J Med 62:581, 1977.
69. Phillips MJ, Knight RK, Green M: Fiberoptic bronchoscopy and diagnosis of pulmonary lesions in lymphoma and leukemia. Thorax 35:19, 1980.
70. Feldman NT, Pennington JE, Ehrie MG: Transbronchial lung biopsy in the compromised host. JAMA 238:1377, 1977.
71. Poe RH, Utell MJ, Israel RH, et al: Sensitivity and specificity of the non-specific transbronchial lung biopsy. Am Rev Resp Dis 119:25, 1979.
72. Smiddy JF: Flexible fiberoptic bronchoscope. Ann Intern Med 75:971, 1971.
73. Tucker GF, Olsen AM, Andrews AH Jr, et al: The flexible fiberscope in bronchoscopic perspective. (Editorial). Chest 64:149, 1973.
74. Zavala DC: Bronchial biopsy in diffuse lung disease. Chest 73:729, 1978.
75. Zavala DC, Rhodes ML, Richardson RH, et al: Fiberoptic and rigid bronchoscopy. The state of the art. (Editorial). Chest 65:605, 1974.
76. Drew WL, Finley TN, Golde DW: Diagnostic lavage and occult pulmonary hemorrhage in thrombocytopenic immunocompromised patients. Am Rev Resp Dis 116:215, 1977.
77. Drew WL, Finley TN, Mintz L, et al: Diagnosis of *Pneumocystis carinii* pneumonia by bronchopulmonary lavage. JAMA, 230:713, 1974.

78. Kelley J, Landis JN, Davis GS, et al: Diagnosis of pneumonia due to Pneumocystis by subsegmental pulmonary lavage via the fiberoptic bronchoscope. Chest 74:24, 1978.
79. Stover DE, Lange M, Armstrong D, et al: The efficacy of bronchoalveolar lavage in the diagnosis of diffuse interstitial pneumonitis in immunosuppressed patients. (Abstr). Am Rev Resp Dis 121:195, 1980.
80. Repsher LH, Schroter G, Hammond WS: Diagnosis of *Pneumocystis carinii* pneumonitis by means of endobronchial brush biopsy. N Engl J Med 287:340, 1972.
81. Nishio JN, Lynch JP: Fiberoptic bronchoscopy in the immunocompromised host: the significance of a "non specific" transbronchial biopsy. Am Rev Resp Dis 121:307, 1980.
82. Fossieck BE, Parker RH, Cohen MH, et al: Fiberoptic bronchoscopy and culture of bacteria from the lower respiratory tract. Chest 72:5, 1977.
83. Wimberly NE, Faling LJ, Bartlett JG: A fiberoptic bronchoscopy technique to obtain uncontaminated lower airway secretions for bacterial culture. Am Rev Resp Dis 119:337, 1979.
84. Hodgkin JE, Anderson HA, Rosenow EC: Diagnosis of *Pneumocystis carinii* pneumonia by transbronchoscopic lung biopsy. Chest 64:551, 1973.
85. Sahn SA, Levin DC: Diagnosis of miliary tuberculosis by transbronchial lung biopsy. Br Med J 2:667, 1975.
86. Scheinhorn DI, Joyner LR, Whitcomb ME: Transbronchial forceps lung biopsy through the fiberoptic bronchoscope in *Pneumocystis carinii* pneumonia. Chest 66:294, 1974.
87. Wallace JM, Harrell JH, Deutsch AL, et al: Bronchoscopy and transbronchial biopsy in evaluation of patients with suspected active tuberculosis (Abstr). Am Rev Resp Dis 121:202, 1980.
88. Hayes DA, McCarthy LR, Friedman M: Evaluation of bronchofiberoptic methods of obtaining samples of lower respiratory tract flora. (Abstr). Am Rev Resp Dis 121:147, 1980.
89. Fletcher EC, Mohr JA, Levin DC, et al: Bacteriologic diagnosis of pneumonia with protected specimen brush and fiberoptic bronchoscopy. (Abstr). Am Rev Resp Dis 121:134, 1980.
90. LeGrand P, Bordelon JY, Gewin WC, et al: The telescoping plugged catheter in suspected anaerobic infections: a controlled series. (Abstr). Am Rev Resp Dis 121:157, 1980.
91. Periera W, Kovnat DM, Kahn MA, et al: Fever and pneumonia after flexible fiberoptic bronchoscopy. Am Rev Resp Dis 112:59, 1975.
92. Aelony Y, Finegold SM: Serious infectious complications after flexible fiberoptic bronchoscopy. West J Med 131:327, 1979.
93. Webb F, Valspinosa A: Outbreak of *Serratia marcescens* associated with the flexible fiber bronchoscope. Chest 68:703, 1975.
94. Flick MR, Wasson K, Dunn LJ, et al: Fatal pulmonary hemorrhage after transbronchial lung biopsy through the fiberoptic bronchoscope. Am Rev Resp Dis 111:853, 1975.
95. Albertini RE, Harrell JH, Kurihara N, et al: Arterial hypoxemia induced by fiberoptic bronchoscopy. JAMA 230:1666, 1974.
96. Albertini RE, Harrell JH, Moser MM: Management of arterial hypoxemia induced by fiberoptic bronchoscopy. Chest 67:134, 1975.

97. Klassen KP, Aniyan AJ, Curtis GM: Biopsy of diffuse pulmonary lesions. Arch Surg 59:694, 1949.
98. Klassen KP, Andrews NC: Biopsy of diffuse pulmonary lesions. A seventeen year experience. Ann Thorac Surg 4:117, 1967.
99. Aaron BL, Bellinger SB, Shephard BM, et al: Open lung biopsy: A strong stand. Chest 59:18, 1971.
100. Baker RK, Lee JM, Carter D: An evaluation of open lung biopsy. Johns Hopkins Med J 132:103, 1973.
101. Gaensler EA, Moister MVB, Hamm J: Open lung biopsy in diffuse pulmonary disease. N Engl J Med 270:1319, 1964.
102. Leight GS, Michaelis LL: Open lung biopsy for the diagnosis of acute, diffuse pulmonary infiltrates in the immunosuppressed patient. Chest 73:477, 1978.
103. Rosen PP, Martini N, Armstrong D: Pneumocystis carinii pneumonia: diagnosis by lung biopsy. Am J Med 58:794, 1975.
104. Scadding JG: Lung biopsy in the diagnosis of diffuse lung disease. Br Med J 2:557, 1970.
105. Singer C, Armstrong D, Rosen PP, et al: Diffuse pulmonary infiltrates in immunosuppressed patients: prospective study of 80 cases. Am J Med 66:110, 1979.
106. Rossiter SJ, Miller C, Chung AM, et al: Open lung biopsy in the immunosuppressed patient. J Thorac Cardiovasc Surg 77:338, 1979.
107. Wolff LJ, Bartlett MS, Baehner RL, et al: The causes of interstitial pneumonitis in immunocompromised children: an aggressive systematic approach to diagnosis. Pediatrics 60:41, 1977.
108. Greene WH: Supportive care of the cancer patient. In Cancer: A Comprehensive Treatise, Vol 5, New York, Becker F, ed. Plenum Press, 223, 1977.
109. Meyers BR, Hirschman SZ, Axelrod JA: Current patterns of infection in multiple myeloma. Am J Med 52:87, 1972.
110. Weitzman S, Aisenberg AC: Fulminant sepsis after the successful treatment of Hodgkin's disease. Am J Med 62:47, 1977.
111. Viola MV: Acute leukemia and infection. JAMA 201:923, 1967.
112. Pierce AK, Sanford JP: Aerobic gram-negative bacillary pneumonias. Am Rev Resp Dis 110:647, 1974.
113. Pennington JE: Infection in the compromised host: Recent advances and future directions. In Seminars in Infectious Disease, Vol 1, eds. Weinstein L, Fields BN, New York Stratton Intercontinental Medical Book Corp, 1978.
114. Notter DT, Grossman PL, Rosenberg SA, Remington JS: Infections in patients with Hodgkin's disease: A clinical study of 300 consecutive adult patients. Rev Infect Dis 2:761, 1980.
115. Peterson PK, Balfour HH Jr, Marker SC, et al: Cytomegalovirus disease in renal allograft recipients: A prospective study of the clinical features, risk factors and impact on renal transplantation. Medicine 59:283, 1980.
116. Ramsey PG, Rubin RH, Tolkoff-Rubin NE, et al: The renal transplant patient with fever and pulmonary infiltrates: Etiology, clinical manifestations, and management. Medicine 59:206, 1980.
117. Sotman SB, Schimpff SC, Young VM: *Staphylococcus aureus* bacteremia in patients with acute leukemia. Am J Med 69:814, 1980.

118. Klastersky J, Cappel R, Debusscher L, et al: Pneumonia caused by gram-negative bacilli in hospitalized patients presenting malignant disease. Eur J Cancer 7:329, 1971.
119. England AC III, Fraser DW, Plikaytis BD, et al: Sporadic Legionellosis in the United States: The first thousand cases. Ann Intern Med 94:164, 1981.
120. Gump DW, Frank RO, Winn WC, et al: Legionnaire's disease in patients with associated serious disease. Ann Intern Med 90:538, 1979.
121. Saravolatz LD, Burch KH, Fisher E, et al: Pneumonia in acute leukemia. Ann Intern Med 90:533, 1979.
122. Harding SA, Donowitz G, Walker G, et al: Opportunistic pneumonia: a clinicopathological study of five cases caused by a new acid-fast bacterium. (Abstract 487). Proceedings of the 19th Interscience Conference on Antimicrobial Agents and Chemotherapy, Boston, Massachusetts, 1979.
123. Myerowitz RL, Pasculle AW, Dowling JN, et al: Opportunistic lung infection due to "Pittsburgh pneumonia agent." (Abstract 486). Proceedings of the 19th Interscience Conference on Antimicrobial Agents and Chemotherapy, Boston, Massachusetts 1979.
124. Sickles EA, Greene WH, Weirnik P: Clinical presentation of infection in granulocytopenic patients. Arch Intern Med 135:715, 1975.
125. Bodey GP: Infections in cancer patients. Cancer Treatment Rev 2:89, 1975.
126. Arroyo JC, Nichols S, Carroll DG: Disseminated *Nocardia caviae* infection. Am J Med 62:409, 1977.
127. Avram MM, Nair SR, Lipner HI, et al: Persistent nocardemia following renal transplantation. JAMA 239:2779, 1978.
128. Young LS, Armstrong D, Blevins A, et al: Nocardia asteroids infection complicating neoplastic disease. Am J Med 50:356, 1979.
129. Louria DB: Fungus infections of the lungs. In Textbook of Pulmonary Diseases, 2nd ed. Baum GL, Boston, Little, Brown 219, 1974.
130. Neu HC, Silva M, Hazen E, et al: Necrotizing *Nocardia* pneumonitis. Ann Intern Med 66:274, 1967.
131. Kaplan MH, Armstrong D, Rosen P: Tuberculosis complicating neoplastic disease: a review of 201 cases. Cancer 33:850, 1974.
132. Miller JW, Horne NW: Tuberculosis in immunosuppressed patients. Lancet 1:1176, 1979.
133. Silver RT: Infections, fever and host resistance in neoplastic diseases. J Chronic Dis 16:677, 1963.
134. Chang H, Rodriquez V, Narboni G, et al: Causes of death in adults with acute leukemia. Medicine 55:259, 1976.
135. Mirsky HS, Cuttner J: Fungal infections in acute leukemia. Cancer 30:348, 1972.
136. Bach MC, Adler JL, Brenan J, et al: Influence of rejection therapy on fungal and nocardial infections in renal-transplant recipients. Lancet 1:180, 1973.
137. Pennington JE: Successful treatment of aspergillus pneumonia in hematologic neoplasia. N Engl J Med 295:426, 1976.
138. Gallis HA, Berman RA, Cate TR, et al: Fungal infection following renal transplantation. Arch Intern Med 135:1163, 1975.
139. Dubois PJ, Myerowitz RL, Allen CM: Pathoradiologic correlation of pulmonary candidiasis in immunosuppressed patients. Cancer 40:1026, 1977.

140. Masur H, Rosen PO, Armstrong D: Pulmonary disease caused by candida species. Am J Med 63:914, 1977.
141. Young RC, Bennett JE, Geelhoes GW, et al: Fungemia with compromised host resistance. Ann Intern Med 80:605, 1974.
142. Weiner MH, Yount WJ: Mannan antigenemia in the diagnosis of invasive candida infection. J Clin Invest 58:1045, 1976.
143. Miller GG, Witwer MW, Braude AI, et al: Rapid identification of Candida albicans septicemia in man by gas-liquid chromatography. J Clin Invest 54:1235, 1974.
144. Young RC, Bennett JE, Vogel CL, et al: Aspergillosis: The spectrum of the disease in 98 patients. Medicine 49:147, 1970.
145. Aisner J, Schimpff SC, Wiernik PH: Treatment of invasive aspergillosis: relation of early diagnosis and treatment to response. Ann Intern Med 86:539, 1977.
146. Gold JWM, Fisher B, Yu B, et al: Diagnosis of invasive aspergillosis by passive hemagglutination assay of antibody. J Infect Dis 142:87, 1980.
147. Holmberg K, Berdischewsky M, Young LS: Serologic immunodiagnosis of invasive aspergillosis. J Infect Dis 141:656, 1980.
148. Weiner MH: Antigenemia detected by radioimmunoassay in systemic aspergillosis. Ann Intern Med 92:793, 1980.
149. Aisner J, Schimpff, SC, Bennett JE, et al: *Aspergillus* infections in cancer patients: association with fireproofing materials in a new hospital. JAMA 235:411, 1976.
150. Greene WH, Andriole VT: An outbreak of nosocomial invasive aspergillosis (Abstr). Program and Abstracts of the 20th Interscience Conference on Antimicrobial Agents and Chemotherapy. New Orleans LA, 1980.
151. Emmons CW, Binford CH, Utz JP, Kwon-Chung KJ: Medical Mycology. Philadelphia, Lea and Febiger, 254, 1977.
152. Hutter RVP: Phycomycetous infection (mucormycosis) in cancer patients: A complication of therapy. Cancer 12:330, 1959.
153. Meyer RD, Rosen P, Armstrong D: Phycomycosis complicating leukemia and lymphoma. Ann Intern Med 77:871, 1972.
154. Meyers JD, Spencer HC, Watts JC, et al: Cytomegalovirus pneumonia after human marrow transplantation. Ann Intern Med 82:181, 1975.
155. Medoff G, Kobyashi GS: Pulmonary mucormycosis. N Engl J Med 286:86, 1972.
156. Lehrer RI, Howard DH, Sypherd PS, et al: Mucormycosis. Ann Intern Med 93:93, 1980.
157. Aisner J, Schimpff SC, Sutherland JC, et al: *Torulopsis glabrata* infections in patients with cancer. Am J Med 61:23, 1976.
158. Pankey GA, Daloviso JR: Fungemia caused by *Torulopsis glabrata*. Medicine 52:395, 1973.
159. Valdivieso M, Luna M, Bodey GP, et al: Fungemia due to *Torulopsis glabrata* in the compromised host. Cancer 38:1750, 1976.
160. Goodwell B, Jacobs JB, Powell BD, et al: *Pneumocystis carinii:* the spectrum of diffuse interstitial pneumonia in patients with neoplastic diseases. Ann Intern Med 72:337, 1970.
161. Jarnum S, Rasmussen EF, Ohlsen AS, et al: Generalized *Pneumocytis carinii* infection with severe idiopathic hypoproteinemia. Ann Intern Med 68:138, 1968.
162. Perera DR, Western KA, Johnson HE, et al: *Pneumocystis carinii* pneumonia in a hospital for children. JAMA 214:1074, 1970.

163. Walzer RP, Pearl DP, Krogstad DJ, et al: *Pneumocystis carinii* pneumonia in the United States. Ann Intern Med 80:83, 1974.
164. Johnson HD, Johnson WW: *Pneumocystis carinii* pneumonia in children with cancer. JAMA 214:1067, 1962.
165. Repsher LH, Levin DC, Matthay RA, et al: Transbronchial lung biopsy via the fiberoptic bronchoscope in the diagnosis of diffuse pulmonary infiltrates in the immunosuppressed host. Natl Cancer Inst Monogr 43:127, 1976.
166. Hughes WT: *Pneumocystis carinii* pneumonia. N Engl J Med 297:1381, 1977.
167. Hughes WT: *Pneumocystis* pneumonia: A plague of the immunosuppressed. Johns Hopkins Med J, 143:184, 1978.
168. Doppman JL, Geelhoed GW: Atypical radiographic features in *Pneumocystis carinii* pneumonia. Natl Cancer Inst Mongr 43:89, 1976.
169. Western KS, Perera DR, Schultz MG: Pentamidine isethionate in the treatment of *Pneumocytis carinii* pneumonia. Ann Intern Med 73:695, 1970.
170. Ryning RW, Mills J: *Pneumocystis carinii, Toxoplasma gondii,* cytomegalovirus and the compromised host. West J Med, 130:18, 1979.
171. Vietzke WM, Gelderman AH, Grimley PM, et al: Toxoplasmosis complicating malignancy. Experience at the National Cancer Institute. Cancer 21:816, 1968.
172. Remington JS: Toxoplasmosis in the adult. Bull NY Acad Med 50:211, 1974.
173. Krick JA, Remington JS: Toxoplasmosis in the adult—An overview. N Engl J Med 298:550, 1978.
174. Aranjo FG, Remington JS: Antigenemia in recently acquired acute toxoplasmosis. J Infect Dis 14:144, 1980.
175. Hughes WT, Feldman S, Cox F: Infectious diseases in children with cancer. Pediat Clin North Am 21:583, 1974.
176. Duvall CP, Casazza AR, Grimley PM, et al: Recovery of cytomegalovirus from adults with neoplastic disease. Ann Intern Med 64:531, 1966.
177. Thomas ED, Storb R, Clift RA, et al: Bone-marrow transplantation. N Engl J Med 292:832, 1975.
178. Naragi S, Jackson GG, Jonasson O, et al: Prospective study of prevalence, incidence, and source of herpes virus infections in patients with renal allografts. J Infect Dis 136:531, 1977.
179. Betts RB, Hanshaw JB: Cytomegalovirus in the compromised host. Annu Rev Med 28:103, 1977.
180. Cheeseman SH, Rubin RH, Stewart JA, et al: Prophylactic interferon in renal transplantation: Effects on cytomegalovirus and *Herpes simplex* virus infection. N Engl J Med 300:1345, 1979.
181. Friedman HM: Cytometalovirus: Subclinical infection or disease? (Editorial). Am J Med 70:215, 1981.
182. Pollard RB, Egbert PR, Gallagher JG, et al: Cytomegalovirus retinitis in immunosuppressed hosts. I. Natural history and effects of treatment with adenine arabinoside. Ann Intern Med 93:655, 1980.
183. Fiala M, Payne JE, Berre TV, et al: Epidemiology of cytomegalovirus infection after transplantation and immunosuppression. J Infect Dis 132:421, 1975.
184. Winston DJ, Ho WG., Howell CL, et al: Cytomegalovirus infections associated with leukocyte transfusions. Ann Intern Med 93:671, 1980.
185. Geiser CF, Bishop Y, Myers M, et al: Prophylaxis of varicella in children with

neoplastic disease: Comparative results with zoster immune plasma and gamma globulin. Cancer 35:1027, 1975.

186. Triebwasser JH, Harris RE, Bryant RE, et al: Varicella pneumonia in adults. Medicine 46:409, 1967.
187. Dolin R, Reichman RC, Mazur MH, et al: Herpes zoster-varicella infections in immunosuppressed patients. Ann Intern Med 89:375, 1978.
188. Reboul F, Donaldson SS, Kaplan HS: Herpes zoster and varicella infection in children with Hodgkin's disease. Cancer 41:95, 1978.
189. Huberman M, Fossick BE Jr, Bunn PA Jr, et al: Herpes zoster and small-cell bronchogenic carcinoma. Am J Med 68:214, 1980.
190. Feld R, Evans WK, DeBoer G: Herpes zoster in patients with small-cell carcinoma of the lung receiving combined modality treatment. Ann Intern Med 93:282, 1980.
191. Nahmias AJ, Roizman B: Infection with herpes-simplex viruses 1 and 2. N Engl J Med 289:781, 1973.
192. Whitley RH, Soong SJ, Dolin R: Adenine arabinoside therapy of biopsy proved herpes simplex encephalitis: NIAID collaborative anti-viral study group. N Engl J Med 297:289, 1977.
193. Zahradnik JM, Spencer MJ, Porter DD: Adenovirus infection in the immunocompromised patient. Am J Med 68:725, 1980.
194. Cheeseman SH, Henle W, Rubin RH, et al: Epstein-Barr virus infection in renal transplant recipients: Effects of anti-thymocyte globulin and interferon. Ann Intern Med 93:39, 1980.
195. Mathur U, Bentley DW, Hall CB: Concurrent respiratory syncytial virus and influenza A infections in the institutionalized elderly and chronically ill. Ann Intern Med 93:49, 1980.
196. EORTC International Antimicrobial Therapy Project Group: Three antibiotic regimens in the treatment of infection in febrile granulocytopenic patients with cancer. J Infect Dis 137:14, 1978.
197. Lau WK, Young LS, Black RE, et al: Comparative efficacy and toxicity of amikacin/carbenicillin versus gentamicin/carbenicillin in leukopenic patients. A randomized prospective trial. Am J Med 62:959, 1977.
198. Vincenti F, Amend W, Feduska N, et al: Improved outcome following renal transplantation with reduction in the immunosuppression therapy for rejection episodes. Am J Med 69:107, 1980.
199. Krick JA, Stinson EB, Remington JS: Nocardia infection in heart transplant patients. Ann Intern Med 82:18, 1975.
200. Goodman JS, Koenig MG: *Nocardia* infections in a general hospital. Ann NY Acad Sci 175:5521, 1970.
201. Winston DJ, Lau WK, Gale RP, Young LS: Trimethoprim sulfamethoxazole for the treatment of *Pneumocystis carinii* pneumonia. Ann Intern Med 92:762, 1980.
202. Medof G, Kobayashi GS: Strategies in the treatment of systemic fungal infections. N Engl J Med 302:145, 1980.
203. First International Symposium on Ketoconazole. Rev Infect Dis 2:519, 1980.
204. Hirsch MS, Swartz MN: Antiviral agents. N Engl J Med 302:903,949, 1980.
205. Dunnick JK, Galasso GJ: Update on clinical trials with exogenous interferon. J Infect Dis 142:293, 1980.

206. McIntosh K, Wilfert C, Chernesky M, et al: Summary of a workshop on new and useful techniques in rapid viral diagnosis. J Infect Dis 142:793, 1980.
207. Lang DJ: Cytomegalovirus immunization: status, prospects and problems. Rev Infect Dis 2:449, 1980.
208. Steele RW, Myers MG, Vincent MM: Transfer factor for the prevention of varicella-zoster infection in childhood leukemia. N Engl J Med 303:355, 1980.
209. Gershon AA: Live attenuated varicella-zoster vaccine. Rev Infect Dis 2:393, 1980.

11

Chest Trauma

Alan R. Hopeman, M.D.

It is not possible in a short chapter on chest trauma as a facet of pulmonary emergencies to cover all phases of the diagnosis and management of chest trauma; recent books have addressed this subject more widely.[1-4]

Trauma follows cardiovascular disease and cancer among causes of death in the United States. Furthermore, it is estimated that 25 percent of the 50,000 annual trauma deaths are caused directly by chest trauma, and that in an additional 50 percent of deaths, chest trauma plays an important contributing role.

Only a few papers have attempted to detail the types of chest injury occurring in the entire spectrum of chest-injured patients. However, it is apparent that there is wide disparity between the types of chest injuries treated in various hospitals. Military wartime chest injury is largely penetrating chest trauma. Most civilian hospitals, especially those with extensive trauma services, report a large incidence of penetrating gunshot and stab injuries of the chest, in addition to the blunt chest injuries.

Examples of the wide variation in individual hospital chest trauma case-loads are a review of 685 cases of chest trauma from the University of Colorado Health Sciences Center which included 635 blunt chest injuries,[5] and a 1-year unpublished tabulation of chest injuries at the Denver General Hospital, in connection with a trauma grant application, which demonstrated an almost equal incidence of penetrating and nonpenetrating chest trauma in over 150 patients. On the basis of such facts it is impossible to establish an overall incidence of the types of chest trauma.

The physiologic impact of trauma on the patient with a solitary chest injury ranges from minimal, in patients whose homeostatic mechanisms will restore them to health regardless of the treatment undertaken, to life-threatening from the moment of injury. Prompt action by the medical team is often the determinant of success or failure in the resuscitation and survival of the latter type of patient.

When the additional physiologic burden of multiple-system trauma in the severely injured patient is considered, the odds against survival rise precipitously, and the importance of prompt evaluation and correct decision-making are apparent.

While serious chest injury compresses the time for completing an evaluation and starting treatment, each patient must have a rapid, near-complete, and systematic evaluation as soon as life-threatening problems are detected and management is begun. When possible, a brief history should be obtained from the patient or any family members or friends who accompany the patient to the emergency room. This should include details of the injury and any past medical history of such diseases as diabetes, drug sensitivities, and heart, renal, or liver disease which may modify treatment.

In the unconscious patient and in the absence of friends or family members, emergency rescue personnel may be able to furnish useful information about the injury, including the state of consciousness and vital signs of the patient when found and en route to the hospital, evidence of external bleeding at the scene of the injury, or details of the trauma. Clothing should be cut away to allow for a complete physical examination.

EVALUATION OF THE PATIENT

Evaluation of the conscious and the unconscious patient must be described separately because of the problems imposed by altered consciousness caused by injury, alcohol, or drugs. Inappropriate responses to common stimuli in patients with psychiatric disease in whom the accident has resulted in such fright, terror, or anxiety that the patient cannot cooperate with the physician, may make the evaluation more difficult. Unfortunately, persons with psychiatric problems and intoxicated individuals often are involved in auto-pedestrian accidents, and the high incidence of alcohol intake in persons injured in motor vehicle accidents is common knowledge.[6]

The Conscious Patient

A quick, overall appraisal should be made to assess the general neurologic status of the conscious patient. A common mistake is to shake the patient and ask him or her to move an extremity. A simple twitch of a muscle group may convince the examiner that the extremity is intact. A more foolproof method is to direct the patient to move the fingers, without touching the patient. The patient who can do this appropriately is clearly receiving, integrating, and sending the correct responses. Sensation and reflexes can be checked quickly. If sensation is altered, a more detailed neurologic evaluation must be done, especially when the sensory loss is in an injured extremity.

Evidence of general injury should also be noted. Swelling or distortion of body parts, as well as lacerations, usually are obvious. If the patient's neurologic status permits, and spine injury has been ruled out, a careful examination of the back should be done. Stab wounds, especially from ice picks and similar thin blades, as well as small caliber gunshot wounds, may be so small that there is little or no evidence of external bleeding.

Extremities that have no apparent injury should be tested for full range of motion to rule out joint damage. Injured extremities will be best evaluated by radiologic examination. The peripheral pulses, especially on injured extremities, should be checked. Also, even though motor evaluation may be difficult, sensation should be assessed and recorded.

In the conscious patient, examination of the eyes, ears, nose, and oral cavity can be accomplished rapidly. If there are no symptoms of neck injury, such as neck pain or extremity numbness, and if the patient can flex his or her chin onto the chest without discomfort, serious neck injury would be unusual. Any symptom of neck injury requires immobilization of the neck by a four-poster collar or similar device. Sandbagging of the head to prevent lateral movement is an adequate substitute in the emergency room, but collar fixation is necessary if the patient is to be moved.

Chest evaluation includes observation of chest-wall motion with breathing; the motion should be assessed for depth and symmetry. Tactile evaluation of the chest wall is also extremely important. If crepitus or a "popping" sensation is felt over areas of rib, cartilage, or sternum, it is clear that severe chest-wall disruption has occurred. Tactile evaluation is particularly important in evaluating cartilage injury, which cannot be seen on a radiograph, and sternal injury which is often difficult to detect on routine chest films.

Auscultation may be helpful in detecting pneumothorax. The evaluation of breath sounds may provide evidence of fluid within the alveoli from a lung contusion, of the aspiration of gastric contents, or of blood in the pleural space. In some instances of ruptured diaphragm, bowel sounds heard during chest auscultation may be the first hint of this particular injury.

Evaluation of the abdomen should follow the chest examination. Splenic injury should be considered when there are rib fractures of the lower left chest. Confusion may arise when rib fractures per se produce upper abdominal tenderness without abdominal injury. Flank tenderness suggests kidney injury. Hematuria of any magnitude will point toward kidney, ureteral, bladder, or urethral injury and will require an intravenous pyelogram. In a patient who cannot void, a catheter will be necessary. When there is possible urinary tract injury, a catheter should be left in place in order to monitor the character and volume of urine output or to perform a cystourethrogram.

With severe blunt abdominal injury or any penetrating wound of the abdomen, peritoneal lavage should be done. All patients with gunshot or stab wounds that have entered the abdomen should have peritoneal lavage. For this reason, all patients with penetrating injuries (stab or gunshot) of the chest below the nipple line who are not definite candidates for laparotomy have peritoneal lavage in our hospital.[7] Patients with gunshot wounds that clearly enter the abdomen or gunshot wounds of the lower chest with abdominal findings are routinely subject to laparotomy. Those with stab wounds with stable vital signs and equivocal or

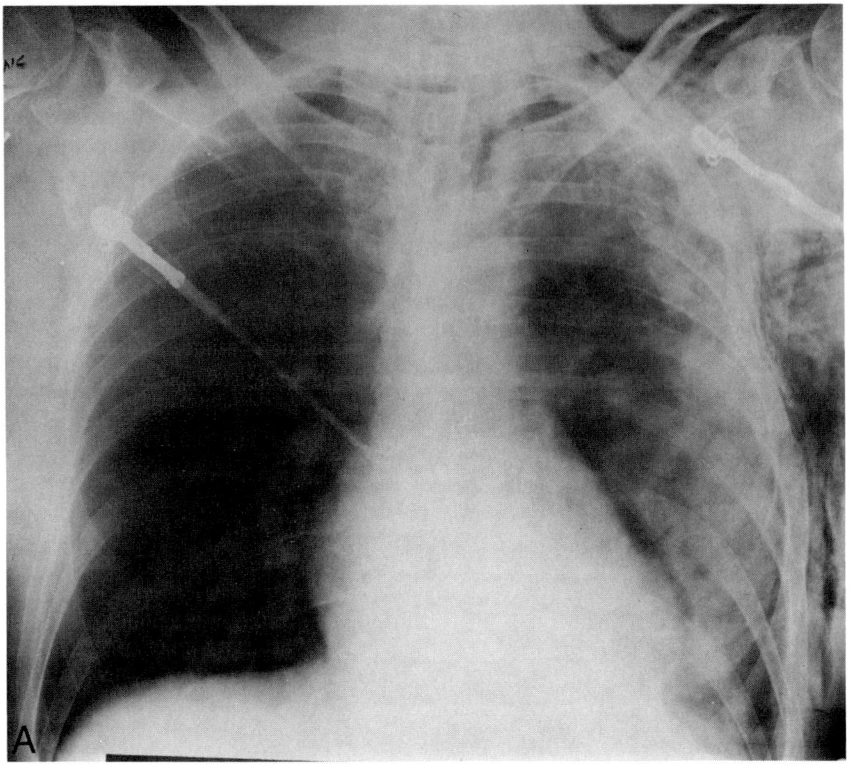

Figure 11–1. (A) Anteroposterior admission chest radiograph of a 57-year-old female who was driving an automobile that was hit on the left. She sustained double fractures of the second to the eighth left ribs and a pelvic fracture. Note alveolar infiltrate on left, which represents a pulmonary contusion, subcutaneous emphysema, and mediastinal air.

negative peritoneal lavage are observed. Occasionally, repeat lavage may be useful if there are subtle changes in the clinical picture. Peritoneal lavage is done almost routinely in the unconscious patient and in patients who cannot cooperate with examination because of alcohol, drug ingestion, or anxiety.

Peritoneal lavage fluid is analyzed for red blood cells, white blood cells, amylase, and bile. Results of analyses of lavage fluid are interpreted differently for blunt injuries and for lower thoracic penetrating (stab or gunshot) injuries.[8] If the effluent has more than 100,000 red blood cells/μl, prompt abdominal exploration is indicated after blunt injury. Using this criterion, there are positive findings in over 90 percent of cases with a false-negative rate of 4 percent (4 percent of patients with <100,000 RBC/μl have severe visceral injury). While the contents of a perforated viscus should evoke an intense outpouring of white blood cells into the peritoneal cavity, this response is delayed for at least 3 hours post-injury. Elevated amylase and bile levels suggest a perforated viscus and are most useful in diagnosing a duodenal injury with leakage into the peritoneum.

If the injury is a stab or gunshot penetration of the lower chest, >5000 RBC/μl

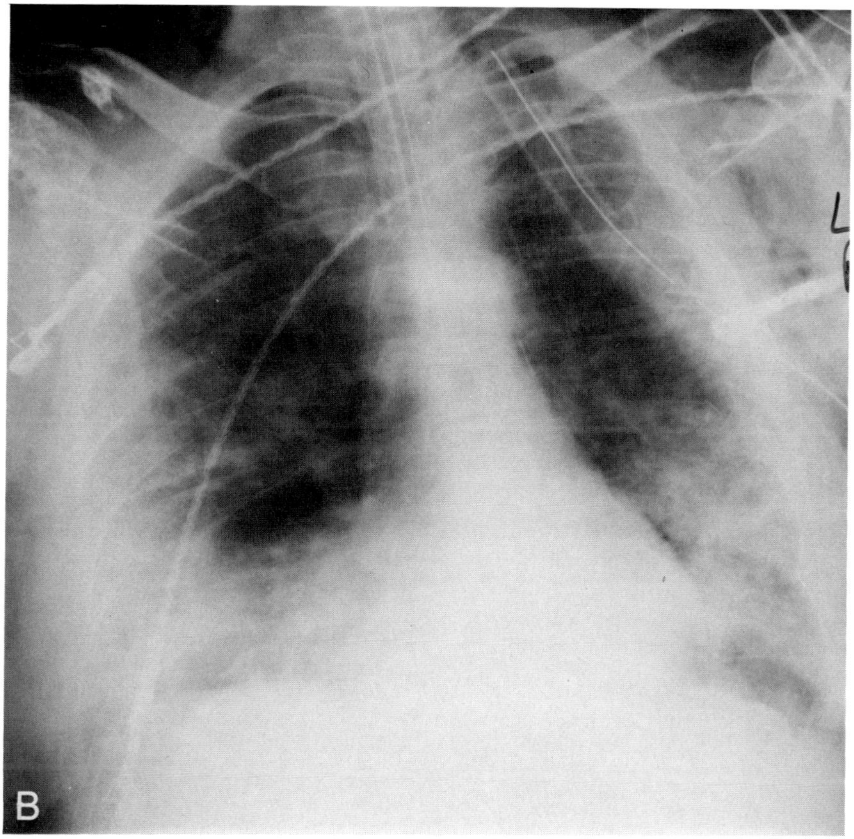

Figure 11–1 (continued). (B) The patient developed respiratory failure (ARDS) 48 hours following the trauma. Anteroposterior chest radiograph at 60 hours demonstrates the bilateral alveolar infiltrates characteristic of ARDS, in this instance secondary to pulmonary contusion and the fat emboli syndrome.

in the peritoneal lavage (approximately 1 cc whole blood/1000 cc infusate) dictates a laparotomy. This finding suggests at least a diaphragmatic injury that alone warrants operative repair, since delayed herniation of abdominal viscera is well known, and may be accompanied by obstruction or strangulation of hollow viscera and severe respiratory compromise. This is especially true if the diaphragmatic injury is small as opposed to large, since in the latter case early herniation with respiratory restriction occurs with less risk of obstruction or strangulation.

The Unconscious Patient

Severe neurologic injury rendering the patient unconscious or semiconscious, or spinal injuries rendering the patient analgesic compromise an initial examination for associated injuries. Neck injury must be ruled out in all such patients, and they must be protected against motion of the neck by a four-poster collar until it is clear that the spine is intact. Thoracic and lumbar spine films will be necessary for screening for such injuries. Associated chest and abdominal injuries may be difficult to detect, dictating that peritoneal lavage in lower chest injury or suspected abdominal injury should be done almost routinely.

Associated head and chest or abdominal injuries may require simultaneous operation if there is sufficient time to evaluate the head injury by computerized axial tomography (CAT) prior to emergency laparotomy or thoracotomy. This combination injury poses difficult management problems because the abdominal injury requires massive fluid replacement and the head injury is best managed with a normal or slightly low intravascular volume.

Life-threatening abnormalities seen in trauma patients are airway obstruction, hemorrhage, and shock. These frequently are associated with severe chest trauma.

AIRWAY THERAPY

Initial emergency room treatment in severe chest trauma usually includes the provision of an adequate airway by oral endotracheal tube, nasal endotracheal tube, or tracheostomy (see chapter 2). A serious consideration in the awake patient is whether or not there are symptoms or signs suggesting cervical spine injury. In the unconscious patient, spinal injury must be assumed to have occurred until the stability of the cervical spine is assured by adequate radiographs of the cervical spine down to the C7 level. In the unconscious patient with a compromised airway, oral endotracheal intubation carries a high risk of spinal cord injury. Careful endotracheal intubation may be done by the nasal route, with lateral motion of the head controlled by sandbags. If this is not successful, cricothyrotomy or tracheostomy should be done, making sure that the head is not extended during the procedure.

Additional indications for tracheostomy are associated massive facial injuries with airway obstruction by secretions or hemorrhage, the loss of soft-tissue support by bony injury, or direct obstruction by injured tissues. Fractures or transections of the larynx or cervical trachea are absolute indications for establishing an airway by standard or temporary end tracheostomy.

Tracheobronchial rupture or a traumatic esophago-respiratory fistula are uncommon but challenging injuries. Direct penetrating injuries of the intrathoracic trachea and major bronchi, although rare, present difficult airway management problems which must be individualized and handled with ingenuity. Long endotracheal tubes or divided endotracheal tubes such as the Carlens or Robertshaw tube may provide an adequate pre-operative airway.

HEMORRHAGE

Overt external hemorrhage is rare in chest trauma, being seen only in patients with massive blunt or penetrating chest wounds. At the same time that an airway is established, preparations for managing hemorrhage are made by the insertion of from two to four large-bore venous catheters at least one of which should be in position to monitor the central venous pressure.

Upper extremity or central (subclavian or internal jugular vein) sites are preferred for venous catheterization, especially in the patient with possible intra-abdominal venous injury, when lower extremity sites may be of less value. Multiple extremity fractures or upper thoracic bony injury may make the selection of adequate venous access sites difficult. A urinary catheter is mandatory to assess the effects of hypovolemia, impaired cardiac output, or associated urinary tract injury. Continuous electrocardiographic monitoring may detect associated cardiac injury or changes in intravascular volume status, oxygenation, CO_2 homeostasis or acid-base balance.

Marked intrapleural accumulation of either blood or air may necessitate the insertion of unilateral or bilateral chest tubes at the 5th or 6th interspace in the mid-axillary line. Initially, large amounts of blood are often lost through the tube, with cessation of the bleeding as the lung expands to fill the pleural space. This is presumed to indicate that the bleeding is from the low-pressure pulmonary circuit and that the large amount of tissue thromboplastin in lung tissue encourages hemostasis. The loss of the equivalent of 3 or 4 units of blood may be tolerated well by the healthy individual who receives adequate fluid replacement. Continued bleeding or the resumption of bleeding requires early thoracotomy, with localization and repair of the bleeding site. The bleeding will often be found to come from a systemic vessel, such as the internal mammary artery or an intercostal artery.

While thoracotomy is necessary for the control of bleeding in only 5 to 7 percent of patients with isolated chest injuries, the patient with massive intrapleural bleeding must be operated upon promptly, since the mortality in this group of patients ordinarily exceeds 50 percent. The bleeding in such patients commonly comes from multiple rib fractures with massive chest wall injury, and major pulmonary lacerations, including those to central pulmonary vessels and systemic arteries (the bronchial, intercostal, and internal mammary).

Massive intra-abdominal injury with hemorrhage requires immediate left thoracotomy, with aortic cross-clamping prior to laparotomy, often in the emergency room. The aorta, lying posterior to the heart in the lower chest, is identified by finger dissection. If possible, an umbilical tape should be passed around the aorta to facilitate cross-clamping, but it may be necessary to cross-clamp the aorta through palpation alone. The risks of cross-clamping are those of injury to an intercostal branch of the aorta, a compromise of blood flow to the spinal cord, and interference with renal blood flow. If hypotension is controlled, the cross-clamp should be removed as promptly as possible to restore spinal and renal blood flow and to lessen the adverse effects of increased afterload on left ventricular function. After laparotomy and the identification of bleeding sites, a more distal location for vascular cross-clamping, which still achieves the goal of controlling bleeding, may be substituted for the thoracic cross-clamp site. Rapid abdominal bleeding necessitating cross-clamping may rarely come from the spleen alone but is more commonly associated with severe liver injury, with major vessel injury, such as that to the aorta or vena cava, or with injury to multiple organs.

SHOCK

Shock in the chest trauma patient may come from several causes.[9] Hypovolemic shock is the most common type of shock in such patients. If the sole cause of shock is a low intravascular volume, treatment is direct and usually successful. Intravenous crystalloid and blood should be administered rapidly to restore a near-normal intravascular volume. If blood loss continues, the bleeding must be stopped. If the blood loss is in the chest, a thoracotomy will be required.

Unfortunately the cause and treatment of shock in the trauma patient is rarely simple; types of shock other than hypovolemic shock are seen alone or together in chest trauma. Septic shock is rare in the trauma patient during the early phases of resuscitation and treatment. Neurogenic shock is seen commonly in patients with associated brain or spinal cord injury. Hypoxic shock of a primary type may be induced by pulmonary contusion, tracheobronchial laceration, the obstruction of airways by blood or secretions, the aspiration of gastric contents, rupture of the diaphragm, flail chest, or loss of respiratory drive following a head injury. Later, local or systemic sepsis may contribute to the development of the adult respiratory distress syndrome.

Cardiogenic shock frequently occurs in the chest trauma patient. Injury to the heart itself may decrease the cardiac output as a result of contusion of the myocardium. Arrythmias from injury to heart muscle or direct injury to conduction pathways may be seen and are especially prominent in patients with preexisting coronary artery disease. Frank myocardial infarction may occur in such patients. Flow alterations produced by cardiac tamponade will reduce the cardiac output. The metabolic effects of chest injury, such as a reduced oxygen content of the blood and acidosis, may depress cardiac function even in the uninjured heart.

CARDIAC FUNCTION

The monitoring of cardiac function is enhanced by inserting an arterial line to measure the arterial pressure and to serially sample blood gases to insure that oxygenation and ventilation are adequate. The continuous ECG allows the assessment of rhythm disturbances. Measurement of the urine volume reflects cardiac function once it is established by the central venous pressure that there is adequate filling pressure. The central venous pressure should reflect the increased venous pressure if cardiac tamponade is present.

A useful adjuvant in the management of severely traumatized patients is the use of the Swan-Ganz catheter to measure the left-sided filling pressures since the pulmonary artery wedge pressure reflects the left atrial pressure. Despite the ease and speed of insertion of a Swan-Ganz catheter under ideal conditions, its placement is not recommended during the phase of acute resuscitation of the injured patient. After resuscitation, the insertion can be accomplished by the internal jugular vein route from the head of the operating table, even with drapes in position. Pressure readings from proximal (right atrial) and distal (pulmonary artery) ports, as well as the pulmonary artery wedge pressure, are useful in diagnosing cardiac tamponade, and help in managing the patient with myocardial contusion. If patients with myocardial contusions have associated injuries and receive large amounts of fluid, the injured heart may not be able to compensate. The Swan-Ganz catheter measurements allow the physician to provide an adequate filling pressure without overload, and to move to other measures to support the failing myocardium. These measures may include digitalization or the use of vasopressors or of agents capable of reducing afterload. Such agents can be used properly by employing a bedside computer that analyzes hemodynamic data and provides information about left ventricular stroke work, peripheral and pulmonary resistances, and respiratory parameters necessary for appropriate therapeutic decisions.

PREPARATION FOR OPERATION

All patients with severe injuries who require life- or limb-saving operations must have certain minimum requirements satisfied before undergoing anaesthesia. The airway must be controlled, and for practical purposes this means that an endotracheal tube is in position. There must be adequate fluid paths (from two to four), and two of these should be in the upper body, with one preferably in a position to record the central venous pressure. Also important is the introduction of a urinary catheter to assess urinary tract injury, monitor urine output, and prevent massive bladder distension during fluid resuscitation.

A nasogastric tube has lower priority, except in low-thoracic penetrating injuries. The tube is ordinarily easy to pass, and should be introduced promptly, since it will prevent or reduce the major gastric dilatation often incurred during early resuscitative efforts. If laparotomy is required, the abdominal exploration will be aided by decompression of the stomach. Patients often have major respiratory distress produced by acute gastric dilatation.

Rectal or esophageal temperature probes are essential to monitor the body core temperature. In major injury with massive blood loss, large open wounds, and massive volume replacement, profound hypothermia may develop. Hypothermic patients are hemodynamically fragile and often acidemic, and their blood coagulation may be affected adversely by altered platelet function. It is our policy to maintain for emergency use a warm trauma operating room which includes a warming mattress on the bed, readily available temperature probes and sterile, warm irrigation fluids, and warm blankets. A heated aerosol for ventilating the patient can avoid the loss of body heat by respiration. Blood warmers are used for all transfusions.

Chest tubes should be inserted into the pleural space where there is evidence of pneumothorax or hemothorax if the patient is going to operation for other causes, since it is difficult to detect and manage an air leak or bleeding into the pleural space under the operating room drapes. Continued bleeding from such chest tubes may serve to direct attention to a major source of hemorrhage not previously thought to be important.

With these measures completed, it should be possible to correct hypovolemia and provide adequate ventilation prior to anaesthesia and operation in all but the most critically injured patients, on whom operation may be required to control hemorrhage before the blood volume can be restored.

Patients may attain a state of compensation from hemorrhage as blood tamponades within the space occupied by a bleeding organ, such as the abdomen, thigh, or chest. This tenuous balance is often lost upon the induction of anaesthesia, the release from a compressive suit (MAST), or opening of the surgical space (abdomen or chest). The anaesthesia and surgical teams must be prepared to replace volume rapidly if bleeding resumes.

Cardiac tamponade, on the other hand, results in reduced ventricular filling and a low cardiac output. Temporary compensation for this can be achieved by raising the venous pressure above normal to increase cardiac filling. Prompt relief of the tamponade and control of the bleeding point will allow rapid return of the cardiac output to normal levels; the expanded intravascular volume should be reduced as the blood pressure rises.

ANTIBIOTICS

Most chest surgeons believe that antibiotics should be utilized in all instances of penetrating chest injury. In a double-blind prospective study, Grover and associates[10] demonstrated a reduced incidence of pneumonia, positive wound and pleural cultures, and empyema in patients treated with antibiotics. In addition, hospitalization was shorter and fewer operations were required in the treated group. In contrast to these findings, Oparah and Mandal[11] reported an incidence of empyema of only 0.5 percent in 200 penetrating stab wounds of the chest in patients who did not receive antibiotics.

Although literature on the subject is limited, it is believed that the contused lung has increased susceptibility to pneumonia, on the basis of the high incidence of pneumonia reported in chest trauma patients, especially those with flail chest.[12] It is probably prudent to treat patients with severe blunt chest trauma with antibiotics. Most thoracic surgeons use a cephalosporin for broad-spectrum coverage. The antibiotic should be given as soon as the determination has been made that the patient has sustained severe chest injury, and before surgery.

In summary, antibiotics should be administered to all patients with penetrating injury of the chest, and to patients with nonpenetrating trauma who have pulmonary parenchymal injury. Any patient requiring thoracotomy should receive antibiotic therapy. Antibiotic coverage for chest tubes is probably not necessary in nonpenetrating trauma when a chest tube is inserted for a readily corrected pneumothorax or hemothorax. However, if there is residual hemothorax on the post-chest tube radiograph, antibiotic coverage should be given.

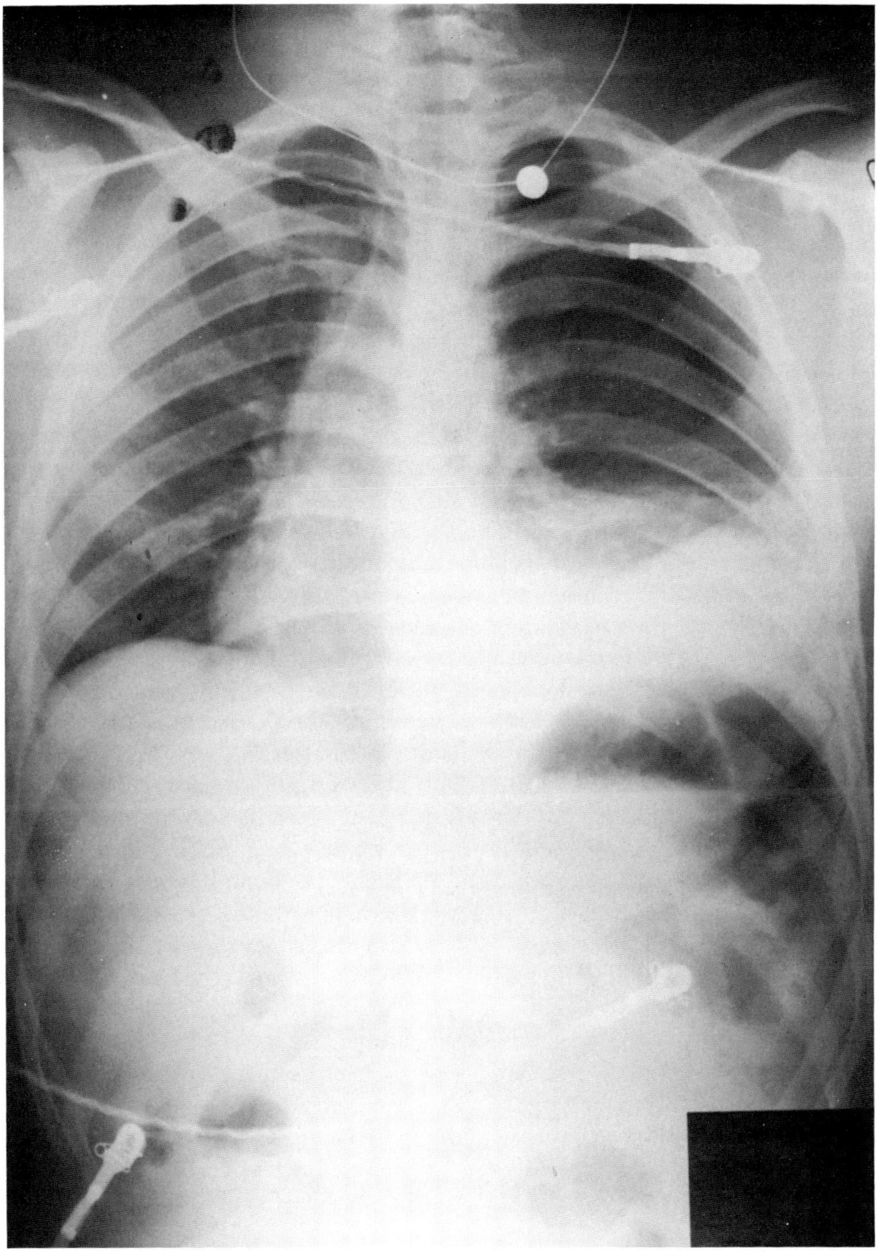

Figure 11–2. A 19-year-old male sustained a long knife stab wound of the right posterior chest. Anteroposterior chest radiograph demonstrated a left hemopneumothorax that was under tension. Left thoracotomy for continued bleeding demonstrated a lacerated intercostal artery.

THE CHEST RADIOGRAPH

The single most important diagnostic aid to the physician caring for a patient with chest injury or multiple trauma is the chest radiograph. In only a few patients with unrelenting hemorrhage and shock or complicated airway problems will it be necessary to proceed to operation without a chest film.

Ideally, the chest radiograph should be taken in the upright position, from a postero-anterior view and at the standard 6-foot distance. This allows a universal standard of comparison so that an evaluation of heart size, mediastinal width, diaphragm height, and other variables can be related to known standards. The detection of pneumothorax, hemothorax, or hemopneumothorax is facilitated by the upright posteroanterior position as compared with an anteroposterior supine film. The lateral film is usually not taken unless the patient can easily assume the upright position.

In the patient who cannot be moved from the supine position because of known or suspected associated injury or an altered state of consciousness, the supine radiograph is very useful but will require altered interpretation. Pleural fluid ordinarily will layer posterior to the lung, and will be seen only as an increased haziness. A small pneumothorax may be difficult to see because of the distribution of a small volume of air over a large anterior lung surface. The only indication of a pneumothorax may be a lucency in the region of the costophrenic angle. Heart and mediastinal shadows will appear widened in the anteroposterior projection as compared with the standard posteroanterior film. In some cases in which a widened mediastinum is seen on the supine film, the patient can be moved to a sitting position with the cassette positioned in front of the patient, and a 6-foot postero-anterior film can be taken; this projection may demonstrate a normal mediastinal or cardiac shadow and preclude further invasive tests. However, if the mediastinum is actually widened, great-vessel injury is of prime consideration in severe blunt chest trauma. Other than mediastinal widening, radiographic findings of aortic rupture include deviation of the trachea to the right, deviation of the nasogastric tube to the left, loss of the aortic knob shadow, a left pleural effusion (blood), rib fractures, and depression of the left main-stem bronchus.[13]

Even in the most serious chest injuries, a posteroanterior and lateral radiograph will give all of the information needed for emergency care of the patient. As mentioned earlier, the lateral radiograph is useful only if the patient can be positioned properly, and for this reason is often unavailable to aid in the diagnosis. Lateral decubitus views may be required later to define whether a collection of fluid in the pleural space is loculated or free-flowing or to differentiate whether an increased density at the base of the lung is due to atelectasis or fluid, or to a combination of both.

Special rib radiographs are often ordered by the physician inexperienced in the care of chest injury, under the impression that such films will aid in the care of the patient and offer legal protection by revealing otherwise missed rib fractures. However, since care of the patient is directed at changes in the underlying lung and not at rib fractures, which universally heal, there is little merit to doing

Table 11–1. Time Course of Chest Radiograph Findings in Blunt Chest Trauma

Injury	Initial Chest Radiograph	Time of Radiographic Appearance from Injury	Radiographic Resolution
Contusion	Consolidation: patchy to homogenous	Early: within 6 hrs.	Rapid: 24–48 hours
Laceration (lung cyst)	Cystic structures 2–14 cm	Immediate to several days depending on associated injury	Slow: 6 weeks to months
Hematoma	Homogenous, well-demonstrated mass	Same as laceration	Same as laceration
Hemothorax	Pleural fluid	Immediate	Several days
Pneumothorax	Air in pleural space	Immediate	Several days
Pneumonia	Consolidation	Several days	Days to weeks
Aortic rupture	Mediastinal widening, other findings	Immediate	Fatal initially in 80%; will rupture by 10 weeks in 90%
Esophageal rupture	Left pleural effusion, subcutaneous and mediastinal emphysema, mediastinal widening	Hours to days	Days to weeks
Diaphragmatic rupture	Silhouette sign of diaphragm and abnormal shadows in chest	Immediate or months- or years	Persists until surgery
Tracheobronchial fracture	Mediastinal and subcutaneous air and pneumothorax	Immediate, 10% have no radiographic findings	Bronchial obstruction and atelectasis occur late.
Adult respiratory distress syndrome	Bilateral alveolar infiltrates	48 to 72 hours	Days to weeks

special films for rib or sternal injuries. These special films are expensive, involve positioning which may be painful to the patient, require additional time in the emergency setting, and will not reveal costal cartilage injury more readily than the routine chest radiograph. Such cartilaginous injuries are detected only by careful physical examination, which will elucidate a popping sensation under the fingers with breathing or coughing.

Once obtained, the chest radiograph must be studied carefully to delineate changes in the mediastinum (which contains the heart, major vessels, trachea and major bronchi, and esophagus), the lung parenchyma, the pleural spaces, the diaphragms, and the bony thorax. Foreign bodies such as teeth or dentures may be seen displaced into the esophagus, trachea, or bronchi. The path of missiles may be marked by fractures or small fragments of metal broken off upon contact with some bony structure and spreading along the subsequent path of the missile.

Traumatic aortic aneurysm, which is characterized by disruption of the intima and media with the thin but intact adventitia containing the blood, carries the threat of rupture into the pleural space with exsanguination and constitutes an indication for emergency aortography (see the discussion below of traumatic aortic rupture).

Pneumomediastinum may be due to rupture of the trachea or major bronchi, or of the esophagus (see the discussions of tracheobronchial rupture and esophageal rupture), but is more commonly due to injury to the parenchyma of the lung without disruption of the pleura, so that alveolar air is released subpleurally and dissects along the vascular sheath to the hilum of the lung and into the mediastinum.

The time of appearance of chest radiograph findings following a thoracic injury will help the physician in diagnosing the types and extent of the injury. The time course of resolution may also be helpful in retrospectively defining the exact nature of the injury (Table 11–1).

PULMONARY PARENCHYMAL INJURY

Penetrating wounds of the lung invariably result in injury to the pulmonary parenchyma. The most common such injuries result from stab wounds or low-velocity gunshot wounds. High-velocity rifle wounds may produce extensive damage to the solid tissues of the chest wall, but do not have a profound explosive effect on the lung itself because of the low density of lung tissue. Peripheral lung-field injuries are tolerated well. Central injuries involving the hilum and major hilar structures may require early thoracotomy and control of hilar vessels, followed by suture of the major arteries or veins, or by pulmonary resection when these vessels cannot be reconstituted.

Owing to the presence of high levels of thromboplastin in lung tissue and relatively low pressures in the pulmonary circuit, bleeding from the lung will commonly stop promptly once the lung is expanded to the chest wall with a chest tube having an underwater seal.

Stab wounds produce a lung laceration with varying amounts of bleeding. Gunshot wounds produce the same injuries plus an element of pulmonary contusion. This contusion is seen to be increased when the wounding missile strikes the bony chest wall, transmitting its kinetic energy to the underlying lung. Shotgun injuries at close range, with multiple wounding pellets, may create extensive chest wall destruction. Indriven bone fragments, wadding from the shotgun shell, and bits of clothing often produce major underlying lung contusion and destruction despite the small size of the individual wounding fragments.

Any penetrating injury of the lung affords the possibility of introducing air into the pulmonary veins for return to the left side of the heart. The risk of this is probably enhanced by vigorous positive pressure breathing during acute resuscitation. There is controversy as to how often this occurs, but there is no question that occasional patients who present with what would seem to be a nonlethal pulmonary parenchymal injury are not salvaged.

Blunt injuries produce lacerations or contusion of the lung. Lacerations may bleed extensively and produce pulmonary hematomas. The pulmonary contusion, associated with and surrounding the pulmonary laceration, may mask the laceration. For this reason, pulmonary lacerations and their associated hematomas are often diagnosed retrospectively, after the contusion has resolved. In a chest radiograph, the pulmonary laceration and associated hematoma are seen as an elliptical radiodensity. Depending upon the amount of blood and air in the pulmonary laceration "cavity," either an air-fluid level or a crescent of air may be seen. Resolution times vary widely, and the hematoma may present as a solitary nodule months following the injury.[14]

Pulmonary contusion is the most frequent radiographic finding in patients with severe blunt chest injury. Radiographic manifestations of this appear during the first few hours and resolve over several days. There are two predominant patterns: (1) patchy, stringy densities, probably representing blood along the distal broncho-pulmonary sheaths; and (2) a homogenous density representing blood and fluid in alveoli. Patients with blunt chest trauma compatible with pulmonary contusion and who do not follow the expected sequence of resolution should be evaluated for infection, an endobronchial obstruction, pulmonary hematoma, or recent hemorrhage.[15,16]

A difficult differential diagnosis in the patient with chest trauma is that of pulmonary contusion versus aspiration pneumonitis (see Chapter 12). Patients presenting after motor vehicle accidents often have high blood alcohol concentrations and full stomachs. A blow to the abdomen during the accident may cause vomiting and aspiration, leading to a chemical pneumonitis with an outpouring of fluid into the alveoli. Pulmonary contusion may cause alveolar filling and presents an identical radiographic picture. Aspiration is more likely to be diffuse rather than localized to the traumatized area of the lung. Minor degrees of aspiration and contusion both clear rapidly, while major aspiration may evidence parenchymal changes for several days.

While the pulmonary alveolar changes in contusion and aspiration occur almost immediately after injury, hemorrhagic changes tend to occur later. Patients who develop the adult respiratory distress syndrome (ARDS) following chest trauma do so only after a latent period. The diffuse alveolar infiltrate on the chest roentgenogram in this syndrome usually does not appear until 48 to 72 hours following injury, although unfavorable changes in blood gases often precede the radiographic findings. The time of appearance of ARDS radiographically is the time that pulmonary contusion should resolve (see Table 11–1).

Radiographic parenchymal changes seen on the initial chest radiograph are consistent with the type of injury. Penetrating injury can produce a hematoma or tract within the lung, bleeding into the pleural space, pneumothorax, or a combination of these. Blunt trauma with laceration of the lung can produce the same changes. Contusion of the lung will produce changes only in the lung itself, although both laceration and contusion may occur simultaneously. A diffuse alveolar infiltrate occurring 48 to 72 hours after a long-bone fracture or massive soft tissue trauma and accompanied by hypoxemia, confusion, and pettichiae is characteristic of the fat embolism syndrome.

THE PLEURAL SPACE

Air in the pleural space (pneumothorax) may come from the lung itself, from injury to major or minor air passages, through the chest wall in penetrating trauma, and rarely from therapeutic misadventures during the placement of central venous catheters. Occasionally abdominal air gains access to the pleural space from small passages through the normal diaphragm or from major diaphragmatic injury. Pneumothorax following trauma must be presumed to be due to the trauma, although apical cystic lung disease, which is usually associated with primary spontaneous pneumothorax, may be a predisposing factor.

Blood enters the pleural space from the lung or its hilar vessels, from systemic chest wall vessels (such as the internal mammary or intercostal vessels), from the heart or great vessels, and when a traumatic aortic aneurysm ruptures into the pleural space. Rarely, a stab wound will injure an extrathoracic systemic vessel and penetrate the chest wall, allowing bleeding into the chest with effective sealing of the external stab wound. We have encountered three such cases, in two of which there was bleeding from large muscular arteries of the chest wall, and one in which there was bleeding from a totally transected subclavian vein.

The presence of pneumothorax, hemothorax, or a combination of both may or may not require a chest tube when identified on the chest radiograph, depending on the degree of lung collapse or the amount of fluid or air in the pleural space. The patient with small accumulations of air ($<$ 10 percent pneumothorax) or fluid ($<$ 100 cc) may be observed closely. In any patient who requires operation for another injury, however, it is prudent to insert a chest tube to prevent the development of a large pneumothorax or to monitor sudden blood loss from the chest while operative drapes are in position.

Special attention to the relative volumes of the pleural spaces will help in the appraisal of lung collapse or the rare incidence of torsion of a pulmonary lobe.

Chest Drainage

Control of pneumothorax or hemothorax after trauma is best achieved by large-bore (36 to 40 French) chest tubes. Ordinarily a single tube placed in the mid-axillary line at the level of the seventh intercostal space is sufficient. If this does not result in prompt emptying of the pleural space, additional tubes may be inserted, with the location of the insertion dictated by the position of residual air or fluid on the chest radiograph. Lower initial tube insertions carry the risk of traversing the diaphragm, especially if that structure is elevated by intra-abdominal bleeding. It is especially important in trauma patients, who may be uncooperative or semiconscious, that the chest tube be firmly fixed to the chest wall with a large suture to prevent its inadvertent removal.

The crisis of tension pneumothorax (see Chapter 9) can be managed by insertion of a large-bore needle into the second anterior interspace. More definitive treatment requires chest tube insertion connected to an underwater seal device, although the complete evacuation of blood and air from the pleural space may require the additional application of chest suction.[17] If the leak is large, an electric chest suction apparatus which can provide a high vacuum and overcome a high-volume leak may be necessary. An ideal machine should produce a vacuum of up to 80 cmH_2O with a volume flow in excess of 20 liters per minute.[18]

Convenient, disposable, commercial chest-suction control units are available. The limitations of these are their high cost and limits on the pressure and volume of the suction they provide. The maximum pressure in such control units does not exceed -25 cmH_2O, and the volume flow is limited, so that an additional chest tube, with an additional collection control unit, may be necessary to manage a high-volume leak. In patients with a large hemothorax, these units are filled rapidly. The units cannot be emptied while maintaining sterility. For these reasons, simple chest-bottle drainage systems of moderate cost are best suited for the early management of hemopneumothorax.

THE CHEST WALL

The chest radiograph is most helpful in detecting chest wall injuries. Pneumothorax may result from penetration of the chest wall with leakage of air resulting from a positive atmospheric pressure relative to the pressure of the pleural space. An oblique fracture of a rib may puncture the lung or pinch a portion of lung into the fracture site, producing an air leak.

Hemothorax may result from such chest wall injuries as intercostal or internal mammary artery lacerations. In this circumstance the bleeding will be arterial and from the higher pressure systemic circuit, so that it is less likely to be stopped by the expedient of attaining full lung expansion with a chest tube than if the bleeding were from a pulmonary vessel.

The chest radiograph will demonstrate a large majority of rib fractures and detect the underlying lung injury. Where there is massive chest wall injury with multiple fractured ribs and gross displacement of rib fragments not corrected by endotracheal intubation and assisted ventilation, stabilization of alternate fractured ribs may allow early removal of the patient from the ventilator and chest wall healing in a normal configuration.

Special attention should be paid to the location, number, and multiplicity of fractured ribs. Specific points of attention are fractures of the well-protected first and second ribs.[19] Fracture of these structures indicates severe trauma, and some authors have reported an increased incidence of thoracic aortic aneurysm, brachial plexus injury, Horner's syndrome, tracheobronchial fracture, injury to the subclavian artery, and high mortality in these patients.[20,21] However, Yee[22] has demonstrated that isolated first rib fractures are of low prognostic significance in vascular injury, and he recommends arteriography only for specific indications.

Fracture of numerous upper ribs posteriorly frequently is seen when the scapula is forcefully driven into the chest wall, creating a line of posterior rib fractures and associated ipsilateral clavicular fracture. Posterior rib fractures produce less instability because of muscular support but suggest more severe trauma.

It is well known that muscle pull can induce first-rib fracture, since contralateral fracture of the first rib is often found coincidentally within a few days after an upper-rib-tailoring thorocoplasty. The muscle strains imposed by trauma probably account for first-rib fractures where there is minimal displacement and no associated vascular or nerve injury.

Multiple lower left rib fractures are often associated with splenic injury, and such fractures should alert the physician to the possibility of acute or delayed rupture of the spleen.

Sternal fractures are best diagnosed on a properly penetrated lateral chest radiograph. Special sternal views are often not as good for this purpose. The fractures are often stable and cause no trouble except for local tenderness and mild deformity. Unstable sternal fractures, which cause severe pain and dyspnea, should be stabilized to improve ventilation. Severe sternal displacement without evidence of rib fractures implies separation of the costochondral junctions or fracture of the anterior chest wall cartilages.

Rib Fractures

Simple fractured ribs per se are of minor importance in the emergency setting, since they will ultimately heal; the important factor is the injury to the underlying lung. However, this reasoning fails in a practical way, since even a single rib fracture is sometimes accompanied by severe and unrelenting chest wall pain which limits motion and more importantly prevents deep breathing and coughing, so that secretions may not be cleared properly and atelectasis and pneumonia may result.

The chest wall pain caused by a rib fracture will to some extent be relieved by restricting chest wall motion with sandbags, strapping with elastic supportive tape or belts, or by taping with a non-yielding tape. However, although the pain relief is welcomed by the patient, this treatment promotes the development of atelectasis.

Intercostal nerve block to the involved segment of rib is the most useful method of treating chest wall pain from simple fractures, allowing normal chest wall motion with coughing and deep breathing.

For several adjacent rib fractures, intercostal nerve block of the involved rib or ribs plus one uninvolved rib above and below, utilizing 0.5 to 1 percent lidocaine hydrochloride, will give almost instantaneous relief lasting for several hours. In some cases this treatment breaks up a severe pain cycle that has limited coughing, permitting the patient to cough vigorously and eliminate retained bronchial secretions. Further blocks may or may not be necessary; their need can be resolved by the patient and doctor at the bedside. Longer effect may be attained by following an initial small lidocaine injection with an injection of 0.5 percent bupivicaine hydrochloride, which has a longer effect. Bupivicaine is not satisfactory for the initial injection because its action is delayed for several minutes and the block is not well tolerated.

The technique of the nerve block is simple. Several skin wheals are raised posterior to the fracture sites to allow approach to each rib from an inferior position, so as to allow the tip of the needle to enter the intercostal bundle (nerve, artery, and vein), which lies protected behind the inferior aspect of the rib. The needle is introduced to contact the outer surface of the rib, and is "walked off" until it is in the region of the intercostal bundle. Aspiration always must be attempted before injection, in order to avoid intravascular injection. When properly located, a 1 ml injection is as effective as several milliliters, and a number of spaces can be injected without risk of toxicity. The addition of epinephrine has no merit, and is contraindicated in patients with cardiac disease. Immediately after a successful nerve block the patient should be encouraged to cough under the benefit of the analgesia afforded by the block. Such inducement may include nasotracheal suctioning for maximum benefit.

As greater numbers of ribs are fractured, the chest becomes increasingly unstable and more complex treatment becomes necessary.

Flail Chest

Understanding this abnormality depends upon recognizing that fractures of ribs and of chest wall cartilages between the costochondral junctions and the articulations with the sternum are of equal importance. In addition, transverse or oblique fractures across the sternum may contribute to chest wall instability. Flail chest occurs when multiple fractures along the chest wall or double fractures of several adjacent ribs occur, leaving a large segment of the chest wall unsupported. The finely coordinated chest wall muscle movements which contribute to normal breathing then become unsychronized. In normal breathing, each rib-cartilage unit is hinged anteriorly and posteriorly like a bucket handle, and all of these units move as one to increase the chest volume as the units swing up and out during inspiration, and to decrease the chest volume as the ribs drop down and in as the inspiratory muscles relax. In the flail chest, a free segment of chest wall may be depressed during inspiration and move outward during expiration, altering the chest wall action to the extent of the size of the involved area.

An additional detrimental effect of a unilateral flail segment is thought to be the so called "pendel-luft." This occurs when the normal, efficient chest wall motion of the uninvolved side continues to move air normally in and out of the tracheobronchial tree, but also causes air to move back and forth across the carina within the tracheobronchial tree. Under such circumstances, alveolar ventilation on the injured side is compromised severely, since the air is moving back and forth within the lung and is not mixing with newly inspired tracheal air. This phenomenon probably occurs to a lesser extent when chest wall motion is restricted by pain and splinting. However, despite its popularity in standard texts, the theory of the nature of pendel-luft has not been substantiated experimentally.[23]

Any mechanism that stabilizes the flail segment will improve respiratory mechanisms in the flail chest. In the past, treatment has included compression and immobilization of the flail segment by sandbags or compression dressings of adhesive tape, as well as by pulling the flail segment outward with traction devices such as towel clips, wires, and screws attached to the ribs percutaneously. Both of these methods reduced the pain of multiple fracture sites by eliminating motion of the flail segment; however, the compression methods did little to improve ventilation, while the traction methods carried the risk of causing pneumothorax or hemothorax by inducing bleeding from intercostal vessels.

In 1956 Avery and Morch[24] introduced the concept treating flail chest through the use of a ventilator, pointing out that most of the pain of breathing in simple fractured ribs or in flail chest is associated with active inspiration, the expiratory phase being essentially passive when the chest wall musculature relaxes. With the production of alkalemia with hyperventilation and maintenance of a high PaO_2, the patient does not attempt to breath with his own effort. Ventilation with a mechanical apparatus allows the inspiratory phase of breathing to become passive; when necessary this is further enhanced by the use of narcotics in doses that would be contraindicated in the patient struggling to maintain adequate ventilation independently.

On the basis of the assumption that artificial ventilation would have to be continued until the healing of chest wall fractures had occurred, and that preliminary stabilization by callus formation and fibrous union would be accomplished by 14 days, it was widely accepted that once begun, ventilatory support would have to be continued for 2 weeks. Subsequent experience has indicated that ventilation may be discontinued by following the usual respiratory parameters that reflect the ability of the chest wall to function and the lungs to adequately participate in gas exchange. In many instances this will be accomplished within a few days after injury.

TRACHEOBRONCHIAL RUPTURE

Injuries of the larynx and cervical trachea may be of the penetrating type, with either partial injury or complete transection, or may be caused by direct blunt trauma to the neck. With transection injuries the distal trachea is disposed to retract into the mediastinum, and must be immediately located and intubated, preferably after pulling the trachea back to its normal cervical location. Once the airway is established, tracheal repair can be done provided that a long segment of the trachea has not been crushed.

Laryngeal lacerations often may be repaired, although temporary or permanent cord paralysis may result from injury to the recurrent laryngeal nerve. In most severe laryngeal injuries it is necessary to splint the larynx internally and to perform a low tracheostomy. This treatment must usually be done over a period of many weeks or months.

The entire trachea is subject to injury from penetrating trauma, but such injuries are rare. The classic injury to the lower trachea is that of rupture of the distal trachea or proximal main bronchus following blunt trauma; this usually occurs within 2 to 3 cm above or below the carina,[25] and is associated with fracture of the first three ribs and a high mortality rate. The mechanism of injury is that of a shearing force on the area of the tracheal bifurcation as the sternum is compressed toward the spine. Experimental rupture of the bronchus requires an increase in the airway pressure in addition to the shearing force. The injury often occurs without any associated chest wall skeletal injury.

The diagnostic triad in tracheobronchial rupture is that of hemoptysis, pneumothorax, and extensive subcutaneous and mediastinal emphysema although in 10 percent of patients there will be no clinical findings at presentation.[27] After neutralization of the pneumothorax or pneumothoraces with chest tubes, the diagnosis can be confirmed by bronchoscopy, at which time injured cartilage will be identified. Prolonged bronchoscopy is unnecessary and usually impossible.

Once the diagnosis of tracheobronchial rupture is established, the patient should be taken to the operating room for a right thoracotomy. A long endotracheal tube of the smallest size that will adequately ventilate the patient should be used. Once the chest is opened, this tube can be advanced into the uninjured bronchus, and the injured bronchus can be repaired. If the tube interferes with repair, intermittent periods of effective ventilation, interspersed with short periods of deliberate apnea with the tube pulled up a short distance from the operative area, will provide satisfactory conditions for suturing the bronchus. The right-sided approach allows easy access to the bifurcation of the trachea and the proximal bronchi through division of the mediastinal pleura and interruption of only the azygous vein. Attempts to reach the bifurcation area through the left thoracotomy approach are hindered by the aortic arch immediately crossing the operative field and not lending itself to easy retraction. The recurrent laryngeal nerve also obstructs this approach to some extent.

Unless the lower respiratory tract is colonized at the time of injury with bacteria, as in bronchiectasis, chronic bronchitis, or acute pneumonia, the lung may remain uninfected after the injury, even when recognition of the injury is delayed. At some time after the injury, bronchial and vascular changes in the lung suggest that lung function will not be restored, and resection may then be recommended; it is for this reason that early recognition and repair of a tracheobronchial rupture is important.

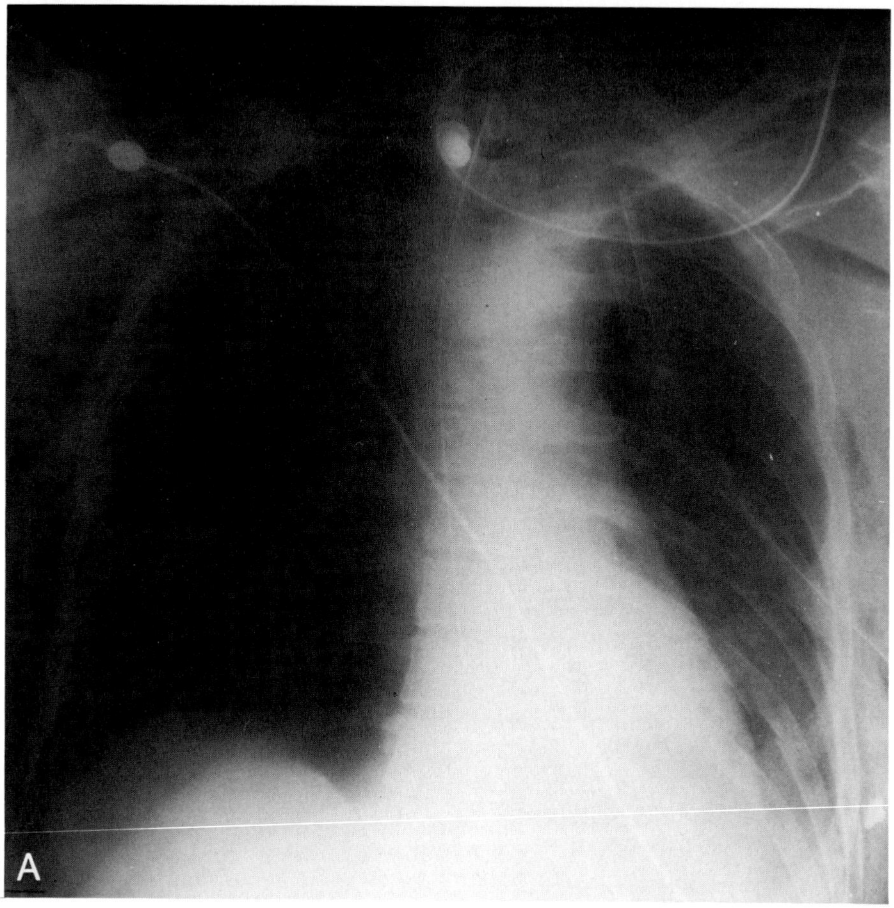

Figure 11–3. (A) Anteroposterior chest radiograph of a 29-year-old male driver injured in a head-on automobile accident. The wide superior mediastinum led to an aortogram.

LUNG TORSION

Torsion of a lung or a lobe of the lung after severe blunt injury to the chest is rare, usually occurring in children, probably because of their very compressible thoracic cage.

The diagnosis should be suspected from a chest radiograph, since the pattern of pulmonary vascular markings is altered in a predictable manner, with a reversal of the usual upper- and lower-lung zone pattern. If the torsion is not relieved, the vascular supply is compromised and alveolar filling ensues, producing a "ground-glass" radiographic density.[28]

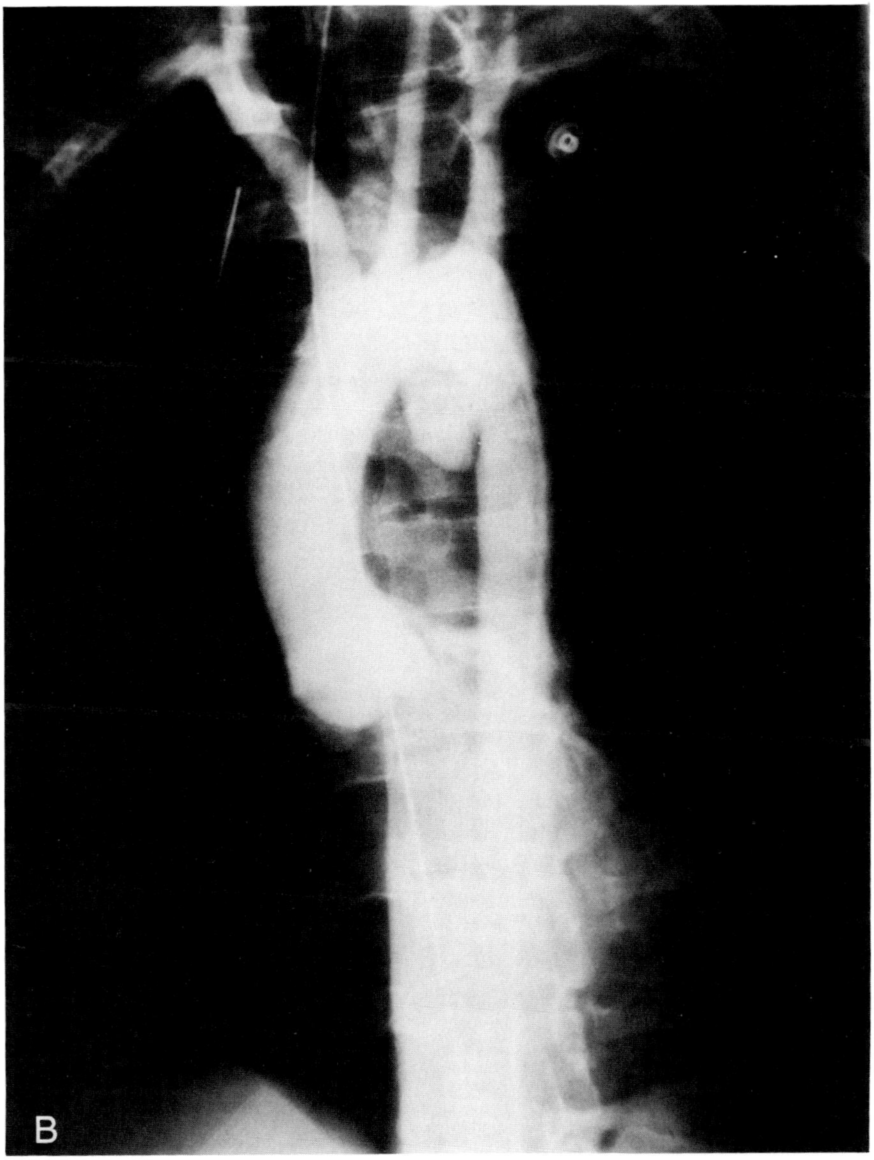

Figure 11–3 (continued).B) Aortogram demonstrated aortic rupture at the isthmus. The hematoma was contained by the adventitia with tear of the intima and media.

CARDIAC TAMPONADE

One of the more subtle diagnostic dilemmas in a stable, hospitalized patient is that of establishing firmly the presence of cardiac tamponade. This difficulty is compounded in the acutely traumatized patient who may be hypovolemic, acidotic, agitated, or bleeding acutely from an associated injury. The central venous pressure (CVP) reading is important, but often so unreliable as to give inadequate data at best and incorrect information at worst. Physical findings may be masked by hemothorax, pneumothorax and, in the agitated patient, a pulsus paradoxus would be possible to assess.

In the relatively stable patient with normal lung examination results, reduced heart tones, a documented elevated CVP, and a falling blood pressure, a strong suspicion of tamponade must be maintained, and aspiration of the pericardial sac may be done. Trinkle reported a 6 percent false-positive rate and a 19 percent false negative rate in the diagnosis of tamponade in 47 trauma patients.[29]

In former years, removal of blood from the pericardium with improvement in the clinical picture allowed a further period of waiting and even repeated aspiration of the pericardial sac before surgery. In recent years, however, it has become apparent that open operation and control of the bleeding point is the safest and most satisfactory method of managing tamponade. Pericardiocentesis should be applied only as a temporizing therapeutic measure in moribund patients exhibiting tamponade during transport to the operating room.[29]

CARDIAC INJURY

Details of the management of cardiac injury are beyond the scope of this chapter. It should be recognized, however, that both blunt and penetrating injuries of the heart may result in laceration of the chambers, valves, conduction tracts, and coronary arteries.[30] Chamber injuries may result in tamponade or exsanguinating hemorrhage, depending on the integrity of the pericardium, and ordinarily will require prompt surgical intervention if there is to be any hope of salvage. The operative approach will depend upon the wounded sites. If a skilled perfusion team is readily available, there is sometimes an indication for the use of cardiopulmonary bypass, which offers the additional advantages of recycling the shed blood. On the other hand, time is of the essence in these serious injuries, and the patient may die during the extra time required for cannulation for bypass. The requirement for total heparinization, with its attendant effect on bleeding from other sites in the patient with multiple injuries limits the use of cardiopulmonary bypass except in extraordinary circumstances. Blood-salvaging autotransfusion devices, which heparinize the blood as it is suctioned from the field and wash and filter it with dilution removal of most of the heparin, are currently available. The product of the equipment is a high-hematocrit fluid with washed cells. However, blood lost in massive amounts can only partially be salvaged because of the restrictions of a single suction tip and the time required for the washing, centrifugation, and return of the blood product. An additional disadvantage of autotransfusion devices is that the wisdom of salvaging blood contaminated with gastrointestinal contents—especially in injuries in which there is spillage from the lower gastrointestinal tract—has not been established.

Injuries to cardiac valves ordinarily result in partial valvular insufficiency which may be well tolerated for long periods of time. If the patient can be stabilized, it is usually better to work through the early post-trauma period without an operation and to plan valve replacement or repair electively once total heparinization for cardiopulmonary bypass is judged to be safe.

Conduction abnormalities are seen commonly in cardiac contusion. Dangerous arrythmias usually can be controlled with the use of a temporary transvenous pacemaker. Occasionally, a severe contusion may result in a permanent depression of ventricular function, although complete recovery is more common after a period of observation and limited activity.

Coronary artery laceration will usually require prompt exploration because of continued bleeding. Small peripheral vessels may be ligated safely with little overall effect on cardiac function. However, the ligation of central vessels may result in a large area of myocardial infarction, with a threat to the patient's life. Patients have survived such injury with placement of a venous bypass graft from the aorta to the distal coronary artery. This requires a prompt decision to operate and to support the circulation with cardiopulmonary bypass during the operation.

TRAUMATIC AORTIC RUPTURE

The most common location of rupture of the aorta is the aortic isthmus, the site of the ligamentum arteriosum, which is the remnant of the ductus arteriosus. Rupture of the aorta is due to a high-speed deceleration injury with the patient in the upright position. It is common in auto accidents and is found in a large percentage of deaths from aircraft accidents, which usually occur at very high speeds. The mechanism of injury is thought to be the relative forward mobility of the heart, ascending aorta, and aortic arch, with the immobility of the descending aorta, which is secured to the posterior chest wall by the small but numerous intercostal vessels. An upright deceleration injury therefore creates a shearing force at the point at which the mobile aortic arch meets the fixed descending aorta—the aortic isthmus. Since the aortic wall in the area of attachment of the ligamentum arteriosum differs histologically from the rest of the aortic wall, a natural weakness in this area may contribute to the rupture.

It is estimated that 20 percent of patients who sustain a rupture of the aortic intima and media in auto accidents are brought to hospitals. During this period the blood flow is contained by the adventitia and mediastinal pleura. One-quarter of these (5 percent of the total) will attain the stage of chronic aneurysm formation at 3 months without a free rupture. Thus, 15 percent of the group are at risk for a free rupture of the aorta and sudden death in the hours, days, or weeks after injury. Prompt diagnosis in the earliest post-injury period may allow the repair of a rupture by direct anastamosis or vascular graft.

Other aortic injuries include avulsion of the innominate artery from the aorta, rupture of the ascending aorta, rupture of the descending aorta distal to the aortic isthmus, and occasional avulsion of the left carotid or left subclavian artery from the aorta.

Innominate artery avulsion is attributed to a natural desire to protect the face when an automobile is nearing impact with a tree, bridge abutment, slowed vehicle ahead, or some other immovable object. Turning the head to the left puts the innominate artery in a stretched position, and impact to the anterior chest forces the heart and ascending aorta downward, putting maximum stress on the area of the innominate artery take-off. Exsanguination is prevented by containment of the hematoma by the aortic and innominate adventitia and mediastinal soft tissues. Sternal fracture is a common associated injury.

Patients with ascending aortic tears are rarely salvaged, since much of the ascending aorta is intrapericardial. These injuries were commonly reported when jumping from heights was a more usual method of self destruction than it is today. With the aortic arch suspended by its major vessels, a downward pull of the heart in deceleration puts marked stress on the ascending aorta. If the adventitia does not contain the blood flow, sudden exsanguination with immediate tamponade occurs. Correction of this particular type of aortic injury requires extracorporeal circulation unless the tear is small and can be controlled by finger pressure until the aorta can be sutured.

Descending aortic tears seem to violate the rule that survival depends on preservation of the intact adventitia, since these injuries are usually seen in association with posterior rib fractures; however, it can be speculated that a sharp rib fragment has perforated the aorta resulting in a partial tear which is then sealed over by the adventitia and parietal pleura.

Left common carotid and subclavian tears, which are rare, must have a similar mechanism of injury to that in innominate artery avulsion.

The hallmark of aortic rupture is the wide superior mediastinal shadow seen on a chest radiograph. Associated upper rib injuries may be found, and a superior pleural cap shadow may be seen. The diagnosis is confirmed by aortography.

If there is free bleeding into the pleural space, the prognosis is extremely grave. Under these circumstances exploration must be done without an arteriogram. This presents special problems because rupture may occur at more than one site. The preferred operative approach for an innominate vulsion or ascending aortic injury is through a median sternotomy. The preferred approach for the other sites of aortic rupture discussed above is a left thoracotomy. The decision about which approach to take is made from the arteriogram. If the latter cannot be done, the approach is through a left anterior chest incision, to get to the more common site of rupture, carrying the incision across the sternum into the right anterior chest if necessary.

If the traumatic hematoma created by an aortic rupture is contained and does not itself rupture during anesthesia and thoracotomy with vascular control of the injury area, the prognosis becomes relatively good. Recurrent laryngeal nerve injury sometimes occurs at the time of injury or coincident to the repair because of the close proximity of this nerve as it loops around the aortic isthmus.

Although some surgeons believe that the aorta can be cross-clamped safely for adequate periods to allow the repair of an injury, most surgeons are concerned that a spinal cord ischemic injury may result from inadequate distal flow during the operation. Extracorporeal circulation with left atrial-to-femoral artery, femoral vein-to-femoral artery, or left ventricular-to-femoral artery flows has been utilized successfully. This technique is a partial bypass system and requires the heart to maintain flow to the ascending aorta and arch during the operation; this provides coronary and cerebral blood flow.

In recent years, pump bypass techniques which require heparinization have been largely supplanted by plastic shunt techniques using heparin-impregnated or other non-clotting shunts.[31] These offer the advantage of a smaller blood loss than that which occurs in the heparinized patient, as well as simplicity of cannulation and easier hemodynamic management during operation.

Occasionally a dissection of the aorta will be seen in association with a traumatic aortic aneurysm. This suggests that the patient had arteriosclerosis of the aorta prior to the injury or that there was an underlying abnormality in the aortic media predisposing to dissection.

To summarize, the patient with uncontrolled bleeding into the pleural space or spaces requires emergency thoractomy with the goal of suturing an aortic tear and salvaging the patient. It has been suggested that brief electrical fibrillation of the heart and even deliberate temporary "exsanguination" of the patient may assist this effort. The patient who has bled extensively into the pleural space often has a fatal injury. The patient whose hematoma remains contained until control is achieved has an excellent chance of survival. Any patient who demonstrates a widened superior mediastinum, with or without upper rib injuries and an apical pleural cap of hematoma, requires immediate aortography for diagnosis and prompt surgical intervention.

THE DIAPHRAGM

Under normal circumstances the diaphragm will be higher on the right than on the left, and the chest radiograph will demonstrate the density of the liver below the right diaphragm and the gastric air bubble beneath the left diaphragm. The diaphragm may be disrupted by either a blunt or a penetrating chest injury, but is more commonly disrupted in association with abdominal trauma with or without chest injury.[32,33] Penetrating injuries occur with about equal frequency to the right or left diaphragm, but blunt rupture of the diaphragm is more likely to occur on the left, presumably because the right diaphragm is protected by the mass of the liver. In large ruptures of the diaphragm, gas-filled abdominal contents (stomach, small or large bowel) may move promptly into the pleural space and be recognized readily on the chest radiograph. The spleen may be visualized as a solid mass along with the omentum. Small tears of the diaphragm occurring with stab or gunshot wounds may not allow the prompt herniation of abdominal contents. However, because the normal pleural pressure is negative and the abdominal pressure is constantly positive, herniation will ultimately occur. Usually this will take the form of a gas-filled viscus which may strangulate months or years later, necessitating prompt surgical intervention.

The risks of diaphragmatic repair rise greatly if the bowel is compromised and the bowel wall loses its integrity. For this reason, every patient with severe injuries should have an upright postero-anterior radiograph prior to hospital discharge if it was not possible to obtain one on admission. Cystic changes in the lungs of patients with chronic pulmonary disease may present a difficult differential diagnosis on the chest radiograph. Because the diaphragm is a vascular structure, positive findings for blood on a peritoneal lavage study might be expected with diaphragmatic injury. However, we recently have seen two patients with major diaphragmatic tears who had negative findings on peritoneal lavage.

On rare occasions the diaphragm may tear in the area in which it is tightly adhered to the inferior pericardium, and abdominal contents may herniate directly into the pericardium.

Rupture of the diaphragm most commonly results in a radial tear, but circumferential tears may avulse the diaphragmatic attachments to the chest wall. Because of the threat of increasing herniation and respiratory compromise, operative reduction and repair is mandatory. Laparotomy for trauma should always include careful inspection of the diaphragm for undetected injury. The entire surface of the diaphragm must be examined, since multiple tears are sometimes found.

ESOPHAGEAL INJURIES

The esophagus may be traumatized in any segment by a penetrating injury. Cervical esophageal injuries are the most common, since the thoracic esophagus is comparatively well protected. Any trauma suspected of causing esophageal injury dictates the need for a contrast-swallow radiograph. Undetected esophageal injury may produce mediastinitis, from the esophageal leak with an exudation of tissue fluid into the mediastinum.

Blunt injury of the esophagus most commonly occurs from a blow to the upper abdomen forcing gastric juices or food under high pressure into the lower esophagus and tearing the lower esophagus in a linear fashion.[15] This is a rare but commonly fatal injury, probably because of the forceful injection of acid gastric contents into the mediastinum, with the production of a severe chemical and bacterial mediastinitis.

Prompt esophageal repair and extensive mediastinal and pleural drainage, in conjunction with early antibiotic coverage (especially for anaerobes) offer the best hope for patients with an injured esophagus. Proximal temporary loop esophagostomy is useful for diverting oropharyngeal secretions away from the injured area, and temporary gastrostomy will aid in preventing gastric contents from entering the lower esophagus.

Traumatic esophago-respiratory fistula is an uncommon injury which may be induced by a severe compression injury of the chest. The common wall between the membranous trachea and the anterior esophagus is violated by a combination of internal (airway and esophageal) and external pressures. Usually this injured wall remains intact for a period of time, with the later appearance of a fistula as necrosis of the avascular tissue occurs. Infection probably plays an important role in the formation of the fistula. The management of an esophago-respiratory fistula is complex, and usually involves bringing vascularized tissues, such as intercostal muscle pedicles, from the chest wall to support whatever repair is necessary. Early recognition will allow esophageal exclusion to reduce mediastinal soiling, as well as preventing constant aspiration of esophageal contents into the unprotected tracheobronchial tree.

ASSOCIATED INJURIES OF SPECIAL IMPORTANCE

Two associated injuries are of special concern in the chest-injured patient: massive facial injury and head injury.

Patients with massive facial injury may have marked compromise of the airway by two major mechanisms: (1) the accumulation or aspiration of blood and oropharyngeal secretions; and (2) massive early edema of the injured parts. Teeth or dentures may be displaced into the airway or the esophagus. Severe bony injury of the maxilla or mandible may result in loss of support for the soft tissues surrounding the airway, allowing major airway collapse. While bleeding may be severe, exsanguination is rare. Airway control must be achieved by endotracheal tube or by emergency tracheostomy to prevent suffocation.

The chest-injured patient who has an associated head injury presents special problems in management. The head injury may impair the respiratory drive so that the patient may have apneas or disordered breathing which requires mechanical ventilation. In addition, the unconscious or semiconscious patient may breathe with a low constant tidal volume and have a poor cough reflex which impairs bronchial clearance. Airway obstruction at the oropharyngeal level can occur because of relaxation of the musculature involved in maintaining a patent airway. Management of the airway must receive early attention in the patient with head injury and is even more critical when there is associated chest injury.

Other associated injuries of special importance in conjunction with chest trauma are abdominal injury with its attendant elevation of the diaphragm and restriction of ventilation and long-bone fractures with its potential for producing the fat embolism syndrome characterized by marked hypoxia. When superimposed on altered ventilation and perfusion from a primary chest injury, the additive detrimental effect of these injuries on lung function assumes major importance.

SUMMARY

Injury to the thorax and its contents constitutes a major cause of death following trauma. Early diagnosis and treatment offer the best chance for survival from the primary chest injury or common associated injuries. Treatment is simple and effective in minor isolated chest trauma, but complex and sometimes ineffective in major chest trauma with associated injuries. Appropriate minute-to-minute early care may mean the difference between success and failure.

REFERENCES

1. Kirsh MM, Sloan H: Blunt Chest Trauma, 1st ed. Boston, Little, Brown, 1977.
2. Trinkle JK, Glover FL: The Management of Thoracic Trauma Victims, 1st ed. Philadelphia-Toronto, JB Lippincott, 1980.
3. Daughtry DC: Thoracic Trauma, 1st ed. Boston, Little, Brown, 1980.
4. Roe BB: Perioperative Management in Cardiothoracic Surgery, 1st ed. Boston, Little, Brown, 1981.
5. Ashbaugh DG, Peters GN, Halgrimson CG, et al: Chest trauma: Analysis of 685 patients. Arch Surg 95:546, 1967.
6. Zuska JJ: Wounds without cause. Bull Am Coll Surg 66: 5, 1981.
7. Moore JB, Moore EE, Thompson JS: Abdominal injuries associated with penetrating trauma. Am J Surg 140:724, 1980.
8. Fischer RP, Beverlin BC, Engrav LH, et al: Diagnostic peritoneal lavage. Am J Surg 136:701, 1978.
9. Trinkle JK: Shock—The metabolic response to trauma. In Management of Thoracic Trauma Victims, 1st ed. Trinkle JK, Grover FL. Philadelphia, JB Lippincott, 1980.
10. Grover FL, Richardson JD, Fewel JG, et al: Prophylactic antibiotics in the treatment of penetrating chest wounds. J Thorac Cardiovasc Surg 74:528, 1977.
11. Oparah SS, Mandal AK: Penetrating stab wounds of the chest: Experience with 200 consecutive cases. J Trauma 16:868, 1976.
12. Trinkle JK, Richardson JD, Franz JL, et al: Management of flail chest without mechanical ventilation. Ann Thorac Surg 19:355, 1975.
13. Flaherty TT, Wegner GP, Crummy AB, et al: Nonpenetrating injuries to the thoracic aorta. Radiology 92:541, 1969.
14. Wiot JF: The radiologic manifestations of blunt chest trauma. JAMA 231:500, 1975.
15. Reynolds J, David JT: Injuries of the chest wall, pleura, pericardium, lungs, bronchi and esophagus. Radiol Clin North Am 4:383, 1966.
16. Stevens E, Templeton AW: Traumatic nonpenetrating lung contusion. Radiology 85:247, 1965.
17. Roe BB: Physiologic principles of pleural space drainage, with special reference to high-flow high-vacuum suction. Am J Surg 96:246, 1958.
18. Emerson DM, McIntyre J: A Comparative study of the physiology and physics of pleural drainage systems. J Thorac Cardiovasc Surg 52:40, 1966.
19. Richardson JD, McElveinn RB, Trinkle JK: First rib fracture: A hallmark of severe trauma. Ann Surg 181:251, 1975.
20. Harrison WH, Jr, Gary AR, Couves CM, et al: Severe non-penetrating injuries to the chest: clinical results in the management of 216 patients. Am J Surg 100:715, 1960.
21. Wilson JM, Thomas AN, Goodman PC, et al: Severe chest trauma: Morbidity implication of first and second rib fracture in 120 patients. Arch Surg 113:846, 1978.
22. Yee ES, Thomas AN, Goodman PC: Isolated first rib fracture: Clinical significance after blunt chest trauma. Ann Thorac Surg 32:278, 1981.

23. Maloney JV, Jr, Schmutzer KJ, Raschke E: Paradoxical respiration and "pendel-luft." J Thorac Cardiovasc Surg 41:291, 1961.
24. Avery EE, Morch ET, Benson DW: Critically crushed chests: A new method for treatment with continuous mechanical hyperventilation to produce alkalotic apnea and internal pneumatic stabilization. J Thorac Surg 32:291, 1956.
25. Kirsh MM, Orringer MB, Behrendt DM, et al: Management of tracheo-bronchial disruption secondary to nonpenetrating trauma. Ann Thorac Surg 22:93, 1976.
26. Burke JF: Early diagnosis of traumatic rupture of the bronchus. JAMA 181:96, 1962.
27. Chesterman JT, Satsangi PN: Rupture of the trachea and bronchi by closed injury. Thorax 21:21, 1966.
28. Daughtry DC: Traumatic torsion of the lung. N Engl J Med 256:385, 1957.
29. Trinkle JK, Toon RS, Franz JL, et al: Affairs of the wounded heart: Penetrating cardiac wounds. J Trauma 19:467, 1979.
30. Marynard A, Brooks HA, Froix CJL: Penetrating wounds of the heart: report of a new series. Arch Surg 90:680, 1965.
31. Kirsh MM, Kahn DR, Crane JD, et al: Repair of acute traumatic rupture of the aorta without extracorporeal circulation. Ann Thorac Surg 10:227, 1970.
32. Hood RM: Traumatic diaphragmatic hernia. Ann Thorac Surg 12:311, 1971.
33. Wise L, Connors J, Hwang YH: Traumatic injuries to the diaphragm. J Trauma 13:946, 1973.

12

Bronchopulmonary Aspiration

Thomas A. Neff, M.D.

INTRODUCTION

One of the literal definitions of the word aspiration is "breathing or sucking" into the lungs. Many descriptive medical terms are used for this often emergent condition: aspiration pneumonia, gastric aspiration, massive aspiration, Mendelson's syndrome, adult respiratory distress syndrome secondary to aspiration, post-anesthetic pneumonia, and sometimes even "cafe coronary." It seems obvious from this array of terms that bronchopulmonary aspiration is a complex, varied medical condition. To correctly understand, diagnose, and manage this condition it is essential to scrutinize the factors that determine the clinical picture that follows aspiration. These factors can be grouped into three major categories: (1) bronchopulmonary anatomy; (2) type of aspirate; and (3) host factors (Table 12–1). For completeness, the table lists six relatively distinct clinical syndromes. Strictly speaking, the inhalation of noxious gases is a form of aspiration, and will be discussed in Chapter 13. Only large airway obstruction, acute pneumonitis due to gastric aspiration, and near-drowning are common pulmonary emergencies. Large airway obstruction is adequately dealt with in Chapters 1, 2, and 3. The main focus of this chapter will be on major life-threatening gastric aspiration, although specific aspects of the management of near-drowning victims will be included.

GASTRIC ASPIRATION INCIDENCE

Obtaining exact figures on the incidence of gastric aspiration is difficult. Mendelson[1] reported 66 cases in 44,016 parturient women, for an overall incidence of 0.15 percent per delivery. Two more current series, from the Mayo Clinic[2] and Parkland Memorial Hospital,[3] were selected from review of these institutions' "directly observed" experience. Both series used rigid criteria for unequivocal gastric aspiration; these criteria included either direct observation of the event, or seeing or removing gastric contents from the trachea, or both of the last two. These rigid entry criteria admittedly underestimate the frequency of gastric aspiration, especially episodes of lesser magnitude. Nevertheless, the Mayo Clinic (a referral institution) series reported 88 major episodes over a 3-year period, while the Parkland (an acute-care oriented hospital) series selected 50 cases of pulmonary aspiration of gastric contents from 227 cases of aspiration pneumonia during a 5-year period. In summary, gastric aspiration is a frequent occurrence today in all institutions caring for sick patients.

COMMON CAUSES

The tragic paradox of gastric aspiration is that it is usually preventable but only "partially" treatable, through nonspecific medical support (see "Management"). Therefore, when it occurs in the hospital setting, as it frequently does, one usually can retrospectively identify physician and nursing error. Prevention must start with an increased awareness of the predisposing factors to gastric aspiration. Some of these host factors are listed in Table 12–1.

The classic original paper of Mendelson[1] reports on 66 parturient patients receiving general anesthesia (an oxygen-ether mixture administered via an opaque face mask). Although obstetric anesthesia practice has changed greatly since the 1930s and 1940s—the era of Mendelson's report—several important lessons from such anesthesia practice still are applicable today. First, patients lying supine with their "laryngeal reflexes" abolished by general anesthesia (or by other mechanisms, such as alcoholic coma) are at great risk for aspiration. Women in labor have additional risk factors. Spontaneous labor usually begins when these women have not been "NPO," and once labor begins, prolonged gastric retention of food and liquids is common. Today, patients who receive general anesthesia for delivery or emergency surgery have an endotracheal tube in place, but they are still at considerable risk for aspiration.[2,3] Of the 54 patients undergoing operation who had major aspiration in Arms'[2] series, 6 (11 percent) had this during anesthesia induction (peri-intubation), while 14 (26 percent) had it during anesthesia recovery (probably immediately postextubation). In Bynum's[3] series of 50 cases of severe gastric-content aspiration, 13 (26 percent) aspirated in relation to general anesthesia; 6 were obstetric patients, 6 were emergency surgery cases while only 1 was an elective surgery case. Patients undergoing general anesthesia for obstetric or emergent reasons are at great risk for major gastric aspiration. All such patients requiring urgent endotracheal intubation can be managed more safely with the nasotracheal technique with the patient sitting during intubation (see Chapter 2). The nasotracheal tube should be passed through the larynx after topical anesthesia, if possible, before the administration of intravenous medication which partially or totally suppresses the "laryngeal reflex." The same sitting position can be used for both elective and emergent endoscopy. Figure 12–1 shows the chest roentgenogram sequence of a patient who vomited and aspirated during endoscopy for acute upper GI bleeding.

Table 12–1. Aspiration Syndromes with Determinant Factors

Clinical Picture (Syndrome)	Location of Anatomy/Pathology	Type of Aspirate	Host Factors "Clinical Setting"
Large "upper" airway obstruction ("cafe coronary")	Hypopharynx Larynx Trachea	Food bolus Large amounts of liquids Foreign bodies	Intoxicated adults. "Oral"-aged children 1-3 years. Patients with bulbar neurologic disease
Smaller "lower" airway obstruction and reaction Chronic bronchitis (frequent) Asthma (occasional) PND (rare) Atelectasis (acute) Bronchiectasis (chronic)	Mainstem bronchi to bronchioles	Small (1-50 ml) often repeated amounts of food, liquid, oral secretions, and gastric reflux	As above, and patients with senility, CVA, organic brain syndromes, psychoses, gastric reflux, and laryngeal dysfunction
Acute chemical pneumonitis (gastric aspiration or Mendelson's syndrome)	Bilateral alveolar infiltrates and conduction airways	Toxic fluid, usually large volumes (50–300 ml) gastric content with pH <2.5; hydrocarbons (gasoline)	Anesthesia, coma, seizures, supine position, vomiting, "iatrogenic" tubes (nasogastric, endotracheal and "scopes")
Bacterial infections Lung abscess Necrotizing pneumonia with or without empyema	Localized to lung parenchyma; dependent distribution	Mouth secretions and flora (small amounts)	Pyorrhea and/or gingivitis and as in large upper airway obstruction and smaller lower airway obstruction
Foreign body "pneumonia" (lipid pneumonia [often cryptic])	Lung parenchyma; usually basilar, but can be any location	Especially vegetable particles, animal fats, and bones	As in smaller lower airway obstruction; forced feeding and tube feeding
Pulmonary edema (near-drowning)	Glottic spasm and/or generalized alveolar flooding	Fresh or sea water	Obvious

In almost every article on gastric aspiration in which patient data are given, there is revealed the predisposing factor of a diminished or abolished protective laryngeal reflex—reflex glottic closure—by coma, stupor, or primary bulbar neurologic disease. Alcohol and sedative drug overdose, seizures, cerebrovascular accidents (CVAs), central nervous system trauma, and cardiopulmonary arrest are the most common factors responsible for this. During the acute precipitating episode, and especially during emergency care and transportation, most patients unfortunately are positioned supine. Cameron[4] appropriately stressed the need to get coma patients off their backs and into the lateral decubitus or prone postures with their feet 6 to 12 inches higher than their heads (Fig. 12–2). This one manuever probably would negate the need for the rest of this chapter, or relegate it to a historical perspective!

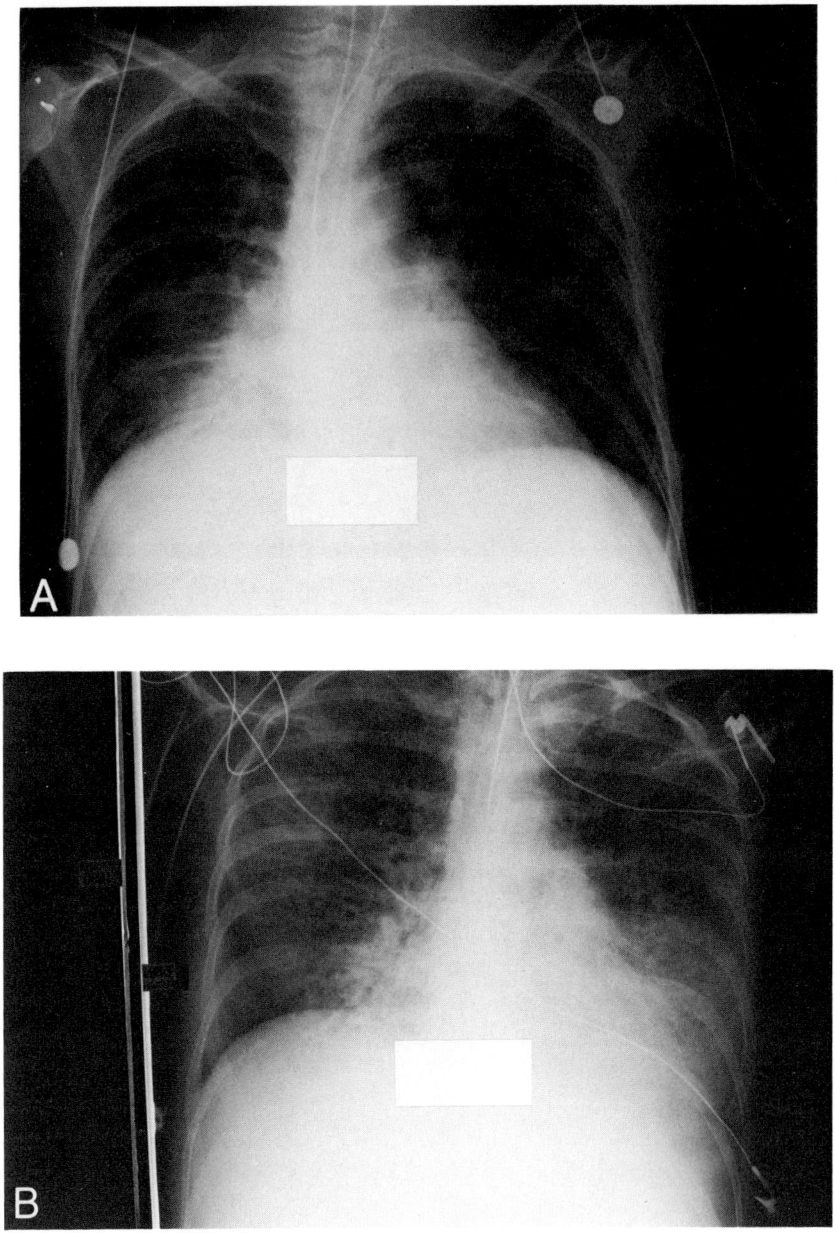

Figure 12–1. This 43-year-old woman presented on July 7, 1980 with severe decompensated alcoholic liver disease, ascites, and a normal chest roentgenogram. Immediately after upper GI endoscopy on July 9, 1980, the patient was noted to vomit while lying supine. She aspirated blood and gastric contents, immediately became apneic and had a cardiopulmonary arrest. Endotracheal intubation was performed with difficulty; the chest roentgenogram, dated July 9, 1980 was obtained 1 hour after the aspiration (A). Note diffuse alveolar infiltrates, greatest in the right lower lung zone. Over the next 24 hours the patient developed progressive severe bilateral aspiration pneumonia and despite intensive respiratory support died 1 day after the chest roentgenogram dated July 15, 1980(B).

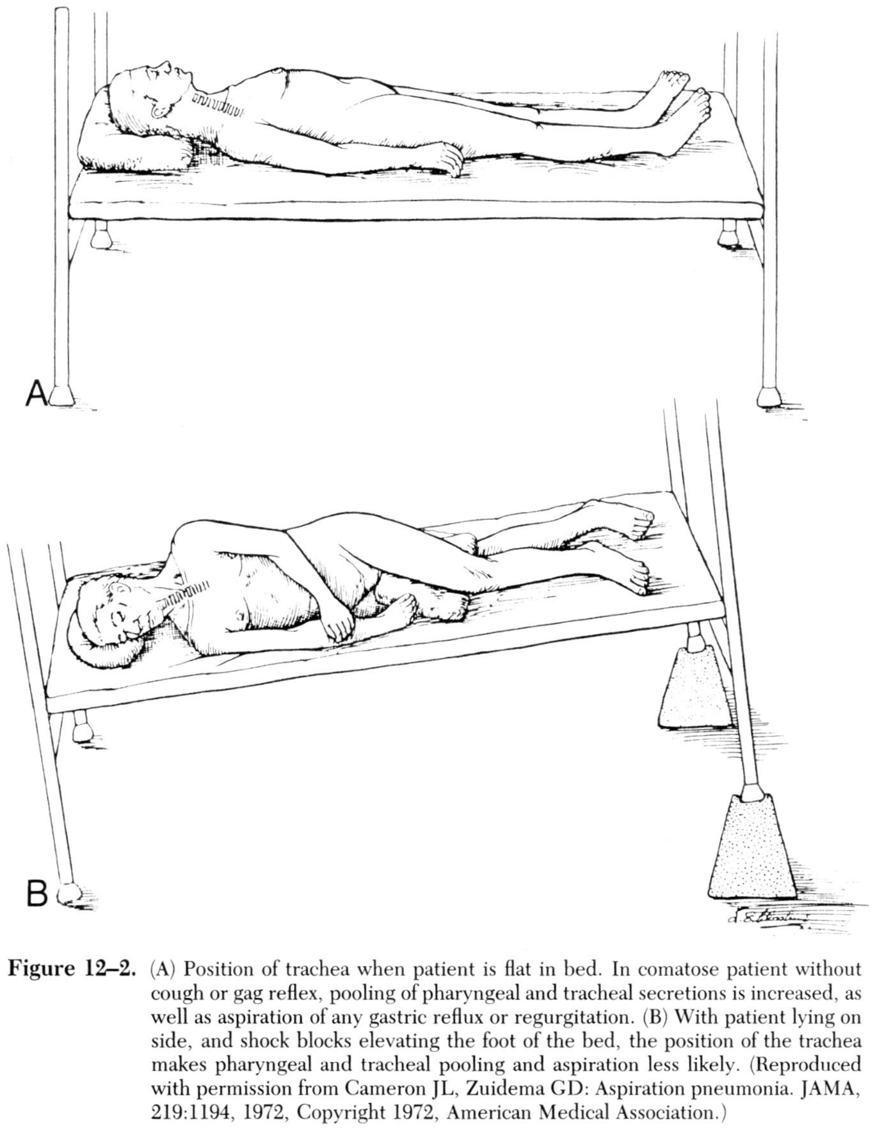

Figure 12–2. (A) Position of trachea when patient is flat in bed. In comatose patient without cough or gag reflex, pooling of pharyngeal and tracheal secretions is increased, as well as aspiration of any gastric reflux or regurgitation. (B) With patient lying on side, and shock blocks elevating the foot of the bed, the position of the trachea makes pharyngeal and tracheal pooling and aspiration less likely. (Reproduced with permission from Cameron JL, Zuidema GD: Aspiration pneumonia. JAMA, 219:1194, 1972, Copyright 1972, American Medical Association.)

DIAGNOSIS AND CLINICAL PICTURE

As mentioned in the section on incidence, the diagnosis of gastric aspiration is made most accurately from: (1) witnessing of the event by a reliable observer; (2) observing gastric contents in the trachea or bronchi at laryngoscopy (intubation) or bronchoscopy; (3) indirect observation of gastric material obtained from tracheobronchial suction; and (4) at autopsy. Probably more often, however, and especially for less than massive episodes, the diagnosis must be made indirectly, by being alert to its possibility in patients with the predisposing risk factors mentioned earlier, and by integrating the symptoms, signs, chest roentgenogram, and laboratory data.

The clinical syndrome of gastric aspiration has three anatomic/pathologic components: (1) large airway obstruction; (2) medium and smaller airway obstruction, "reaction", or both; and (3) pneumonia. Any patient may manifest any one or a combination of the three.

Large Airway Obstruction

Especially in older patients (and in infants also) who were not observed during the event, the first indication of aspiration often is sudden apnea or even a cardiopulmonary arrest. These patients usually are misdiagnosed as having a primary cardiac event or, occasionally, a massive pulmonary embolus. If they survive the first few minutes and are observed within the hour, they often are dyspneic, cyanotic and hypotensive. The initial impression usually is one of cardiogenic shock, massive pulmonary embolus, and even septic shock.

Medium and Small Airway Obstruction

From bronchographic experience, we know that Dionisil, a relatively inert, oily liquid, is cleared by mucociliary action and coughing as quickly as 5 to 15 minutes after tracheal or bronchial instillation. This is true even after the cough reflex has been partially suppressed by a narcotic and by topical anesthesia. A mixture of gastric acid and food particles certainly is a more "potent" cough stimulus than Dionisil, but by injuring the mucociliary escalator, such a mixture probably retards tracheobronchial clearance. Wolfe[5] reported that 90 percent of patients with proven gastric aspiration had substantial subsegmental endobronchial mucosal erythema visualized at bronchoscopy from within a few minutes up to 48 hours after the event. Since the author did not see this change in a somewhat comparable control group, he concluded that this bronchoscopic finding was highly suggestive of aspiration. The clinical correlate of this endobronchial pathology is an "asthma-like" reaction; this was observed in 92 percent of Mendelson's patients (the remaining 8 percent had a large airway syndrome of suffocation or "massive collapse". Bynum[3] observed wheezing in 32 percent of 50 patients with aspiration. My experience is similar; rales, and especially rhonchi and wheezes, usually are heard from the first few hours up to 24 hours after a large aspiration. Major atelectasis visible on a chest roentgenogram occurs infrequently[1,3] (in about 5 percent of cases), and usually is indicative of large food particles in the airway, which may be one of the rare indications for therapeutic bronchoscopy (see Management).

Pneumonia (See Also Pathophysiology)

The clinical picture of pneumonia is nonspecific and, unfortunately, often misleading in that the population risk for aspiration also is frequently at risk for bacterial pneumonia. However, before a patient can develop aspiration pneumonia, the gastric contents must transit the smaller airways; therefore, the combination of an acute asthma "attack" (especially in the nonasthmatic patient) and an acute pneumonia in a hospitalized patient is highly suggestive of aspiration. If pneumonitis is going to develop following aspiration, alveolar infiltrates usually are present by the time the initial chest radiograph is obtained (within 1 hour); these infiltrates often progress during the first 24 to 48 hours. If no infiltrate is observed by 24 hours after a "suspected" episode of aspiration, probably no substantial chemical injury has occurred. In contrast, lung abscess may take days to develop after small amounts of bacterial aspiration.

A highly characteristic radiographic finding in gastric aspiration is multiple-lobe involvement with acute alveolar or alveolar-interstital infiltrates. Bynum[3] found more than three of six lung zones involved in 64 percent of his patients initially, and follow-up radiographs revealed that this extent of involvement increased to 72 percent.

An early but nonspecific test to determine if substantial alveolar injury has occurred involves obtaining an arterial blood gas sample with the patient breathing 100 percent oxygen for 20 minutes. If the PaO_2 is greater than 550 mmHg at sea level (450 mmHg at 5000 feet), no clinically important shunt exists and it is highly probable that no substantial alveolar injury has occurred (no chemical pneumonitis will develop). When interpreting the results of arterial blood gas analysis, it is important to remember that this test is quite sensitive but absolutely nonspecific. The blood gas determination indicates the severity of the respiratory process but nothing about the etiology!

In summary, the diagnosis of gastric aspiration, except when directly observed, is best made on the grounds of reasonable probability so that early treatment can be instituted.

PATHOPHYSIOLOGY

Extensive experimental work has been done in an attempt to elucidate the pathophysiologic processes following gastric aspiration. This work correlates reasonably well with the human clinical and pathologic data available. For an extensive, detailed discussion of this subject, the reader is referred to the recent review by Wynne.[6] In brief, important factors that determine the type and extent of lung injury in aspiration are: (1) the pH of the aspirate fluid; (2) the toxicity of the aspirate fluid; (3) the amount and kind of particulate matter in the aspirate; (4) the amount of total aspirate; and (5) the distribution and depth of penetration into the lungs of the aspirate.

Mendelson's original paper reported comparable injury from the introduction of unneutralized gastric contents and 0.1 N hydrochloric acid into rabbit lungs. Teabeaut[7] and Awe[8] have confirmed the principle that the pH of the aspirated fluid is critical. With a pH greater than 2.5 there is no chemical burning of tissue, while the severity of the injury increases as the pH decreases until it becomes maximal at a pH of 1.5. Even "neutral" pH fluids (water, saline) introduced into the lung will cause a rapid but reversible edema and vascular congestion,[7] with airway narrowing or closure, and hypoxemia.[9] Acid fluids cause an immediate (in seconds to minutes) severe reaction[10] which progresses rapidly to irreversible cellular and tissue necrosis. The clinical report of Lewis[11] correlates with this laboratory work. Immediately following aspiration, gastric contents were obtained by nasogastric tube suction and the pH measured. All 4 patients with a gastric pH of below 1.75 died, while only 1 of 4 with a pH of 1.75 to 2.4 died. In addition, of 5 patients with a pH greater than 2.4, 2 had a nonlethal pneumonitis while 3 had no evidence of pneumonitis. At autopsy, the pathology of gastric aspiration pneumonitis usually can not be distinguished from that in many other forms of acute severe lung injury except by visualizing gross stomach contents in the airways in cases of acute death, and food particles with granulomatous pneumonia microscopically in cases that have survived longer.[12]

The physiologic abnormalities from gastric aspiration are predictable from knowledge of the pathology. This has been well studied in both animals and humans. Hypotension and decreased cardiac output are secondary to loss of intravascular fluid volume[11] from a profound capillary leak, which causes flooding of the pulmonary interstitium and eventually the alveolar spaces with a protein rich fluid.[8,13] It is known that with a high-protein leak into the alveolar spaces, there is a change in surfactant.[14] This in turn causes a marked loss in pulmonary compliance. Lewis[11] measured dynamic pulmonary (lung and thoracic) compliance in six patients during the period of most severe pneumonitis, and found it to be from 0.014 to 0.025 L/cmH_2O (normal 0.1 L/cmH_2O). Compliance remained low even after clinical, arterial blood gas, and chest roentgenographic evidence of improvement had occurred.

Marked hypoxemia is a constant finding in all patients with severe aspiration pneumonitis; the PaO_2 in 12 of Lewis' patients breathing ambient air was 44 $\pm$ 18 mmHg (mean $\pm$ SD). This was proven to be due largely to venous admixture—a shunt effect—in that the arterial PaO_2 only increased to 223 $\pm$ 158 mmHg after the breathing of 100 percent oxygen for 15 to 30 minutes. The $PaCO_2$ initially tends to be low secondary to hyperventilation from hypoxic drive, and probably more importantly from mechanical and irritative stimuli to the large airways and lung parenchyma. An elevated $PaCO_2$ means hypoventilation secondary to either acute or chronic airways obstruction, or both, and is a bad prognostic sign. In general, aspiration pneumonia is just one of the specific etiologies of the new popular collective category known as adult respiratory distress syndrome (ARDS) previously described by Petty and Ashbaugh.[15]

Role of Bacterial Infection

In a recent review on aspiration pneumonia, Bartlett[16] states that "there is no evidence that bacteria play any role in the initial events that follow aspiration of gastric acid." This certainly appears to be the majority opinion, as summarized by Wynne.[6] The incidence of infection later in the course of gastric aspiration is variable ranging from 8 of 66 (12 percent),[1] through 13 of 50 (26 percent),[3] to 43 of 88 (49 percent),[2] and to 15 of 18 (83 percent)[11] cases. Infection does not appear to be prevented by prophylactic (given immediately after the episode of aspiration) antimicrobial therapy.[3,11] Since there are too many uncontrollable variables in humans who have aspiration, no absolute answer on the role of "prophylactic" antibiotic therapy is anticipated. Bacterial isolates in patients who develop infection following gastric aspiration most frequently include both anaerobes and aerobes, specifically *Staphylococcus aureus* and Gram-negative bacilli. This is the same pattern that is found in hospital-aquired aspiration pneumonia.[16,17] As mentioned earlier, most authors' criteria for selection of patients with gastric aspiration for study essentially limits the population to "in-hospital" patients.

MANAGEMENT

The main theme of management of gastric aspiration is its prevention. Treatment after the event has occurred should be considered in two phases: (1) acute emergency support; and (2) subacute "specific" modalities, such as steroids, antibiotics, and bronchoscopy. If a physician is present at the moment of aspiration, or within minutes thereafter, the principles of cardiopulmonary resuscitation (see Chapters 1 and 2) apply: establish or insure an adequate airway, oxygenate the patient, and support the circulation. The placement of an endotracheal tube always should be considered. Elevating the patient's head and body during endotracheal tube insertion may prevent repeat aspiration. With endotracheal tube placement, therapeutic and diagnostic suctioning can also be done. The person placing the endotracheal tube should record as accurately as possible the amount and type of aspirate seen and removed from the trachea and bronchi. Immediate endotracheal suctioning and coughing is probably much more effective in relieving obstruction than bronchoscopy 30 to 60 minutes later (see section on subacute "specific" modalities). After the initial suctioning has been completed, lavage with small amounts (5 to 10 ml) to a total of 20 to 30 ml of slightly alkaline isotonic solution (normal saline with 1 amp $NaHCO_3$ 44 mmol added/L) probably is appropriate. Lavage with larger volumes of saline may wash the aspirate more distally into the alveoli and is contraindicated. Administering 100 percent oxygen until the PaO_2 is measured, and then titrating the FIO_2 to maintain the arterial saturation in the 90 to 95 percent range, is appropriate. If an FIO_2 of greater than 0.4 (0.5 at 5000 feet) is required to maintain an arterial oxygen saturation of 90 percent or greater, mechanical ventilation, including positive end expiratory pressure (PEEP) ventilation, is indicated.

The details of further respiratory care management of the patient with aspiration ARDS are similar to those for other forms of ARDS (see Chapters 4 and 6). Immediately following aspiration, the central venous pressure (CVP) and intravascular volume are normal (at their levels before aspiration). Over the ensuing hours, pulmonary capillary leakage develops, producing the typical alveolar infiltrates (noncardiac pulmonary edema) seen in a chest radiograph, and a plasma volume deficit of approximately 500 to 1000 ml.[11] Therefore, limited volume re-expansion with 500 to 1000 ml of fluid, preferably colloid (whole blood or plasma), is indicated. The limited use of crystalloid may be acceptable, but large volumes appear to be deleterious.[11] Maintaining the CVP below 10 cmH_2O, or the pulmonary artery capillary wedge pressure below 10 mmHg, and maintaining a near normal intravascular oncotic pressure, is preferred to minimize the noncardiac pulmonary edema.

Placing a nasogastric tube after the airway has been protected may be of both prognostic and prophylactic value. It will allow measurement of the gastric content pH and will empty the stomach as completely as possible and allow the instillation of 30 ml of liquid antacid every 1 to 2 hours. Intravenous cimetidine every 6 hours also can be used to reduce gastric pH.[18] Many authors have shown that a nasogastric tube connected to suction is rarely completely effective and may be an increased-risk element for further aspiration.[2]

Subacute "Specific" Measures

Because experimental reports are contradictory and the human experience is anecdotal, the use of corticosteroids in gastric aspiration remains controversial. Wynne[5] reviewed their use in depth and concluded that "one who uses steroids in the treatment of this disorder must weigh their unproven benefits against possible complications." My recommendation is to give 100 mg of methylprednisolone intravenously (or its equivalent) immediately and every 6 hours for three additional doses after an observed, clinically "significant" gastric aspiration. This means that the patient demonstrates objective signs and symptoms of the aspiration, such as respiratory distress, wheezing, rales, a decrease in the PaO_2, or a new infiltrate on a chest roentgenogram. If steroids are not given within the first 12 hours, experimental and theoretical evidence strongly suggests that they are not helpful; their use after this time lapse is inappropriate and contraindicated.

Antibiotic Therapy

The role of infection in gastric aspiration was reviewed in the section on pathophysiology. On the basis of this information, I do not recommend the use of any antibiotic immediately after gastric aspiration. The one exception to this might be in a patient with a bowel obstruction.[10,19] It is important to remember that the inflammatory responses of fever, leukocytosis, a purulent sputum, and pulmonary infiltrates are not specific for a bacterial process, and when present acutely only represent a chemical-induced pneumonitis. If a patient is still febrile with a persistent or progressive pneumonitis 24 to 48 hours after an episode of gastric aspiration or if the patient develops a new fever, leukocytosis, or infiltrate, blood and sputum cultures should be obtained. In patients with an endotracheal tube in place, a carefully interpreted, deep-suction Gram-stain specimen probably is more reliable than a routine culture. With analysis of the Gram stain and while culture results are pending, the initiation of a "nosocomial" regimen in a severely ill patient is recommended.[16,17] Two to 3 g of oxacillin every 6 hours, or an equivalent dose of methicillin or nafcillin (clindamycin or a cephalosporin can be used in a penicillin-allergic patient), as well as 7.5 mg/kg every 12 hours of amikacin or an equivalent aminoglycoside will provide broad spectrum nosocomial coverage. If no specific flora, such as *Staphylococcus aureus* or aerobic Gram-negative bacilli, is obtained, a change to "anaerobe" doses of penicillin—2 to 6 million units/day—seems appropriate.[16]

The indications for bronchoscopy after aspiration are twofold: First, it may be helpful diagnostically, as mentioned previously.[5] Secondly, it is indicated when clinical (absent breath sounds) or radiologic (lobar atelectasis) evidence of a major bronchial obstruction exists.

Sequelae

Death is the ultimate "complication" of gastric aspiration. Patients may die acutely from upper airway obstruction in the first few minutes. If the patient survives the initial insult, he or she may succumb to progressive respiratory failure (ARDS) or severe pulmonary sepsis (necrotizing pneumonia with empyema). Fortunately, the majority of patients recover rapidly, although in two recent series the overall mortality was still 38 percent[3] and 30 percent.[2] The underlying status of the patient's health at the time of aspiration is obviously important. In Mendelson's[1] series of "basically healthy young pregnant women," only 2 of 66, or 3 percent died, while in Cameron's[20] experience with sick hospitalized patients the mortality rate was 62 percent. Any patients surviving ARDS or pulmonary sepsis of any cause may have some chronic pulmonary function abnormalities, but severe long-term sequelae in patients surviving aspiration pneumonia are rare.[21]

Near-Drowning

Drowning is currently the third most common cause of accidental death in the United States, with more than 10,000 people dying annually. Bradley[22] defines drowning "as death by acute asphyxia during submersion, whether or not liquid has entered the lungs." Actually, the best evidence suggests that from 80 to 90 percent of drowning and near-drowning victims aspirate water and its impurities (sand, diatoms, and so forth), as well as some of their own regurgitated gastric contents. A minority of victims (10 to 20 percent) may develop severe reflex laryngospasm leading to asphyxia. In addition, most victims other than those previously rendered unconscious by trauma or stuporous from drugs (such as alcohol) struggle violently, causing tremendous and often maximal oxygen consumption. These two factors of asphyxia—hypoxia and hypercarbia—as well as marked oxygen consumption, uniformly lead to severe acidosis in near-drowning victims.

THERAPY

After the victim of a near-drowning episode is rescued from the water, the basic principles of cardiopulmonary resuscitation (CPR) are applied (see Chapter 1). Immediate CPR (mouth-to-mouth breathing and external cardiac massage if needed) at the scene is much more "neurologically saving" than even the most sophisticated ventilation management applied belatedly at the hospital. If the patient remains unconscious, placement of an endotracheal tube (see Chapter 2) is indicated, and 100 percent oxygen should be delivered. After the airway is secured, nasogastric tube placement for draining swallowed water and air from the earlier mouth-to-mouth breathing is always appropriate. Since the victims are almost always acidemic, it is empirically sound to give one ampule (44 mEq) of sodium bicarbonate i.v. stat. Obtaining an arterial blood gas result as soon as feasible is indicated, but withholding the first ampule of bicarbonate pending "slow" results is unwise. Careful monitoring and appropriate "titration" of the patient's PaO_2, $PaCO_2$, and pH is the mainstay of the ICU management of near-drowning. Management of the patient's hemodynamic status (vascular volume, cardiac output), is similar to that in other forms of acute, non-cardiac pulmonary edema (see Chapters 4 and 6). A positive end expiratory pressure (PEEP) of 5 to 20 cmH_2O is helpful if the patient has ARDS. The use of antibiotics for near-drowning-induced ARDS is not indicated unless the patient has aspirated overtly contaminated water or develops a specific infection later in the course. The use of corticosteroids usually is restricted to cases with marked bronchospasm not responding to intravenous aminophylline and beta-agonists.

Special attention to barotrauma of the ear (ruptured tympanic membrane, which is frequent in diving accidents) should be given, since this condition puts the patient at risk for bacterial otitis media. This etiology may otherwise be overlooked as a source of fever in the comatose patient. The literature suggests that most of the cardiopulmonary and metabolic abnormalities in near-drowning victims respond well to modern intensive care management and leave few permanent residua. In contrast, the original anoxic brain injury is the critical determinate of the final outcome in most cases, and early neurologic consultation for prognosis and management is helpful.

REFERENCES

1. Mendelson CL: The aspiration of stomach contents into the lungs during obstetric anesthesia. Am J Obstet Gynecol 52:191, 1946.
2. Arms RA, Dines DE, Tinstman TC: Aspiration pneumonia. Chest 65:136, 1974.
3. Bynum LT, Pierce AK: Pulmonary aspiration of gastric contents. Am Rev Respir Dis 114:1129, 1976.
4. Cameron JL, Zuidema GD: Aspiration pneumonia. JAMA 219:1194, 1972.
5. Wolfe JE, Bone RC, Ruth WE: Diagnosis of gastric aspiration by fiberoptic bronchoscopy. Chest 70:458, 1976.
6. Wynne JW, Modell JH: Respiratory aspiration of stomach contents. Ann Intern Med 87:466, 1977.

7. Teabeaut JR II: Aspiration of gastric contents. An experimental study. Am J Pathol 28:51, 1952.
8. Awe WC, Fletcher WS, Jacob SW: The pathophysiology of aspiration pneumonitis. Surgery 60:232, 1962.
9. Halmagyi DF, Colebatch HJ, Starzecki B: Inhalation of blood, saliva, and alcohol: Consequences, mechanisms, and treatment. Thorax 17:244, 1962.
10. Hamelberg W, Bosomworth PP: Aspiration pneumonitis: experimental studies and clinical observations. Anesth Analg 43:669, 1964.
11. Lewis RT, Burgess JH, Hampson LG: Cardiorespiratory studies in critical illness. Changes in aspiration pneumonitis. Arch Surg 103:335, 1971.
12. Knoblich R: Pulmonary granulomatosis caused by vegetable particles. Am Rev Respir Dis 99:380, 1969.
13. Greenfield LJ, Singleton RP, McCaffree DR, Coalson JJ: Pulmonary effects of experimental graded aspiration of hydrochloric acid. Ann Surg 170:74, 1969.
14. Petty TL, Reiss OK, Paul GW, et al: Characteristics of pulmonary surfactant in adult respiratory distress syndrome associated with trauma and shock. Am Rev Respir Dis 115:531, 1977.
15. Petty TL, Ashbaugh DG: The adult respiratory distress syndrome. Clinical features, factors influencing prognosis and principles of management. Chest 60:233, 1971.
16. Bartlett JG: Aspiration pneumonia, Clin Notes Respir Dis 18(4):3, 1980.
17. Lorber B, Swenson RM: Bacteriology of aspiration pneumonia. A prospective study of community and hospital-acquired cases. Ann Intern Med 81:329, 1974.
18. Strain JD, Moore EE, Markovchick VJ, et al: Cimetidine for the prophylaxis of potential gastric acid aspiration pneumonitis in trauma patients. J Trauma 21:49, 1981.
19. Vilinskas J, Schweizer RT, Foster JH: Experimental studies on aspiration of contents of obstructed intestine. Surg Gynecol Obstet 135:568, 1972.
20. Cameron JL, Mitchell WH, Zuidema GD: Aspiration pneumonia. Clinical outcome following documented aspiration. Arch Surg 106:49, 1973.
21. Lakshminarayan S, Stanford RE, Petty TL: Prognosis after recovery from adult respiratory distress syndrome. Am Rev Respir Dis 113:7, 1976.
22. Bradley ME, Near-drowning: CPR is just the beginning. Am Rev Respir Dis 2(6):37, 1981.

13

Inhalation Injury of the Lungs

S. Lakshminarayan, M.D.

INTRODUCTION

The vast array of chemicals used in any modern industrialized society poses a potential threat from gases and fumes both to workers and to the rest of the population. This chapter will deal with inhalation injury to the lungs associated with the acute and often accidental inhalation of two of the more common irritant gases, one which is relatively insoluble in water (nitrogen dioxide) and the other which is more soluble in water (chlorine), and with the inhalation of smoke secondary to fire; it will not deal with the effects of atmospheric pollutants, industrial substances, cigarette smoke, and other agents, although Table 13–1 lists the commonly encountered toxic gases and vapors that cause lung damage.

IRRITANT GASES

The irritant gases commonly encountered in accidental exposures are chlorine, phosgene, ammonia, sulfur dioxide, and nitrogen dioxide. Exposure to these gases results in similar pathophysiologic effects. The more soluble gases injure the mucous membranes of the eye, throat, and upper respiratory tract, while the more insoluble gases are distributed more peripherally in the lung and cause a more diffuse lung injury. The effects of nitrogen dioxide inhalation will be discussed as the prototype for inhalation of an insoluble gas.

NITROGEN DIOXIDE

The importance of nitrogen dioxide (NO_2) as a cause of pulmonary tissue damage has become widely recognized in the last 25 years, following the recognition that it was the gas predominantly responsible for lung damage to silo workers.[1] That nitrogen dioxide can cause an acute, potentially fatal pulmonary injury has been

Table 13–1. Toxic Gases and Fumes

Agent	Main Occupations for Exposure	Acute Effects from Exposure to High Concentrations
Nitrogen dioxide	Farming (silo), electroplating, acetylene welding, detonation of explosives	Asphyxia, methemoglobinemia, bronchospasm, pulmonary edema
Carbon dioxide	Mining, underwater construction	Asphyxia
Chlorine	Paper and textile industries	Mucous membrane irritation, pulmonary edema
Nitrogen	Mining, undersea exploration	Asphyxia
Cyanide	Extraction of gold, electroplating, chemical industries, photographic supplies, fumigants	Chemical poison of cellular respiration—blocks cytochrome oxidase
Hydrogen sulfide	Fishing industry, gas production, oil and petroleum refining, waste disposal	Mucous membrane irritation, neurotoxicity leading to respiratory paralysis; poisons cellular enzyme systems, especially CNS cells
Ammonia	Manufacture of fertilizers, explosives & plastics, refrigeration, petroleum refining	Acute mucous membrane irritation, pulmonary edema in a few hours, chemical pneumonitis
Ozone	Arc welding, bleaching of flour, emissions from copying equipment, photochemical air pollutants	Mucous membrane irritation, pulmonary edema in severe cases
Phosgene	Metallurgy, chemical industry, fire fighting	Mucous membrane irritation, pulmonary edema and chemical pneumonitis—like chlorine, ammonia, etc.
Sulfur dioxide	Paper manufacture, refrigeration, food processing, oil refining, bleach and sulfuric acid manufacture	Mucous membrane irritation, epistaxis, pulmonary edema
Hydrogen fluoride	Metal refining, etching	Mucous membrane irritation, pulmonary edema
Formaldehyde	Manufacture of resins, leathers, rubber, metals and woods, laboratory workers, emissions from urethane foam insulation	Mucous membrane irritation, chemical bronchitis and pneumonitis
Vanadium pentoxide	Chemical industry—catalysts	Acute bronchitis and pneumonitis
Mercury	Electrolysis	Tracheobronchitis, pneumonitis, myoneural toxicity
Cadmium oxide	Smelting of ores, welding	Tracheobronchitis, pulmonary edema, emphysema
Manganese	Ore smelting, permanganate manufacture, alloy manufacture	Pneumonitis, neurotoxicity
Chromates	Ore smelting, electroplating	Tracheobronchitis, pneumonia, nasal septal perforation, lung cancer

known since 1804, when a merchant in Lyon, France and his dog were both exposed to massive concentrations of this gas after several crocks of nitric acid were broken in the merchant's shop. Both the merchant and the dog died, and the description of the merchant's illness is very suggestive of acute pulmonary edema.[2] The first grain storage silo was built in the United States in 1874, and unexplained deaths occurring in these structures were first reported in 1914.[3] Initially, these accidents were attributed to asphyxia from high concentrations of carbon dioxide, but in 1949 it was noted that high concentrations of nitrogen oxides were present in silo gas. The term silo filler's disease was first used in 1956 by Lowry, who described milder forms of the disease.[1]

The NO_2 in silo gas is derived from the nitrates within plants. Normally, grain plants have low nitrate concentrations; but this is increased by fertilizers, drought, and long periods of ultraviolet and visible light exposure. During silo storage, plant nitrates are fermented into nitrites and oxygen; the nitrites then combine with organic acids in the silo to form nitrous acid (HNO_2). As the temperature in the silo rises, HNO_2 decomposes into nitrous oxide (NO), nitrogen tetroxide (N_2O_4), and nitrogen pentoxide (N_2O_5). NO_2 and its dimer, N_2O_4, are the gases responsible for pulmonary injury. Fortunately, large amounts of NO_2 are formed from fermenting silage only for the first 5 to 7 days after filling the silo; concentrations ranging from 200 to 4000 ppm have been observed. If ventilation of the silo is adequate, the gases usually disappear quickly.

Nitrogen dioxide also has been released in several industrial settings. Release of the oxides of nitrogen, with injury to workers, has been reported with electroplating, acetylene welding, the combustion of cellulose film and plastics, the detonation of explosives, numerous industrial reactions involving nitric acid, and unusual exposures, such as the burning of shoe polish. In addition, workers handling the oxidizer component of missile fuels (liquid nitrogen tetroxide) can be exposed to nitrogen dioxide.[4] At present, the threshold limit for human industrial exposure to nitrogen dioxide has been set at 5 ppm.[5]

MECHANISMS OF TISSUE INJURY

Nitrogen dioxide reacts with water in the respiratory tract to form nitric acid; the nitrates and nitrites that are formed by the dissociation of this nitric acid cause extensive tissue damage. In addition, nitrogen dioxide is a powerful oxidant. Large concentrations cause acute pulmonary edema, while lower levels induce acute inflammation, bronchoconstriction, and alveolar duct constriction, as well as alveolar epithelial and pulmonary capillary endothelial injury.[6] Peroxidation of lung lipids, with the formation of destructive free radicals, also occurs.[7] Beyond this, a recent study of American astronauts of the Apollo-Soyuz mission in which the crew members developed a diffuse pneumonitis following the accidental inhalation of nitrogen dioxide suggests that considerable collagen degradation occured as a consequence of the inhalation. This was based on increased levels of urinary hydroxylysine glycosides that were noted in the three astronauts, who had been exposed to an average concentration of 250 ppm of nitrogen dioxide for approximately 5 minutes.[8]

CLINICAL PRESENTATION AND TREATMENT OF NO_2 INHALATION

The clinical course of patients exposed to high concentrations of nitrogen dioxide follows the general sequence outlined below.

Superacute Phase

This type of clinical course is relatively rare, occurs immediately, and is probably a consequence of severe hypoxemia from asphyxiation and possibly methemoglobinemia as a result of breathing very high concentrations of nitrogen dioxide. Invariably, these patients are critically ill and often die before they reach a medical facility.

Acute Phase (Bronchospasm and Acute Injury)

This form of inhalation effect is more common than the superacute course; the patient presents with cough, dyspnea, bronchospasm, and weakness, and often nausea, headache, tachycardia, and chest pain which may sometimes be pleuritic. There is frequently a lag period of a few hours between the time of exposure and the development of symptoms. Bronchospasm is a prominent feature of the acute phase. Acute increases in airway resistance follow experimental nitrogen dioxide exposure even at low doses and appear to be mediated by histamine release.[9] If the exposure is severe, the patient develops pulmonary edema and, depending upon the severity of the disease, may require intubation and ventilatory support. A trial of corticosteroid therapy in the acute phase is advocated.[10] The role of prophylactic antibiotics is unclear, but it would be prudent to withhold antibiotic treatment until evidence of infection is documented.

Other specific measures such as the administration of methylene blue to reverse methemoglobinemia, and the use of dimercaprol (BAL) in severe cases, have been proposed, but have not been subjected to clinical trials.[11] Their routine use is not recommended, since the pathophysiology of nitrogen dioxide inhalation is primarily pulmonary rather than hematologic. There is no role for hyperbaric oxygen therapy in the treatment of nitrogen dioxide inhalation, since at least one animal study has shown it to have an adverse effect, with worsening pulmonary injury.[12]

The treatment of pulmonary edema is that of the adult respiratory distress syndrome, since the edema is noncardiogenic (see Chapter 6). Supplemental oxygen, intubation, and ventilatory support in severe cases with the use of positive end-expiratory pressure (PEEP), and the continuation of corticosteroids are the mainstays of treatment.

Subacute and Chronic Phase (Bronchiolitis Obliterans)

If the patient survives, the pulmonary edema clears within a few days and the second phase of the illness begins. During this phase, which lasts from 2 to 5 weeks, the patient usually remains asymptomatic or has mild shortness of breath.

The third phase is characterized by fever, progressive shortness of breath, cough, and occasionally cyanosis. The chest roentgenogram shows multiple, discrete nodular densities or, occasionally, pulmonary edema. During this phase, the patient may develop respiratory insufficiency with severe hypoxemia and CO_2 retention. The course may progress to death from chronic respiratory failure or recovery with chronic obstructive pulmonary disease (COPD). Bronchiolitis obliterans has been noted in patients who die during the third phase. A number of patients who recover are found to have obstructive lung disease of varying severity.[13] Treatment for bronchiolitis obliterans is systemic corticosteroid therapy to reduce the inflammatory process. The prognosis with early, adequate treatment is good unless the inflammatory process has progressed to the irreversible stage. The long-term sequelae of nitrogen dioxide inhalation are probably related to the extent of exposure to the gas and the severity of the bronchiolitis obliterans.

The common, irritant, soluble gas inhalations that occur are those of chlorine and ammonia. Ammonia is very soluble in water while chlorine and sulfur dioxide are less so, but are more soluble than nitrogen dioxide. Chlorine inhalation will be described in detail; the inhalation of other gases causes similar effects.

CHLORINE

Chlorine is a heavy, irritating gas with a yellowish-green color and a specific gravity of 2.49 times that of air. It commonly is used as a bleaching agent in the paper and textile industries, and also as a disinfectant of water and sewage. For industrial use, it is liquefied under pressure and is stored or transported in steel cylinders. When released, 1 liter of liquid chlorine produces 434 liters of chlorine gas at 25°C. Inhalation injuries usually are a consequence of accidental leakage of the gas from containers.

Chlorine reacts with water to produce hydrochloric acid and a number of other reaction products such as hypochlorous acid, perchloric acid, and additional unstable oxidizing agents. This series of reactions in which unstable oxidizing compounds form stable hydrates of organic chlorine produces more tissue damage than is produced by equivalent amounts of hydrochloric acid.[14]

CLINICAL PRESENTATION AND TREATMENT OF CHLORINE INHALATION

Exposure to chlorine causes choking, chest pain, cough, and dyspnea. White or pink sputum is often produced. Physical examination reveals the conjunctivae and oropharyngeal mucosa to be hyperemic. Auscultation of the chest often reveals wheezing and coarse crackles. Pulmonary edema is a common occurrence with severe exposures and may occur either immediately or after a lag period of several hours. Laboratory results show arterial hypoxemia and a high alveolar-to-arterial oxygen difference which may persist for several days. The chest roentgenogram typically shows changes of pulmonary edema. The pathologic changes in fatal cases include focal and confluent areas of edema, with protein-rich fluid in the alveolar spaces, hyaline membranes lining the alveolar spaces, sloughing of the alveolar epithelium from the walls, and thrombi which partially or completely fill the lumen of otherwise normal pulmonary vessels.[15] In addition, mucous membranes of the bronchial and bronchiolar walls may be destroyed or denuded circumferentially. These changes are indistinguishable from those resulting from other soluble gas poisonings, such as occurs in sulfur dioxide or ammonia inhalation.

The treatment of chlorine inhalation consists of removing the patient from the area of the accident, bed rest, and the administration of supplemental oxygen. If the patient has severe nasopharyngeal and laryngeal edema, intubation or tracheostomy may be needed. Severe cases wtih pulmonary edema may require mechanical ventilation and benefit from positive end-expiratory pressure respiration.[16] The role of corticosteroids in the treatment of chlorine inhalation is not definitely established, although there has been one case report suggesting that it may have some beneficial effect.[17] The role of prophylactic antibiotics is not proven, and these drugs probably should be reserved for frank infection after the responsible organism is identified.

Follow-up studies of nonlethal exposures to chlorine have been inconclusive in demonstrating any long-term pulmonary damage. Weil et al.[18] were unable to document persistent physiologic abnormalities in humans accidentally exposed to chlorine gas.

Ammonia is much more water soluble than chlorine, and the brunt of its attack is therefore borne by the skin, conjunctivae, and mucous membranes of the mouth and upper respiratory tract. However, with high concentrations of the gas and with deep inhalations, some ammonia does invade the lower respiratory tract, and changes indistinguishable from those seen with chlorine can be seen.[19] There have been isolated case reports of bronchiectasis following recovery from accidental ammonia inhalation.[20,21]

SMOKE INHALATION

Respiratory burns and smoke poisoning must have been known to humanity ever since Prometheus stole fire from the heavens and brought it to Earth. In the first century A.D., Pliny reported that prisoners against the state were executed by placing them over a green-wood fire. Presumably the ancient Romans knew about the hazards of smoke and about its lethal nature.

The Coconut Grove fire in Boston in 1942 resulted in 492 fatalities. Of the 114 patients admitted to Massachusetts General Hospital, 75 were dead on arrival and 36 of the remaining 39 had severe respiratory problems. This catastrophe brought into focus the problems of respiratory damage as a result of smoke inhalation during fires.[22,23]

In 1978, 2.7 million fires were reported in the United States. The National Fire Data Center estimated that the total number of fires was close to 30 million. Although 840 deaths, 32,000 civilian fire injuries, and 58,000 injuries among firefighters were reported, the National Fire Data Center estimated that the number of fire injuries to civilians was on the order of 200,000. Trunkey observed that approximately 60 percent of deaths as a result of fires were secondary to smoke inhalation injury.[24]

PATHOPHYSIOLOGY

There are two main causes of lung injury due to acute smoke inhalation: (1) thermal injury, and (2) inhalation of toxic gases and particulate matter.

Thermal Injury

In the classical experiments of Moritz et al.,[25] in which dogs were exposed to varying temperatures of inhaled air, it was noted that inhalation of hot air (350 to 500°C) caused injury only to the upper trachea. However, the inhalation of steam caused injury to the entire tracheobronchial tree, owing to the fact that steam contains 4000 times the heat capacity of air. Thus, the upper airway cools inhaled hot air very efficiently and protects the lower respiratory tract from the damaging effects of heat.

Toxic Gases and Particulate Matter

Burning materials can either smolder (pyrolysis), flame (combustion), or both. The products of complete combustion are generally less harmful than those of pyrolysis. However, because fires use oxygen, and the ambient oxygen concentrations in the area of a fire are less than 21 per cent and may be as low as 10 percent, persons in the fire area are asphyxiated, and the fire pyrolyzes. The particulate matter and toxic gases released depend on the types of material being pyrolyzed. Common noxious gases produced in a fire include aldehydes, oxides of nitrogen and sulfur, hydrogen cyanide, and carbon monoxide. Combustion of the newer synthetic materials has dramatically increased the types of chemical injury seen in fires, due to the variety of gases that are produced.[26] The injury caused by the inhalation of noxious gases and that due to carbon monoxide will be dealt with separately, since the former injure the lung directly, while carbon monoxide affects the oxygen carrying capacity of hemoglobin.

Zikria et al.[27] noted that smoke from burning kerosene did not produce pulmonary edema or death in dogs, while wood smoke caused death. The authors attributed the difference to the fact that wood smoke had 20 to 25 times the concentration of aldehyde gases that kerosene smoke did. The initial result of the inhalation of the noxious gases is mucosal swelling and loss of ciliary activity; this progresses to airway occlusion from edema or mucosal sloughing. The mucosal damage impedes effective bacterial clearance, resulting in bacterial tracheobronchitis or pneumonia. The most common infecting organisms are staphylococcus and a variety of gram-negative bacteria such as klebsiella, *E. coli*, and pseudomonas. Additionally, edema fluid collects in the lumina of subsegmental and segmental bronchi and bronchioles, as well as in the alveoli.

The above picture is complicated if the patient also has had sustained thermal injury to the skin. Thermal burns to the skin damage the pulmonary vascular endothelium by several different mechanisms, including disseminated intravascular coagulation (DIC), microemboli, and probable burn toxins.[28,29] The use of large amounts of intravenous fluids to resuscitate the patient promotes the development of interstitial and alveolar edema. As damage at the alveolar level becomes more manifest during the first days following smoke inhalation, ventilation-perfusion abnormalities and intrapulmonary shunting result in hypoxemia and tachypnea. There is some experimental data suggesting that the aldehydes in smoke bind irreversibly with the hydrogen bonds of amino acids and with the RNA of respiratory tissue proteins, causing further tissue damage. Moreover, the various other gases that are released in smoke cause their effects by being either asphyxiating gases or direct chemical irritants.

Carbon monoxide is a colorless, odorless, tasteless gas produced by the burning of carbon-containing material in an area with limited oxygen. Thus, with fires in closed spaces, large amounts of carbon monoxide may be present in the ambient air. Carbon monoxide does not injure the lung, but competes with oxygen for the binding site on the hemoglobin molecule—which has a 210 times greater affinity for carbon monoxide than for oxygen. Further, the combination of carbon monoxide with hemoglobin shifts the oxygen-hemoglobin dissociation curve to the left, impairing oxygen unloading at the tissue level[30,31]; this is a major cause of tissue hypoxia in carbon monoxide poisoning. As a result of decreased tissue oxygen delivery, lactic acidosis often ensues. Upper airway obstruction due to supraglottic or laryngeal edema from the inhalation of hot air and irritating gases adds to the respiratory distress. Acute myocardial infarction may occur in persons with ischemic heart disease, as a result of the tissue hypoxia. Impairment of chemotaxis and phagocytic or bactericidal activity of the alveolar macrophages also has been demonstrated in experimental animals and in humans as a consequence of smoke inhalation, and may be another reason for the increased propensity to infections following smoke inhalation.[32,33]

CLINICAL PRESENTATION IN SMOKE INHALATION

The symptoms of smoke inhalation may range from a nonproductive cough and eye irritation to coma and hypoxemia requiring immediate mechanical ventilation. Surface burns may be evident on the face and other parts of the body. A number of smoke-inhalation victims who develop respiratory symptoms may have associated burns about the face, although only a small percentage of all patients with facial burns develop severe inhalation injury.[34] Cyanosis and cherry red lips due to carbon monoxide inhalation may be difficult to identify in the acute phase of smoke inhalation injury, especially if the patient also has facial burns. The mental status of the patient, and especially the level of consciousness, should be assessed. Following a lag period of several hours, patients who initially had minimal symptoms may frequently develop more severe symptoms such as cough, increased secretions, wheezing, and labored breathing. Physical examination may reveal an inflamed oropharyngeal mucosa, stridor, wheezing, and rales over the chest.

Establishment of a patent airway is the first step in the management of fire victims who have facial burns associated with hoarseness, stridor, and hypoxemia. Usually, patients with these symptoms require prompt endotracheal intubation. Visualizing the upper airway by bronchoscopy or indirect laryngoscopy helps to assess the degree of mucosal injury and laryngeal edema.[35,36] The chest roentgenogram is an insensitive indicator of inhalation injury and may be normal in patients with tracheobronchitis and arterial hypoxemia. Focal or diffuse infiltrates may occur as late as 24 to 36 hours following inhalation, and a pulmonary edema pattern may take as long as 3 to 4 days to develop following smoke inhalation.[37] Recently, the use of radioactive xenon ventilation scanning has been advocated for the early diagnosis of inhalation injury. Abnormal retention of ^{133}Xe in the lung at 90 seconds is considered diagnostic of inhalation injury.[38,39] However, caution must be used in interpreting these scans, since abnormal ventilation scans are commonly seen in patients with pre-existing lung disease.

The blood carboxyhemoglobin level should be measured. Normal, nonsmoking individuals have a carboxyhemoglobin level of less than 2 percent, while cigarette smokers may have levels as high as 5 to 10 percent. In fire victims, severe carbon monoxide poisoning is present when carboxyhemoglobin levels are higher than 30 to 40 percent. When the carboxyhemoglobin level is high, the oxygen-carrying capacity of hemoglobin is impaired, even though the arterial oxygen tension and the calculated oxygen saturation may be normal. It is therefore necessary to measure the oxygen saturation of arterial blood directly, using an oximeter. The half-life of carboxyhemoglobin is 4 to 6 hours, but increased alveolar ventilation and high inspired oxygen concentrations shorten this. During the breathing of 100 percent oxygen at 1 atmosphere pressure, the half-life of carboxyhemoglobin is shortened to approximately 40 minutes. Since carbon monoxide poisoning also can cause myocardial damage, an electrocardiogram should be performed routinely in all victims of smoke inhalation.

MANAGEMENT OF SMOKE INHALATION

Treatment of victims at the scene of a fire is usually done by the emergency paramedical personnel of the fire department. On-the-scene treatment usually comprises removal of the victim from the toxic environment, checking of the victim's pulse and breathing pattern, and the establishment of an airway if indicated. Supplemental oxygen at high flow rates via a face mask should be given to most fire victims. If the patient is suspected of having underlying chronic obstructive lung disease, lower flow rates (2 to 4 L/min) of oxygen should be used so as not to suppress alveolar ventilation.

In the emergency room, following a quick examination of the nasal and oropharyngeal mucosa, more definitive therapy can be started. A carboxyhemoglobin level should be determined and repeated at ½ to 1 hour intervals while the patient receives 100 percent oxygen. A patent airway should be maintained, and this may require a tracheostomy in rare instances in which the amount of laryngeal edema makes endotracheal intubation impossible. Bronchodilators usually are administered when wheezing is detected on auscultation. In patients who develop acute respiratory failure and a clinical picture compatible with ARDS, early intubation and mechanical ventilation with a positive end-expiratory pressure is recommended.

Antibiotics

The routine use of prophylactic antibiotics is to be discouraged in smoke inhalation victims; however, a careful surveillance of the patient's sputum should be done to detect infection at an early stage.

Corticosteroids

The data for the routine use of corticosteroids in inhalation injury is conflicting. Levine et al.[40] did not find a decrease in the pulmonary complications or mortality in treated versus the placebo group. Moylan[41] found that patients treated with corticosteroids actually had a higher mortality than did a placebo-treated group, primarily due to infectious complications. In contrast, experimental studies of rats with acute smoke inhalation have shown that prednisolone and dexamethasone reduced the mortality.[42] Although controlled studies are lacking in humans, it would be reasonable to use a short trial of corticosteroids (for 24 to 48 hours) in those patients with evidence of upper airway obstruction, pulmonary edema, or severe bronchospasm.

Where a specific chemical agent, such as hydrogen cyanide, can be implicated in a case of inhalation injury, specific antidotes such as sodium nitrite and sodium thiosulfate may be required.

DELAYED COMPLICATIONS OF SMOKE INHALATION

Apart from the infectious complications that occur during the course of hospitalization of smoke inhalation victims, further lung damage, such as tracheal stenosis and bronchiolitis obliterans or bronchiectasis, may be seen in some cases after smoke inhalation.[43,44] The repeated exposure of firefighters to smoke has been thought to be associated with a more rapid loss of pulmonary function than could be accounted for by smoking alone.[45,46] However, this is an area of controversy, since other studies have shown that the incidence of small airway disease in fire fighters chronically or repeatedly exposed to smoke in small concentrations was no different than that of the general population.[47,48]

REFERENCES

1. Lowry T, Schuman LM: Silo filler's disease: A syndrome caused by nitrogen dioxide. JAMA 162:153, 1956.
2. Jose-Ramirez R: The first death from nitrogen dioxide fumes: The story of a man and his dog. JAMA 229:1181, 1974.
3. Hayhurst ER, Scott E: Four cases of sudden death in a silo. JAMA 63:1570, 1914.

4. Yockey CC, Eden BM, Byrd RB: The McConnel missile accident: Clinical spectrum of nitrogen dioxide exposure. JAMA 244:1221, 1981.
5. Tabershaw IR, Ohoboni F, Cooper WC: Oxidants: Air quality criteria based on health effects. J Occup Med 10:464, 1968.
6. Buckley RD, Balchum OJ: Chronic exposures to nitrogen dioxide: Effects on oxygen consumption and enzyme activity on guinea pig tissues. Arch Environ Health 10:220, 1965.
7. Thomas HV, Mueller PK, Lyman RL: Lipoperoxidation of lung lipids in rats exposed to nitrogen dioxide. Science 159:532, 1967.
8. Hatton DV, Leach CS, Nicogossian AE, et al: Collagen breakdown and nitrogen dioxide inhalation. Arch Environ Health 32:33, 1977.
9. Guidotti TL: The higher oxides nitrogen: Inhalation toxicology. Environ Res 15:443, 1978.
10. Morrissey WL, Gould IA, Carrington CB, et al: Silo filler's disease. Respiration 32:81, 1975.
11. Prys-Roberts C: Principles of treating poisoning by higher oxides of nitrogen. Br J Anaesth 39;432, 1967.
12. Schechter Y: Deleterious effects of hyperbaric oxygen treatment on mortality and pathological changes in nitrogen dioxide poisoned dogs. Respiration 32:210, 1975.
13. Becklake MR, Goldman HI, et al: The long-term effects of exposure to nitrous fumes. Am Rev Tuberc 76:398, 1957.
14. Kramer CG: Chlorine. J Occup Med 9:193, 1967.
15. Kaufman J, Burkons D: Clinical, roentgenographic and physiologic effects of acute chlorine exposure. Arch Environ Health 23:29, 1971.
16. Conner EH, Dubois AB, Comroe JH: Acute chemical injury of the airway and lungs. Anesthesiology 23:538, 1962.
17. Chester EH, Kaimal J: Pulmonary injury following exposure to chlorine gas: Possible beneficial effects of steroid treatment. Chest 72:247, 1977.
18. Weil HG, George R: Late evaluation of pulmonary function after acute exposure to chlorine gas. Am Rev Resp Dis 99:374, 1969.
19. Montague TJ, MacNeil AR: Mass ammonia inhalation. Chest 77:496, 1980.
20. Kass T, Zamol N: Bronchiectasis following ammonia burns of the respiratory tract. Chest 62:282, 1972.
21. Sobonya R: Fatal anhydrous ammonia inhalation. Hum Pathol 8:293, 1977.
22. Finland M, Davidson SC, Levenson SM: Clinical and therapeutic aspects of the conflagration injuries to the respiratory tract sustained by victims of the Coconut Grove disaster. Medicine 25:215, 1943.
23. Aub JC, Pittman H, Brues AM: The management of the coconut grove burns at the Massachusetts General Hospital. The pulmonary complications—A clinical description. Ann Surg 118:834, 1943.
24. Trunkey DD: Inhalation injuries. Surg Clin North Am 58:1133, 1978.
25. Moritz AR: The effects of inhaled heat on the air passages of the lungs: An experimental investigation. Am J Pathol 21:311, 1945.
26. Petajan JH: An approach to the toxicology of combustion. Products of materials. Environ Health Perspect 17:65, 1976.
27. Zikria BA, Ferrer HM: The chemical factors contributing to pulmonary damage in smoke poisoning. Surgery 71:704, 1972.

28. Pruitt BA, Erickson DR, Morris AH: Progressive pulmonary insufficiency and other pulmonary complications of thermal injury. J Trauma 15:369, 1975.
29. McArdle CS, Finlay WF: Pulmonary complications following smoke inhalation. Br J Anaesth 47:618, 1978.
30. Greenberg AG, Frank H, Peskin GW: The left shifted oxyhemoglobin curve in the burn patient. J Trauma 16:563, 1976.
31. Larkin JM, Brahos GJ, Moylan JA: Treatment of carbon monoxide poisoning: Prognostic factors. J Trauma 16:111, 1976.
32. Demarest GB, Hudson LD, Altman LC: Impaired alveolar macrophage chemotaxis in patients with acute smoke inhalation. Am Rev Resp Dis 119:279, 1979.
33. Skornik WA, Dressler DP: Alveolar macrophage function in immunized burned rats. Arch Surg 108:715, 1974.
34. Wroblewski DA, Bower GC: The significance of facial burns in acute smoke inhalation. Crit Care Med 7:335, 1979.
35. Hunt JL, Agee RN, Pruitt BA: Fiberoptic bronchoscopy in acute inhalation injury. J Trauma 15:641, 1975.
36. Wanner A, Cutchavaree A: Early recognition of upper airway obstruction following smoke inhalation. Am Rev Resp Dis 108:1421, 1973.
37. Putnam CE, Loke J, Matthay RA, et al: Radiographic manifestations of acute smoke inhalation. Am J Roentgenol 129:865, 1977.
38. Agee RN, Long JM, Hunt JL, Petroff PA, et al: Use of ^{133}Xenon in early diagnosis of inhalation injury. J Trauma 16:218, 1976.
39. Moylan JA, Wilmore DW, Mouton DE, et al: Early diagnosis of inhalation injury using ^{133}Xenon lung scan. Ann Surg 176:477, 1972.
40. Levine BA, Petroff PA, Slade CL, et al: Prospective trials of dexamethasone and aerosolized gentamicin in the treatment of inhalation injury in the burned patient. J Trauma 18:188, 1978.
41. Moylan JA: Diagnostic techniques and steroids. J Trauma 19(Suppl): 917, 1979.
42. Dressler DP, Skornik WA, Kupersmith S: Corticosteroid treatment of experimental smoke inhalation. Ann Surg 183:46, 1979.
43. Kirkpatrick MB, Bass JB: Severe obstructive lung disease after smoke inhalation. Chest 76:108, 1979.
44. Perez-Guerra F, Walsh RE, Sagel SS: Bronchiolitis obliterans and tracheal stenosis: Late complications of inhalation burn. JAMA 218:1568, 1971.
45. Loke J, Farmer W, Matthay RA, et al: Acute and chronic effects of fire fighting on pulmonary function. Chest 77:369, 1980.
46. Unger KM, Snow RM, Mestas JM, et al: Smoke inhalation in firemen. Thorax 35:838, 1980.
47. Sidor R, Peters RM: Differences in ventilatory capacity of Irish and Italian fire fighters. Am Rev Respir Dis, 108:669, 1973.
48. Tashkin DP, Genovesi MG, Chopra S, et al: Respiratory status of Los Angeles firemen: One-month follow-up after inhalation of dense smoke. Chest 71:445, 1977.

14

Superior Vena Cava Syndrome

Steven A. Sahn, M.D.

INTRODUCTION

The superior vena cava syndrome (SVCS) results from interference in the return of blood through the superior vena cava to the right atrium. In 1757, William Hunter first described the clinical presentation of a patient with an aortic aneurysm obstructing the superior vena cava.[1] Since its original description in the eighteenth century, the etiology of superior vena cava obstruction has changed markedly. In early reports, SVCS was usually secondary to an infectious process involving the mediastinum, most commonly tuberculosis or syphilis.[2] As staining techniques improved, histoplasmosis was found to be a cause of the syndrome.[3] Today, malignancy accounts for 79 to 97 percent of cases (Table 14–1).[4–9]

The reported etiologies of SVCS are shown in Table 14–2. Lung cancer is now the most frequent single cause, with oat cell carcinoma being the most common histologic type of cancer producing the syndrome.[9] This is due to the propensity of this particular tumor to metastasize to the mediastinum. Lymphoma and metastatic carcinoma and sarcoma constitute the majority of the other malignant lesions that involve the mediastinum and cause superior vena cava obstruction.[9] Benign causes of the syndrome can be vascular abnormalities such as thrombosis secondary to a central venous catheter[10] or transvenous pacemaker,[11] aortic aneurysm[5] and, rarely, Bechet's syndrome.[12] Mediastinitis secondary to histoplasmosis,[13] tuberculosis,[14] and *Nocardia* infection[15] have been described. Obstruction of the superior vena cava also has been noted following radiation therapy to the mediastinum.[16] Mediastinal trauma,[17] thymic tumors,[18] goiters,[19] and even sarcoidosis[20] have been described as etiologies of the SVCS.

Since a malignant etiology is currently the predominant cause of SVCS, there is a tendency, in certain situations, for emergency treatment to be instituted without a specific etiologic diagnosis being ascertained. Statistically, the clinician and radiotherapist will be correct in recommending this therapy in an emergency situation. However, it would be a great disservice to the patient to have radiother-

Table 14–1. Etiologies of the Superior Vena Cava Syndrome (N = 734)

Etiology	No.	%
Malignant neoplasm	540	74
Unclassified neoplasm	28	4
Benign neoplasm	9	1
Mediastinitis[a]	74	10
Aneurysm	34	5
Thrombophlebitis	10	1
Idiopathic	39	5

[a]Histoplasmosis, tuberculosis, pyogenic, syphilis, post-radiation.

(Adapted from Kamiya K, Nakata Y, Naiki K, Hayashi H: Superior vena cava syndrome. Review of the literature and a case report. Vasc Dis 4:59, 1967.)

apy for a thrombosis of the superior vena cava that has been precipitated by a pacemaker wire or central catheter. Thus, it is prudent to attempt to establish a specific etiology in all cases, except acute SVCS with neurologic abnormalities, before proceeding to therapy.

In general, when superior vena cava obstruction is caused by malignant disease, the syndrome is characterized by a rapid onset with prominent symptoms. This is particularly notable with the most common cause of superior vena caval obstruction today, oat cell carcinoma of the lung. The often dramatic syndrome with this tumor apparently is due to the rapid growth of the tumor which does not allow adequate time for collateral channels to develop. With benign causes of superior vena cava obstruction, the presentation is often insidious and less fulminant.

PATHOPHYSIOLOGY

The superior vena cava is the major conduit for return of venous blood to the right side of the heart from the upper thorax, upper extremities, head, and neck. There are several reasons for the vulnerability of the superior vena cava to obstruction by primary lung cancer or cancer metastatic to the lymph nodes: (1) the superior vena cava is a thin-walled structure with low venous pressure; (2) it is situated in a small compartment in the right anterior-superior mediastinum behind the sternum; (3) it is in close proximity to the right mainstem bronchus; and (4) it is encircled by chains of lymph nodes which drain structures of the right thorax and lower part of the left thorax. The right anterior mediastinal lymph nodes lie in front of the superior vena cava, while the paratracheal nodes are situated behind the superior vena cava. The lowermost of these paratracheal nodes lie in close proximity to the arch of the azygos vein, the most vital auxiliary of the superior vena cava.[21–23]

On the basis of these anatomic and physiologic observations, it is not surprising that carcinoma of the lung is the most common cause of the SVCS. Superior vena cava obstruction is found with tumors of the right tracheobronchial tree, particu-

Table 14–2. Reported Etiologies of Superior Vena Cava Syndrome

Malignant Etiology
Lung cancer (especially oat cell)
Metastatic cancer
Lymphoma
Leukemia
Sarcoma
Mediastinal tumor
Benign Etiology
Vascular
Thrombosis secondary to catheter, pacemaker, polycythemia, or peritoneovenous shunt
Idiopathic thrombophlebitis
Aortic aneurysm
Vasculitis
Behcet's syndrome (probably vasculitis)
Mediastinitis
Histoplasmosis
Tuberculosis
Actinomycosis
Nocardiosis
Syphilis
Pyogenic
Post-radiation
Idiopathic
Mediastinal tumors
Thymic
Neural
Teratoma
Bronchial cyst
Dermoid cyst
Goiter
Trauma
Mediastinal hematoma
Gastroscopy
Cardiac
Pericarditis
Atrial myxoma
Pericardial cyst
Mitral stenosis
Surgical correction of transposition of the great vessels
Other
Sarcoidosis
Silicosis

larly such rapidly growing tumors as oat cell carcinoma of the lung. Roswit et al.[24] found superior vena cava obstruction to be present in 15 percent of 40 patients, while Steinberg and Dotter[25] found this complication in 17 percent of 100 patients with lung cancer studied preoperatively by angiocardiography.

In lung cancer, blood flow in the superior vena cava is interrupted either by the primary tumor per se or by metastatic lymph nodes, principally as a result of external compression of the vessel wall. Occasionally, obstruction is caused by intraluminal invasion by the tumor; rarely, obstruction is caused by thrombosis of the vessel.

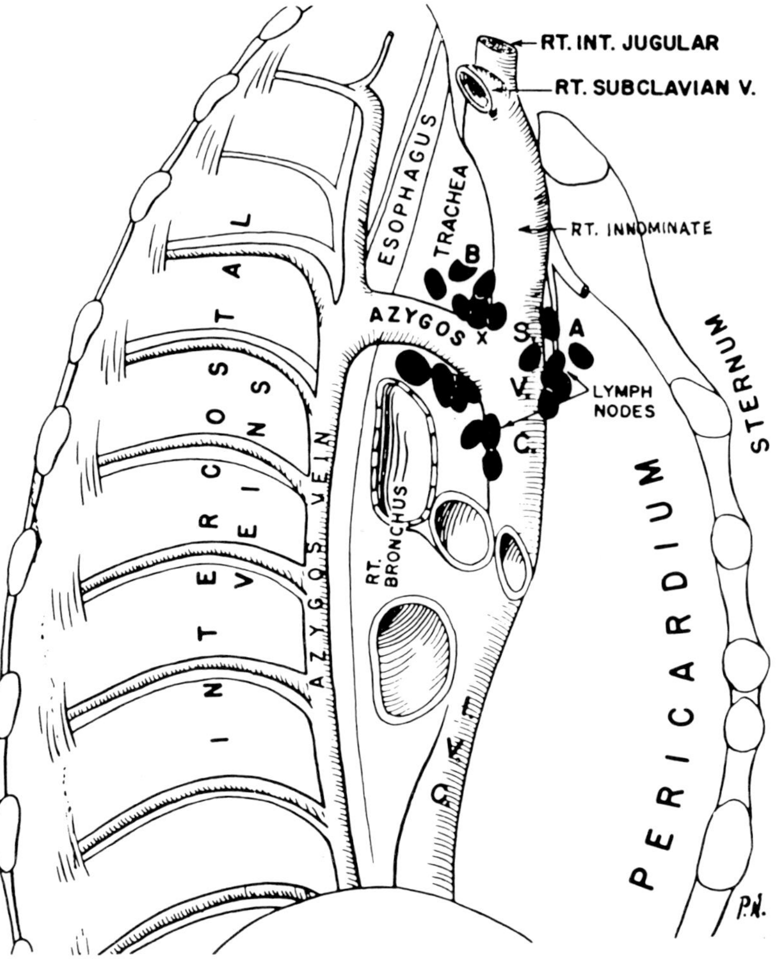

Figure 14–1. Vulnerable location of superior vena cava and azygos system in relation to carcinoma of the right mainstem bronchus and the lymph nodes commonly involved by lung cancer: (A) anterior prevascular nodes and (B) right paratracheal nodes. (Roswit B, Kaplan G, Jacobson HG: The superior vena cava obstruction syndrome in bronchogenic carcinoma. Radiology 61:722, 1953. Reproduced by permission of the Radiological Society of North America.)

When the superior vena cava or its tributaries is compromised, a collateral venous system begins to develop in an attempt to return blood to the right side of the heart from the upper thorax, upper extremities, head, and neck. The effectiveness of this collateral system dictates the clinical status of the patient. Specifically, the collateral system determines the degree of impairment and immediate prognosis. The rapidity of onset and extent of obstruction are further determinants of the magnitude of the clinical signs and symptoms. Rapidly growing anaplastic lesions will cause marked patient discomfort with rapid induction of the complete

TABLE 14–3. Presenting Symptoms in Superior Vena Cava Obstruction (N = 66)

Symptom	No.	%
Facial edema	55	83
Dyspnea	55	83
Cough	46	70
Orthopnea	42	64
Nasal stuffiness	23	35
Hoarseness	23	35
Dizziness	19	29
Tongue swelling	16	24
Headache	2	3
Syncope	2	3
Dysphagia	1	1
Epistaxis	1	1

(Adapted from Lochridge SK, Knibble WP, Doty DB: Obstruction of the superior vena cava. Surgery 85:14, 1979.)

SVCS. In these cases, the collateral circulation is inadequate and could lead to a poor prognosis in the absence of emergent therapy.

When the obstruction is above the level of the azygos vein, this vessel can take over the function of the superior vena cava (Fig. 14–1A). The resulting system of collaterals is less elaborate than when the obstruction is above the azygos, and is seen principally in the prominence of neck, shoulder girdle, and upper thoracic veins. With this collateral system, venous blood from the head and neck will return to the heart first via the external jugular vein and then via a superficial plexus on the anterior chest wall that connects with the perforating branches of the internal mammary and intercostal veins, finally joining the azygos system at the superior vena cava below the site of obstruction.[24]

Obstruction below the azygos arch or including it has much more serious consequences than obstruction above this vein. The venous pressure is higher, the patient has more severe symptoms, and the immediate prognosis is worse. Experimental models in dogs have shown that when an obstruction exists below the azygos vein, the route of venous blood flow into the right heart is more circuitous and involves support of the inferior vena cava.[26] The collecting circulation of the lower abdominal wall, back, and groin is utilized for this purpose, carrying blood to the inferior vena cava via the femoral and iliac veins. The details of this collateral circulation were described by McIntire and Sykes in 1949.[27] There are four important collateral routes for carrying venous blood around the obstruction and to the right side of the heart; they include the internal mammary, vetebral, azygos, and lateral thoracic systems.

CLINICAL PRESENTATION

The presentation of patients with superior vena cava obstruction is variable, owing to the time course of the vascular obstruction. Those with acute obstruction will tend to have a more striking clinical presentation, while in those in whom the

TABLE 14–4. Presenting Signs in Superior Vena Cava Obstruction (N = 66)

Signs	No.	%
Neck vein distention	61	92
Facial swelling	57	86
Arm vein distention	45	68
Upper extremity swelling	42	64
Abnormal mental status	18	47
Glossal edema	16	24
Laryngeal edema	16	24
Rhinorrhea	12	18
Stupor	9	14
Coma	4	6
Upper body plethora	2	3

(Adapted from Lochridge SK, Knibble WP, Doty DB: Obstruction of the superior vena cava. Surgery 85:14, 1979.)

obstruction is more insidious, the physical findings may be more subtle. The SVCS has been misdiagnosed early in its clinical course as congestive heart failure, myxedema, allergic blepharitis, or angioneurotic edema.[28]

When superior vena caval obstruction is acute, the most common presenting symptoms are facial edema, dyspnea, cough, and orthopnea (Table 14–3). The edema of the superior vena cava syndrome is limited to the upper body including the arms, breasts, head, and neck. The edema is pitting and varies with changes in position, being most prominent in the morning and subsiding as the day progresses.[28] The edema tends to increase if there is further obstruction of the superior vena cava and to decrease as new collateral vessels are recruited. Edema of the vocal cords may lead to hoarseness. It is not clear why patients with superior vena cava obstruction are dyspneic, but this may be related to ventilation-perfusion mismatching in the lung because of impaired right ventricular output.

The presenting signs in superior vena cava obstruction are shown in Table 14–4. Venous distention and edema, particularly of the face, are usually the most consistent physical findings.

An important historical point that some patients may relate is that they have noted an increase in their neck size, which probably represents a combination of neck edema and dilated veins.

DIAGNOSIS

The diagnosis of superior vena cava obstruction usually can be made on clinical grounds. If the obstruction is relatively acute, patients present with the classic symptoms and signs that have been discussed previously. The question that remains concerns the etiology of the SVCS. Since malignancy involving the mediastinum is responsible for 80 to 95 percent of cases of superior vena caval obstruction today, the chest radiograph is often the single most helpful examination in suggesting an etiology. Since oat cell carcinoma is the most common cause

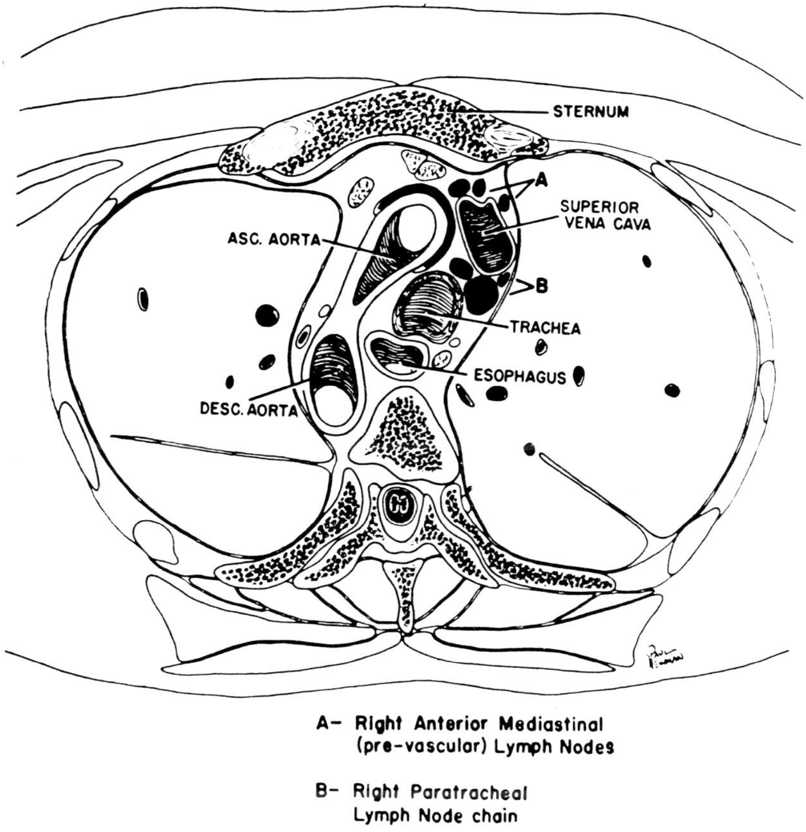

Figure 14–2. Cross-section of superior mediastinal compartment at the level of the first intercostal space. Note the vulnerable position of the superior vena cava in relation to the right anterior mediastinal lymph nodes (A) and right paratracheal nodes (B), which are commonly involved by lung cancer. (Roswit B, Kaplan G, Jacobson HG: The superior vena cava obstruction syndrome in bronchogenic carcinoma. Radiology 61:722, 1953. Reproduced by permission of the Radiological Society of North America.)

of superior vena cava obstruction, the typical chest radiograph may show a central mass lesion, usually less than 4 cm in diameter, with a hilar and mediastinal mass or widening[29] (Figs. 14–3A and B). Metastatic tumors to the lung will commonly show multiple parenchymal lesions in addition to the mediastinal widening. By the time lymphoma involves the mediastinal lymph nodes there is usually evidence of peripheral tumor (Figs. 14–4A and B). A "negative" chest radiograph in association with the SVCS is suggestive of either mediastinal fibrosis or thrombosis secondary to previous central venous catheterization.

If the clinician feels that an instance of acute superior vena cava obstruction is emergent (see p. 2), it is imperative that benign causes of SVCS be ruled out

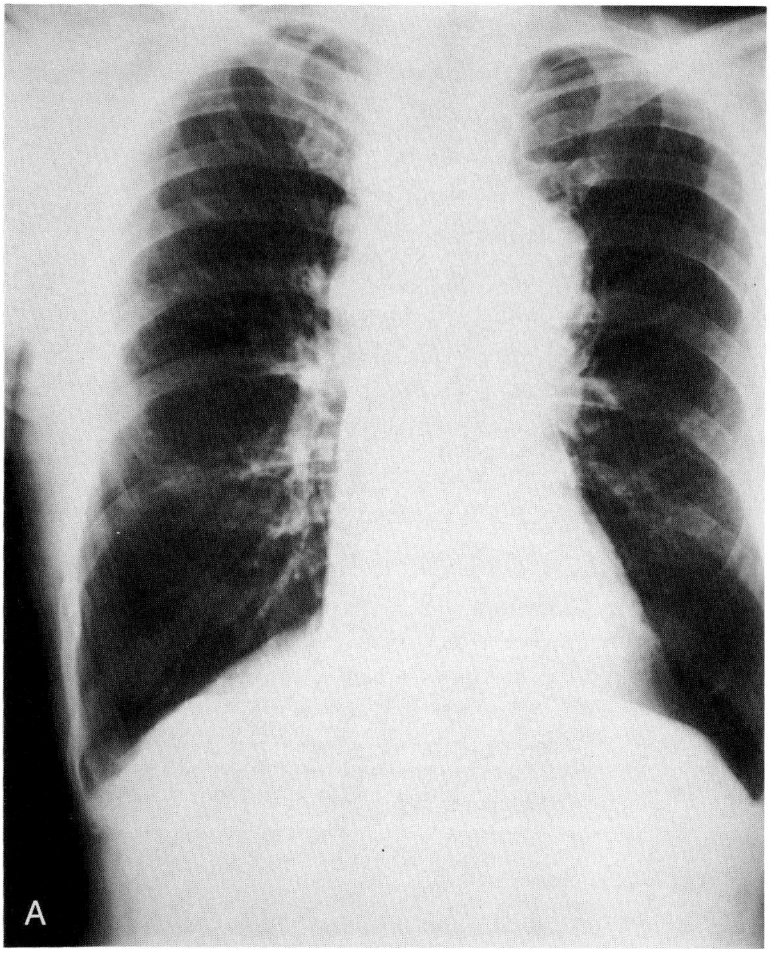

Figure 14–3. (A) Posteroanterior chest radiograph of a 57-year-old male smoker who presented with dysphagia, hoarseness, weight loss, and superior vena cava syndrome. Note the widened superior mediastinum due to metastatic oat cell carcinoma.

before initiating radiotherapy; a history of recent central venous catheterization, placement of a pacemaker, or peritoneovenous shunt should be specifically sought. In most cases, the chest radiograph will provide the most important etiologic clue on whether the syndrome is due to lung cancer, metastatic cancer, cardiac abnormality, goiter, or sarcoidosis. The occurrence of serious neurologic complications, tracheal obstruction, pericardial involvement, or brain metastases with increased intracranial pressure as complications of superior vena caval obstruction may require emergency therapy; however, these instances are unusual. The trend today is to pursue an etiologic diagnosis even to thoracotomy, so that specific therapy can be instituted.

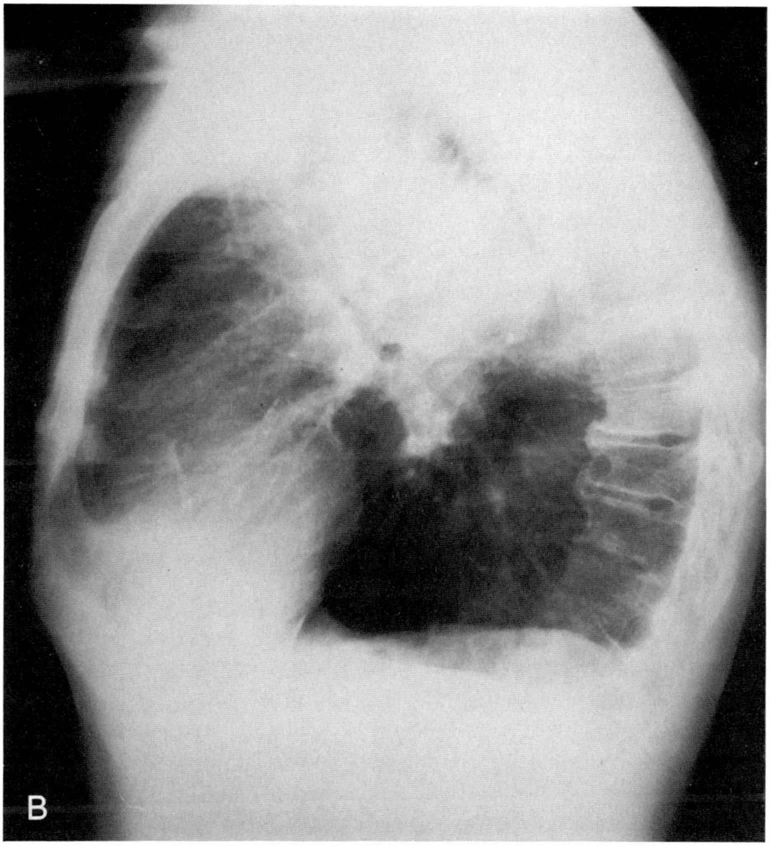

Figure 14–3 (continued). (B) Lateral chest radiograph showing large middle mediastinal mass displacing the trachea anteriorly.

If tissue from a skin lesion, peripheral lymph node, or bone marrow is easily accessible for biopsy, it should be taken and evaluated immediately. There is a high probability that with fiberoptic bronchoscopy an obstructing tumor can be visualized and a biopsy obtained; this procedure, which is done with local anesthesia, should induce a minimum of respiratory distress for the often compromised patient. Venography or venous pressure measurement will confirm the clinical impression and localize the site of an obstruction, but will not provide an etiology. In the acute syndrome due to malignancy, venous studies usually are superfluous and should not be done; however, if the syndrome is insidious and not clinically obvious, or if a benign cause is suspected, then venography is justifiable. Recently, scintiphotographic evaluation techniques have been used to visualize the vena cava and to follow the results of therapy for the SVCS.[30] This technique could be used for diagnostic confirmation in the subtle case. Some advantages of the scintillation camera method over contrast venography are the small volume of material that is injected (only 1 to 2 cc) and minimal discomfort for the patient.

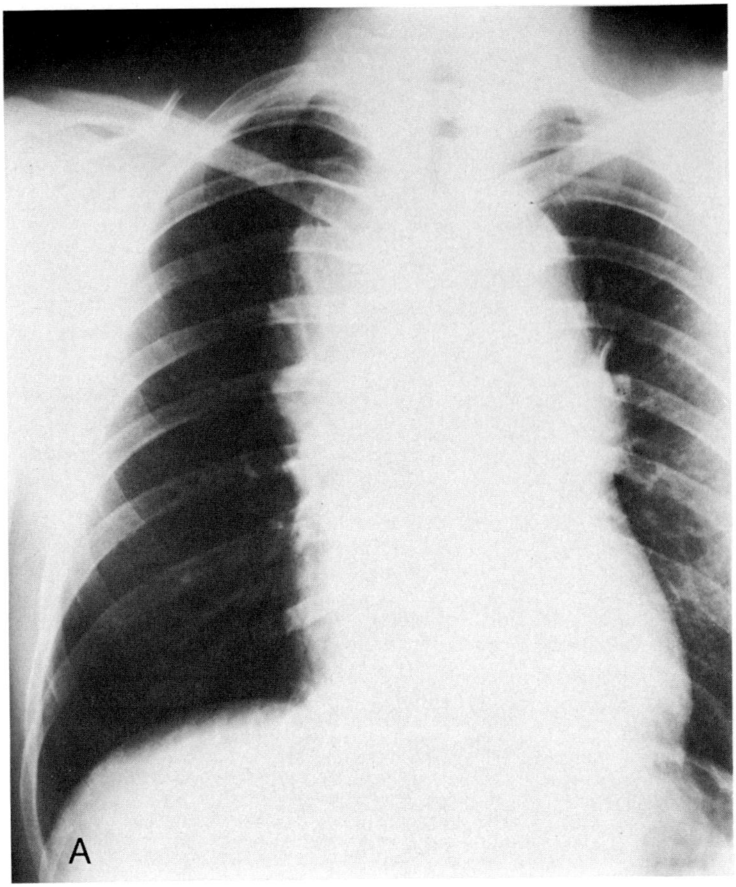

Figure 14–4. (A) Posteroanterior chest radiograph of a 39-year-old male who presented with the superior vena cava syndrome and a pericardial effusion secondary to lymphoma. Note the large superior-anterior mediastinal mass.

Esophagoscopy would be the diagnostic procedure of choice in a clinical situation suggesting carcinoma of the esophagus. Obviously, mediastinoscopy and thoracotomy would provide the highest diagnostic yield, but may be associated with substantial morbidity in rare situations.

Whereas the SVCS was considered by many to always be a medical emergency carrying a high risk with the use of invasive procedures, recent evidence suggests that diagnostic procedures should be planned and carefully performed so that a specific histologic diagnosis can be achieved.[31–33] Shimm et al.[31] reported on 18 patients in whom SVCS was the initial manifestation of disease. Sixteen of the 18 patients had a diagnosis established by bronchoscopy, thoracentesis, pleural biopsy, lymph node biopsy, and thoracotomy without major complications. Schraufnagel et al.[32] reviewed 107 cases of superior vena cava obstruction; 93 invasive

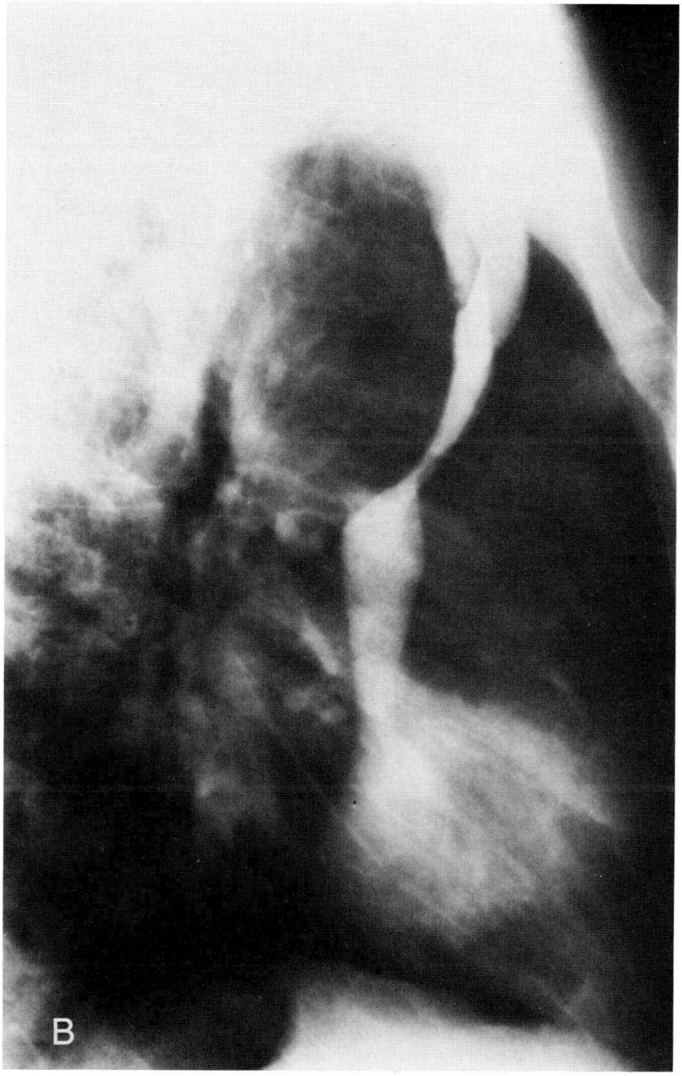

Figure 14–4 (continued). (B) Venography shows the superior vena cava compressed and displaced anteriorly by the mediastinal mass, without intraluminal invasion.

procedures were performed in 62 patients who were diagnostic problems. Thirteen of 29 patients were diagnosed by bronchoscopy, 14 of 21 by superficial lymph node biopsy, 10 of 14 by mediastinoscopy, 3 of 3 by mediastinotomy, and 14 of 15 by thoracotomy. No fatalities were recorded. There were 2 episodes of excessive bleeding (from bronchoscopy and mediastinoscopy) and 1 episode of transient respiratory distress following surgical biopsy for a mediastinal seminoma. In

Kirschner's[34] report of his results from mediastinoscopy in superior vena cava obstruction, a diagnosis was obtained in 14 of 16 patients without complications. Only a few modifications of standard mediastinoscopy are necessary in the patient with SVCS; these include: (1) positioning the patient to at least 45 degrees; (2) placing intravenous lines in the lower extremities; (3) making the initial skin incision cautiously to expose the dilated anterior cervical veins; and (4) retracting laterally rather than ligating the superficial veins. There are no engorged veins in the pretracheal zone.

MANAGEMENT

Two errors are made in the management of patients with SVCS: (1) treating without a specific diagnosis; and (2) pursuing a diagnosis too vigorously in lieu of treatment. The former probably is more detrimental to the patient as more effective therapy becomes available for specific diagnoses. Diagnostic procedures should be planned and range from those that are noninvasive (sputum cytology) to those that are most invasive (thoracotomy) until a specific histologic diagnosis is reached. In the rare occurrence of severe neurologic complications or mediastinal entrapment, emergency radiotherapy without a specific histologic diagnosis should be done. It should be noted, however, that with superior vena cava obstruction, diagnostic procedures can lead to life-threatening complications such as hemorrhage and upper airway obstruction. For instance, interruption of the venous system for the purpose of venography or venous pressure measurement in the presence of a markedly elevated venous pressure could lead to excessive hemorrhage. In addition, because of impaired venous flow, the intravenous administration of drugs will impaired local circulation and may produce inflammation and thrombosis. Thus, great care should be taken in manipulating the veins of the upper extremities.

Radiation has been the cornerstone of therapy in the SVCS.[35-37] Chemotherapy has been advocated in certain situations and may become a first-line therapy in oat cell carcinoma. Surgery has been utilized rarely, and other medical measures are of little value in most cases of superior vena cava obstruction. As noted earlier, the SVCS is one entity in which the radiation therapist may not request a histologic diagnosis before proceeding with therapy. This has inherent problems, since a definitive diagnosis is important because future therapy and the prognosis are influenced by the histologic type and anatomic site of the primary lesion. If such less invasive procedures as sputum cytology, bronchoscopy, and biopsy of palpable supraclavicular lymph nodes have not yielded the diagnosis, the more invasive procedures, mediastinoscopy and thoracotomy, should be performed in almost all patients with SVCS unless the patient is critically ill.

The patient with SVCS should be monitored in an intensive care unit where problems of the upper airway and hemodynamic compromise that result from the syndrome can be handled effectively. Oxygen should be given to correct hypoxemia, and airway patency should be maintained by appropriate measures. Corticosteroids and diuretics probably are of no value in treatment of the syndrome. Diuretics can, in fact, be dangerous, in further lowering intrathoracic blood volume in a state of compromised filling of the right side of the heart. Green et al.[35] have demonstrated the absence of an inflammatory reaction and edema following radiotherapy in SVCS. Thus, the anti-inflammatory effect of corticosteroids would seem to have little benefit in this situation. Because a number of patients with superior vena cava obstruction develop thrombosis in this vessel or its tributaries at some time during their course,[39] anticoagulants and fibrinolytic agents[40] have been used. Residual thrombosis has been found in the vena cava at postmortem examination in a high percentage of cases of SVCS.[39,41]

Three important points must be considered with regard to radiation therapy in tumor-associated SVCS: (1) dose fractionation; (2) total dose; and (3) portal size. Some investigators have suggested that a high initial daily dose (300 to 400 rads) followed by lower, more conventional daily doses (50 to 100 rads) would provide faster resolution than conventional daily doses.[36,38] Others, however, have not found an appreciable difference in the response to conventional and initial high-dose therapy.[9] Furthermore, it appears that high-dose therapy does not cause additional compromise due to edema, and that this form of therapy is relatively safe.[37] Apparently, higher doses of radiation cause enough cellular death and decrease the size of the obstructing mass sufficiently to offset the effects of radiation-induced edema. The total dose of radiation would depend upon the histologic type of the tumor, the extent of disease, the severity of symptoms, and the general condition of the patient. Generally, lower radiation doses are effective in treating lymphoma while higher doses are required for adenocarcinoma or squamous cell carcinoma of the lung, with even higher doses being required for epithelial tumors.[4] If disease is confined to the thorax, a higher radiation dose, with the intent to cure, might be employed, whereas if distant metastasis are present in addition to mediastinal lesions, a lower dose, for palliation only, might be considered. Thus, 3000 to 4000 rads might be considered for lymphomas, while 5000 to 6000 rads would be required for oat cell carcinomas.

In general, chemotherapy should be reserved for those patients who have received a maximum dose of radiation therapy or for patients who do not respond to a course of radiation therapy. The combined use of chemotherapy and radiation therapy has been suggested for a more rapid antitumor effect; however, in experimental and clinical studies, there does not appear to be an effect from the addition of nitrogen mustard to radiation.[9,42,43] It may be that patients with oat cell carcinoma and lymphoma producing superior vena cava obstruction would have a similar or better response to chemotherapy than to radiation therapy. Most clinicians who have treated patients with superior vena cava obstruction believe that the primary method of treatment should be radiation therapy, and that chemotherapy should be withheld until the obstruction has responded to the radiation therapy. However, in two recently published series comprising a total of 29 patients with oat cell carcinoma of the lung and superior vena cava obstruction, treatment consisted of chemotherapy alone, without radiation therapy.[44,45] Every patient had partial disappearance of the SVCS after a median period of 7 days. Twenty-eight of the 29 patients had complete disappearance of the obstruction after 14 days. Thus, there is gathering evidence that chemotherapy alone may be the treatment of choice in SVCS due to oat cell carcinoma of the lung; radiation therapy alone is inadequate for this carcinoma because it does not increase survival.[46] Additionally, radiation therapy may compromise the ability to give the intensive chemotherapy required for oat cell carcinoma.

Surgical procedures have been used in the treatment of superior vena cava obstruction. These have consisted of venectomy or bypassing of the vein by either venous grafts or synthetic material.[6,47] Surgery will provide rapid resolution of the syndrome with definitive removal of the obstruction, and has the additional benefit of establishing a tissue diagnosis. However, the morbidity and mortality associated with surgery in this setting are high. Surgery should be considered only when a SVCS due to malignancy has not responded to either radiotherapy or chemotherapy, or when the patient has received maximum doses of radiation. Surgical success has been reported following bypass grafting in granulomatous mediastinitis and SVCS.[6]

Symptomatic relief of tumor-associated SVCS is achieved in most patients following radiotherapy. The degree of improvement will depend on the histologic type of tumor, being greater with those tumors that are more radiosensitive, such as lymphoma and oat cell carcinoma. Only about 15 percent of patients with lung cancer of all types show no improvement with therapy. In one series of 84 patients with SVCS (most of whom had lung cancer), aproximately 25 percent survived one year and 10 percent survived 2½ years following initial therapy.[7] However, there have been reports of long-term survival in SVCS due to lymphoma and to squamous and oat cell carcinoma.[36,48,49]

Radiation therapy generally is well tolerated by patients with tumor-associated SVCS. There does not appear to be any appreciable difference in the adverse effects of radiation therapy alone from those in radiotherapy combined with chemotherapy (except leukopenia), or from high-dose therapy versus conventional-dose therapy.[9] Dysphagia is usually the most common complaint, with nausea and vomiting being relatively infrequent. Major complications or long-term sequelae of therapy are unusual.

Despite apparent clinical recovery from SVCS after therapy, the involved portion of the superior vena cava is usually neither morphologically nor functionally normal. In an autopsy series, limited patency of the vessel was found despite absence of the clinical syndrome.[39] This fact should not be surprising, since an increase in diameter of the superior vena cava to the extent of only a few millimeters may produce a sufficiently increased blood flow to alleviate the obstructive symptoms. Longacre and Shockman[39] found a high incidence of cardiac metastasis in cancer patients dying with a clinical diagnosis of SVCS. They believe that pericardial or myocardial disease may be directly related to the death of patients with SVCS, and is probably the explanation for the apparent recurrence of the syndrome in many of these patients.

SUMMARY

Superior vena cava obstruction, most commonly caused by oat cell carcinoma, usually is not a medical emergency requiring immediate therapy. The diagnosis can be made at the bedside with the observation of upper body edema, distended neck veins, and increased numbers of collateral vessels in the upper extremities. A chest radiograph often will provide an important clue about the etiology of the vena cava obstruction. The major pitfall in the management of superior vena cava obstruction is treatment before a histologic diagnosis is established. Diagnostic tests may be associated with an increased morbidity in the SVCS and should be carefully selected prior to therapy, beginning with the least invasive test and proceeding to mediastinoscopy and thoracotomy if necessary. Therapy should be instituted without delay once the etiologic diagnosis is established, and generally produces rapid palliation. Radiation therapy has been a cornerstone of therapy for tumor-associated SVCS, but recent advances in chemotherapy may supplant this modality in certain types of tumor, particularly oat cell carcinoma of the lung.

REFERENCES

1. Hunter W: The history of an aneurysm of the aorta with some remarks on aneurysms in general. Med Obs Soc Phys Lond 1:323, 1757.
2. Ochsner A, Dixon J: Superior vena caval thrombosis. J Thorac Surg 5:641, 1935.
3. Grocott RG. A stain for fungi in tissue sections and smears: using Gomori's methenamine-silver nitrate technic. Am J Clin Pathol 25:975, 1955.
4. Lockich JJ, Goodman R: Superior vena cava syndrome: Clinical management. JAMA 231:58, 1975.
5. Kamiya K, Nakata Y, Naiki K, Hayashi H: Superior vena caval syndrome. Review of the literature and a case report. Vasc Dis 4:59, 1967.
6. Lochridge SK, Knibble WP, Doty DB: Obstruction of the superior vena cava. Surgery 85:14, 1979.
7. Urschel HC Jr, Paulson DL: Superior vena caval obstruction. Dis Chest 49:155, 1966.
8. Failor HJ, Edwards JE, Hodgson CH: Etiologic factors in obstruction of the superior vena cava. A pathologic study. Staff Meet Mayo Clin 33:671, 1958.
9. Perez CA, Presant CA, Van Amburg AL III: Management of superior vena cava syndrome. Semin Oncol 5:123, 1978.
10. Kanada DJ, Jung RC, Ishihara S: Superior vena cava syndrome due to a retained central venous pressure catheter. Chest 75:734, 1979.
11. Youngson GG, McKenzie FN, Nichol PM: Superior vena cava syndrome: Case report. A complication of permanent transvenous endocardial cardiac pacing requiring surgical correction. Am Heart J 99:503, 1980.
12. Chajek T, Fainaru M: Behcet's disease with decreased fibrinolysis and superior vena caval occlusion. Br Med J 1:782, 1973.
13. Case records of the Massachusetts General Hospital. N Engl J Med 295:381, 1976.
14. Steinberg I: Superior vena caval syndrome due to tuberculosis. Report of three cases. Am J Roentgenol 98:440, 1966.
15. Rankin RS, Westcott JL: Superior vena cava syndrome caused by nocardia mediastinitis. Am Rev Resp Dis 108:361, 1973.

16. Smith AR, Richards V: Superior vena caval obstruction. Am J Surg 96:353, 1958.
17. Mahajan V, Strimlan V, Van Ordstrand HS, et al: Benign superior vena cava syndrome. Chest 68:32, 1975.
18. Larrieu AJ, Just Viera JO: Superior vena cava syndrome caused by a malignant thymoma. Case Report. Bol Asoc Med PR 65:122, 1973.
19. Ulreich S, Lowman RM, Stern H: Intrathoracic goiter: A cause of the superior vena cava syndrome. Clin Radiol 28:663, 1977.
20. Gordonson J, Trachtenberg S, Sargent EN: Superior vena cava obstruction due to sarcoidosis. Chest 63:292, 1973.
21. Drinker CK: The lymphatic system. Its part in regulating composition and volume of tissue fluid. Stanford University Press 4:73, 1942.
22. McCort JJ, Robbins LL: Roentgen diagnosis of intrathoracic lymph node metastasis in carcinoma of the lung. Radiology 57:339, 1951.
23. Rouviere H: Anatomy of the Human Lymphatic System, Ann Arbor, Edwards Bros., 1938.
24. Roswit B, Kaplan G, Jacobson HG: The superior vena cava obstruction syndrome in bronchogenic carcinoma. Radiology 61:722, 1953.
25. Steinberg I, Dotter CT: Lung cancer: angiocardiographic findings in 100 consecutive proved cases. Arch Surg 64:10, 1952.
26. Carlson HA: Obstruction of the superior vena cava: An experimental study. Arch Surg 29:669, 1934.
27. McIntire FT, Sykes EM Jr: Obstruction of the superior vena cava: a review of the literature and report of two personal cases. Ann Intern Med 30:925, 1949.
28. Angevine CD, Condemi JJ: The facial edema of vena cava syndrome mistaken for angioneurotic edema. J Allergy 38:308, 1966.
29. Byrd RB, Miller WE, Carr DT, et al: The roentgenographic appearance of small cell carcinoma of the bronchus. Mayo Clin Proc 43:337, 1968.
30. Krishnamurthy GT, Blahd WH, Winston MA: Superior vena caval syndrome: scintiphotographic evaluation of response to radiation therapy. Radiology 117:609, 1973.
31. Shimm DS, Logue GL, Rigsby LC: Evaluating the superior vena cava syndrome. JAMA 245:951, 1981.
32. Schraufnagel DE, Hill R, Leech JA, Pare JAP: Superior vena caval obstruction. Is it a medical emergency? Am J Med 70:1169, 1981.
33. Teirstein AS: Diagnostic procedures in patients with superior vena cava syndrome. JAMA 245:956, 1981.
34. Kirschner PA. Mediastinoscopy in superior vena cava obstruction. In *Mediastinoscopy*, eds. Jepsen O, Sorensen HR, Odense, Denmark, Odense University Press, 40-42, 1971.
35. Green J, Rubin P, Holzwasser G: The experimental production of superior vena caval obstruction. Trial of different therapy schedules. Radiology 81:406, 1963.
36. Rubin P, Green J, Holzwasser G, et al: Superior vena caval syndrome. Slow low-dose versus rapid high-dose schedules. Radiology 81:388, 1963.
37. Fisherman WH, Bradfield JS: Superior vena caval syndrome; response with initially high daily dose irradiation. South Med J 66:677, 1973.
38. Davenport D, Ferree C, Blake D, et al: Response of superior vena cava syndrome to radiation therapy. Cancer 38:1577, 1976.
39. Longacre AM, Shockman AT: The superior vena cava syndrome and radiation therapy. Radiology 91:713, 1968.

40. Salsali M, Cliffton EE: Superior vena caval obstruction with carcinoma of the lung. Surg Gynecol Obstet 121:783, 1965.
41. Salsali M, Cliffton EE: Superior vena caval obstruction with lung cancer. Ann Thorac Surg 6:437, 1968.
42. Levitt SH, Jones TK Jr., Kilpatrick JJ Jr, et al: Treatment of malignant superior vena caval obstruction. Cancer 24:447, 1969.
43. Geller W: The mandate for chemotherapeutic decompression in superior vena caval obstruction. Radiology 81:385, 1963.
44. Dombernowsky P, Hansen HH: Combination chemotherapy in the management of superior vena caval obstruction in small-cell anaplastic carcinoma of the lung. Acta Med Scand 204:513, 1978.
45. Kane RC, Cohen MH, Broder LE, et al: Superior vena caval obstruction due to small-cell anaplastic lung carcinoma. JAMA 235:1717, 1976.
46. Roswit B, Patno ME, Rapp R, et al: The survival of patients with inoperable lung cancer: A large-scale randomized study of radiation therapy versus placebo. Radiology 90:688, 1968.
47. Effeney DJ, Windsor HM, Shanahan MX: Superior vena cava obstruction: Resection and by-pass for malignant lesions. Aust NZ J Surg 42:231, 1973.
48. Percarpio B, Gray S: Prolonged survival following the superior vena cava syndrome. Chest 75:639, 1979.
49. Nogeire C, Mincer F, Botstein C: Long survival in patients with bronchogenic carcinoma complicated by superior vena caval obstruction. Chest 75:325, 1979.

Index

Page numbers followed by f represent figures; page numbers followed by t represent tables.